PRAISE FOR *VEGAN FOR LIFE*

"This book explains everything one needs to know about going vegan. Comprehensive and succinct, it is a must-have for nutritionists and anyone contemplating a vegan diet."

 —*Library Journal*

"Armed with this compendium and a vegan cookbook, novices will make an easy, healthy transition to meat, egg and dairy-free meals, while practicing vegans can use it as a guide to the best food choices."

 —*Publishers Weekly*

"Packed with science yet never boring, Norris and Messina—both long-time vegans themselves—put their wealth of knowledge at your fingertips while putting to rest any nutritional issues that concern those aspiring to a plant based-diet . . . No vegan myth goes unbusted . . . *Vegan for Life* is a complete reference guide that deserves a spot in your library or kitchen."

 —*VegNews*

"*Vegan for Life* is full of helpful charts that show specific nutrients found in numerous fruits, nuts and vegetables. I love how easy this makes it to be sure you are getting the proper nutrition in your vegan lifestyle."

 —*Texas Kitchen*

"A book that is both so encouraging and so incredibly necessary right now."

 —*Run Vegan*

"*Vegan for Life* makes going vegan doable. I would definitely recommend this book to vegans, the vegan-curious, and those living with vegan family members."

—*Veggie Voyeur*

"Beyond setting straight some outdated nutrition information, the book will put to rest most nutrition worries you might have."

—*Lone Star Plate*

VEGAN FOR LIFE

ALSO BY VIRGINIA MESSINA

Never Too Late to Go Vegan,
with Carol J. Adams and Patti Breitman

Vegan for Her,
with JL Fields

VEGAN FOR LIFE

EVERYTHING YOU NEED TO KNOW TO BE HEALTHY ON A PLANT-BASED DIET

SECOND EDITION

BY JACK NORRIS, RD,
AND VIRGINIA MESSINA, MPH, RD

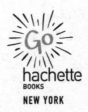

Go
hachette
BOOKS
NEW YORK

Copyright © 2011, 2020 by Jack Norris, Virginia Messina

Cover design by Terri Sirma
Cover images: (top) © Pressmaster/Shutterstock; (bottom) © Photographee.eu/Shutterstock
Cover copyright © 2020 Hachette Book Group, Inc.

Hachette Go, an imprint of Hachette Books
Hachette Book Group
1290 Avenue of the Americas, New York, NY 10104
HachetteGo.com
Facebook.com/HachetteGo
Instagram.com/HachetteGo

Printed in the United States of America

First Edition: May 2020

Published by Hachette Books, an imprint of Perseus Books, LLC, a subsidiary of Hachette Book Group, Inc. The Hachette Go and Hachette Books name and logos are trademarks of the Hachette Book Group.

The Hachette Speakers Bureau provides a wide range of authors for speaking events. To find out more, go to www.hachettespeakersbureau.com or call (866) 376-6591.

The publisher is not responsible for websites (or their content) that are not owned by the publisher.

Print book interior design by Trish Wilkinson.

Library of Congress Cataloging-in-Publication Data has been applied for.

ISBNs: 978-0-7382-8586-3 (trade paperback); 978-0-7382-8585-6 (ebook)

LSC-C

10 9 8 7 6 5 4 3 2 1

To all farmed animals,
and to those who work to end their suffering.

CONTENTS

INTRODUCTION
Going Vegan for Life

A vegan diet is the world's most simple solution to a host of complex problems. Our current food system contributes to a growing health crisis in America, a worrisome loss of global resources, and some of the worst cruelty to animals imaginable. Veganism is a potent response to these problems, and that's a message that is resonating with a growing number of people.

Since we wrote the first edition of *Vegan for Life* a decade ago, interest in plant-based eating patterns, especially vegan diets, has skyrocketed. More and more restaurants, including fast-food establishments, offer vegan entrees. The selection of vegan meats, milks, and cheeses at mainstream grocery stores keeps growing as innovative food companies introduce increasingly delicious products. And the traditional food industry is taking notice, launching their own lines of vegan foods. Answers to just about any question about vegan cooking are usually just a few clicks away on the internet and so are recipes for vegan versions of every dish you can imagine, from pulled pork to macaroni-and-cheese to chocolate layer cake. The result is that eating vegan is easier than ever. But, newcomers to this way of eating, as well as more seasoned vegans, often have questions about what to eat to meet nutrient needs and stay healthy.

In this new edition of *Vegan for Life*, we've updated guidelines and recommendations to reflect new knowledge and a better understanding of nutrition that comes from extensive research on diet and health over the past ten years. In addition to updating recommendations, we've revised sample menus, provided more helpful tips for adopting a vegan diet, and explored vegan perspectives on popular diet trends. We've provided vegan solutions for dealing with chronic illnesses like heart disease, irritable bowel syndrome, and depression.

As dietitians and animal advocates, we are unapologetically pro-vegan, and we want to help as many people as possible take steps toward an animal-free diet. That means that we want you to have the best nutrition advice possible, because a vegan diet isn't a realistic choice if you aren't meeting nutrient needs or eating in a way that supports optimal health. We'll give you all of the basic nutrition information—the absolutely essential facts that you need to safeguard your health while moving toward a vegan diet. We've also provided plenty of practical tips and tools to make the transition easy.

If you are new to veganism, we hope the information in this book will reassure you that a vegan diet is safe and healthy. If you are a longtime vegan, there's plenty of useful information here for you as well. We're going to sort through myths that have caused some vegans to make less-than-optimal food choices and give you ideas on how to make your vegan diet even healthier.

And if you are just dipping your toe in the water, that's fine. Use the information here to start a transition, because even reducing the amounts of animal foods in your diet makes a big difference.

THE COMPELLING CASE FOR A VEGAN DIET

Since 1950, profound changes have taken place on farms, driven by efforts to cut costs and produce cheap meat, milk, and eggs. The changes have given birth to factory farms, where animals are crammed into sheds and cages with virtually no room to move. Modern farming ignores the basic instinctual needs and welfare of individual animals. Many die before they ever make it to the slaughterhouse from disease or injury or because they couldn't access food or water. Conditions at slaughterhouses are cruel as well. Today's farm is less likely to be a friendly family enterprise and more likely to be a factory where efficiency takes precedence over respectful treatment of animals. The plain and simple—and uncomfortable—fact is that production of animal foods (even dairy and eggs) contributes to animal suffering.

Thanks to the work of animal-rights organizations, more people are becoming aware of these abuses. One answer for many has been to seek out foods from animals who were raised more humanely. Many products that boast "humanely produced" type labels come from animals who lived under somewhat better circumstances, but often the differences are negligible. And all of these animals usually go to the same slaughterhouses. Likewise, the term "organic" doesn't translate to "humanely produced." A large percentage of organic animal foods come from animals who were raised on factory farms.

Any truly meaningful welfare improvements can take place only on very small farms where every phase of the animal's life (and death) is monitored. But that's a costly and inefficient way to produce animal foods. Even if people could afford them, there isn't enough land for farms of this type to feed the American population.

In Chapter 1 we'll look at these issues in more depth. We'll also touch on the ways in which meat, dairy, and egg production is wasteful and harmful to the environment. Land that is used to raise food for billions of farm animals could grow food for direct human consumption, saving forests, water, and fossil fuels. A reduced dependence on animal foods is a significant step toward making your carbon footprint smaller.

Finally, those who opt for a plant-based diet are likely to enjoy personal benefits as well. Vegans have lower cholesterol and less hypertension and are less likely to develop diabetes. And vegan diets have been used as part of successful programs for treating chronic disease. We'll look at veganism through life stages, and also its impact on overall health, in the second half of the book.

ARE VEGAN DIETS SAFE?

According to the Academy of Nutrition and Dietetics, appropriately planned vegan diets are safe for all stages of the life cycle.[1] The

A FEW DEFINITIONS

OMNIVORE: In this book, we use the terms "omnivore" and "meat-eater" to describe anyone who chooses to include meat and other animal foods in his or her diet. So, an omnivore is someone who eats plants, meat, dairy foods, and eggs.

PLANT-BASED DIETS: Diets that emphasize plant foods and limit animal foods to varying degrees all fall under the big umbrella term "plant-based." These diets may or may not include small amounts of animal foods. So vegan, vegetarian, "flexitarian," semi-vegetarian, "mostly vegetarian," and traditional Mediterranean are all examples of plant-based diets.

LACTO-OVO VEGETARIAN: Vegetarians who include dairy and eggs in their diet are lacto-ovo vegetarians, sometimes abbreviated as LOV. Historically, most vegetarians in the United States have eaten this way, and some of what we know about vegan diets is actually extrapolated from studies of vegetarians.

VEGAN: The word "vegan" was coined to describe a lifestyle that avoids all animal products for food, clothing, and personal care. It's based on ethical concerns regarding animals. However, a vegan diet—which includes no meat, fish, dairy, or eggs—is chosen by people for a variety of reasons, including issues regarding animal use as well as health and environmental considerations. Since this is a book about nutrition, when we use the word "vegan," we are referring to anyone who consumes a diet that includes only plant foods.

"appropriately planned" caveat has been a source of annoyance among vegan dietitians for nearly three decades. Any diet, vegan or not, has to be well planned. Those who consume animal products don't automatically meet all nutrient needs and can fall short on fiber and other compounds that are abundant in vegan diets. Likewise, vegan diets require more attention to some nutrients like vitamin B_{12} and iron.

OUR JOURNEYS:
HOW WE BECAME VEGAN DIETITIANS

JACK

I was nineteen years old and went on a fishing trip with my dad and grandfather. It consisted of putting out a number of lines at the same time, sitting back, and waiting for one to be tugged on. When a fish was reeled in, they put the fish in an empty water cooler, where it thrashed around for a good long time as it suffocated. I felt horrible and decided not to reel in any fish. I realized that if the fish were human, we would do all we could to save the person from such pain, but since it was a fish, no one cared. Yet the suffering seemed very similar. My grandfather and father were a bit confused by my reaction. Still, it took me another two years to stop eating fish.

The first step I took toward becoming vegan was to stop eating mammals—it was a struggle because meat was very tempting. But soon I discovered some high-protein vegan foods, mostly legumes, which satisfied my cravings. When my chiropractor told me that I could get calcium from greens, I gave up dairy and went vegan in 1988.

After college, I became a full-time activist for animals, co-founded Vegan Outreach (a nonprofit animal advocacy group), and spent two years traveling the country handing out our booklets on veganism to college students. In that time, I came across numerous people who said they had been vegan or vegetarian and had not been healthy. Due to this and all the other nutrition issues surrounding a vegan diet, I decided to become a registered dietitian. I now spend most of my time as the executive director of Vegan Outreach, making sure that we spread vegan living to as many people as possible in order to hasten the day that humans no longer view animals as food.

Vegan Outreach has a college outreach program that visits about 1,000 schools each semester throughout the United States, Canada, Australia, Mexico, and India. We also do outreach at community events such as cat and dog festivals and comic conventions. All our outreach is aimed at directing interested people to sign up for our 10 Weeks to Vegan online challenge.

continues

OUR JOURNEYS: HOW WE BECAME VEGAN DIETITIANS   *continued*

GINNY

I was one of those kids who was always bringing home lost kittens and injured birds. But it took decades for me to make the connection between the food on my plate and the lives of animals. Even when I headed off to college to become a dietitian, veganism wasn't much on my radar. It was another ten years before the little light bulb above my head clicked on.

I had just gotten my master's in public health nutrition and was employed by a small rural clinic in southwest Michigan, where I worked with migrant farm workers, low-income elderly people, and pregnant teens. I was also newly married and experiencing a new-found enjoyment in cooking in my tiny apartment kitchen. Just for fun I was exploring the wonderful vegetarian cookbooks that were starting to become popular. One of those was *Laurel's Kitchen*, and I credit it with opening my eyes to the reality of meat. It was the dedication in that cookbook—which was to a "glossy black calf on his way to the slaughterhouse many years ago"—that triggered a sort of epiphany for me. Something clicked as I realized that the slab of flesh on my plate was once a living, breathing creature. I stopped eating meat then and there.

Several years later, I was hired by the Physicians Committee for Responsible Medicine, a vegan advocacy group in Washington, DC, to work on their nutrition programs. My work there brought another shift in my understanding about how animals, including those used to produce eggs and milk, are treated on farms. I made the decision to adopt a vegan diet. It was a turning point for me not just personally, but also professionally. I knew that I wanted to help other people move toward a vegan diet in ways that would support their health. And that I wanted to be a resource for health professionals who work with the vegan public as well. My work today as a writer, educator, speaker, and consultant continues with that focus—sharing information about vegan nutrition and helping others make a safe and happy journey toward compassionate food choices.

The point is that everyone, no matter what type of diet they eat, needs a little nutrition know-how. But yes, vegan diets can—and do—support optimal health throughout the life cycle. Many of the negative stories about vegans, especially children, who suffer from nutrient deficiencies are actually due to very restrictive types of vegan diets such as macrobiotic or raw foods.

A vegan diet isn't difficult; it's just a different way of meeting nutrient needs. This book is a guide to vegan nutrition and meal planning at all stages of the life cycle as well as for those who wish to adopt a vegan diet to reduce their risk for chronic disease. We've provided steps that translate nutrition information into real food choices and realistic menus for everyone.

Going vegan for life is a choice that has win-win written all over it. It respects the lives of animals and represents a refusal to contribute to their suffering. Many people feel a sense of relief when they become vegan because it reflects how they feel about animals. A plant-based menu is also broadening and will introduce you to new foods and menus; it's very likely to make your diet more interesting, not less. And depending on what your diet is like right now, making the move toward veganism is very likely to improve your health.

If you want to reap these benefits and get started on the path to compassionate and healthy eating, turn the page.

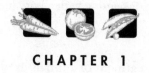

Why Vegan?

For almost all of human history, people ate whatever they could get their hands on; availability, habit, and taste preferences were the factors that drove food choices. That changed a mere century or so ago, when the new science of nutrition revealed that food was more than just something to eat—it was part of an approach to optimal health. Today, our perspective continues to evolve with a growing appreciation for the ways in which food choices affect much more than our own health and well-being. What we eat has far-reaching effects on the welfare and rights of both humans and animals—and on the very future of life on our planet.

The term "vegan" was coined in 1944 by a small group of vegetarians who recognized that animal products like dairy foods involved the same exploitation and slaughter of animals as production of meat. They founded the Vegan Society in the United Kingdom, which defines veganism as:

A philosophy and way of living which seeks to exclude—as far as is possible and practicable—all forms of exploitation of, and cruelty to, animals for food, clothing or any other purpose; and by extension, promotes the development and use of animal-free alternatives for the benefit of humans, animals and the environment. In dietary terms it denotes the practice of dispensing with all products derived wholly or partly from animals.

Although the cruel treatment of animals used in sport and circuses, in cosmetic testing, and for clothing are all important vegan issues, most people who are exploring veganism begin with dietary changes. Factory farming of animals for meat, dairy, and eggs is an especially pressing issue because of the huge numbers of animals involved, the unspeakable ways in which they are treated, and also the impact of this industry on the environment.

LIFE ON A MODERN FARM

Most people would be uncomfortable with the way animals are treated on today's farms, and that's why so much of that treatment occurs behind closed doors. When it is shared with the public at all, it's usually through carefully curated videos and photos and sometimes through meticulously planned public farm tours. These show pictures of clean facilities and animals who appear well cared for and in good health. Investigations by animal protection advocates reveal a different story: crowded conditions, sick and injured animals, and sometimes wanton cruelty by workers.[1]

In response to these investigations, the farming industry has sought to limit access to their facilities through Ag Gag laws. These state-level bills are designed to silence whistleblowers who reveal animal abuses on farms. As we go to press with this book, legal challenges have had some success in getting some of these laws struck down by courts as unconstitutional and a violation of First Amendment rights.

The animal agriculture industry says that the conditions that appear in undercover videos are unusual and are evidence of a "few bad apples." Yet, undercover investigations continue to reveal these conditions. But even without undercover investigations and evidence of illegal practices on some farms, we know that standard legal practices on farms and at the slaughterhouse are cruel. While the industry might downplay the significance of certain practices, they don't deny the use of many of the systems that we talk about in this chapter. In fact, much of the information we share here comes directly from industry publications. The practices that cause suffering among farmed animals are for the most part legal, and are discussed in agricultural trade magazines, among farmers on social media platforms, and on government websites associated with the farming industry.

There is not a single federal law in place to protect animals while they are living on the farm. While a few states have laws regarding the treatment of farmed animals, they are weak and rarely enforced. Farmed animals typically live in huge warehouses that you wouldn't even recognize as farms. They can't breathe fresh air, and they live on concrete or wire that damages their feet.

Most of these farms share three common elements, all aimed at maintaining high efficiency and low costs. These are confinement of animals, breeding for excessive growth, and mutilation.

Confining animals saves on space and also reduces feed requirements since the animals can't move much. Because animals can become aggressive in these unnatural conditions, farmers routinely use different types of mutilation, trimming the beaks of birds or the teeth of pigs for example, so that they are less likely to injure one another.

This drive for efficiency as well as the large number of animals on most farms means that it isn't always possible to consider the welfare of individual animals. On a dairy farm with seventy cows, a farmer is likely to notice a sick animal. But a single egg farm may house tens of thousands of chickens, which means that a sick or injured chicken is likely to go unnoticed. And if someone does see that she is sick, there is no veterinary care for her since that wouldn't be economically feasible. Farmers say that the system wouldn't be viable if it didn't protect the health and well-being of animals. But the truth is that letting some animals die due to overcrowding is more economical than allocating more space and attention to keep them healthy.

Although the practices vary among different types of farms, confinement, mutilation, and selective breeding are common approaches for production of all of the commonly consumed animal foods: eggs, chicken, pork, milk, and beef.

Egg-Laying Hens

The life of an egg-laying hen begins at the hatchery. Because these birds are not bred for their meat, male chicks have no function on an egg farm. Within minutes of emerging from their shells, they are separated out and killed. As with all aspects of animal farming, efficiency is key, since millions of these unwanted birds are hatched every year. Most commonly, the tiny, conscious birds are tossed by a spinning auger into a grinding machine. In other hatcheries, live male chicks are simply loaded into dumpsters and left to suffocate or die.

The female chicks are sent to egg farms, but first they usually have one-third to one-half of their beaks removed. This keeps the chickens from pecking each other in the cramped conditions in which they are housed. Their highly sensitive beaks may be painful for weeks or can cause long-term chronic pain and stress.[2]

Although the practice has been outlawed in some states, most egg-laying hens are housed in cages so small they can't stretch their wings. The United Egg Producers, which is a cooperative of egg farmers in the United States, recommends that the cages provide at least sixty-seven square inches per bird.[3] This is smaller than a piece of 8 × 11 paper, and it is where hens spend their entire lives. The cages aren't particularly comfortable, either. They have wire bottoms that can cause sores and bruises. With thousands and sometimes tens of thousands of chickens living on a typical farm, no attention is paid to individual birds. Many die from dehydration or starvation if they become caught in the wires, if their toenails grow around the wires, or if the mechanized food or water delivery system malfunctions. Others die from inhalation of ammonia from the manure pits below the cages.

Conditions are sometimes better in cage-free facilities where hens are more able to move around but can still live in very cramped conditions. Some of these facilities have "enrichment" features that allow hens to perch. But they suffer many of the same abuses as their caged sisters. While the words "cage-free" may conjure up an image of happy hens scratching around the barnyard, most are housed in huge buildings with no access to the outdoors. And regardless of how they are housed, because they are bred to produce eggs at an unusually high rate, both caged and cage-free hens are at risk for a prolapsed uterus. This occurs when part of the uterus is pushed out of the body. It leads to infection and a painful death.

Selective breeding is not the only way in which animals are forced to produce more. Some egg farms still employ the practice of forced molting, in which birds are starved for up to two weeks after the first laying period so that they'll start producing eggs again.

For birds living in these unnatural, highly stressful conditions, egg production begins to decline after just a year or two. Hens are loaded onto trucks and taken to the slaughterhouse. Their bones are brittle from excessive egg production and many of them suffer fractures as they are ripped out of their cages.[4] Some, referred to as "spent" hens by the industry, are in such poor condition that they can't be used for food. In that case, they might be killed right on the farm. On one farm, "spent" hens were tossed, while conscious, into a wood chipper for disposal. But the most common legal means of killing these hens is by carbon dioxide gassing using gas concentrations of 30 percent or more. Research has shown that at this level, birds feel pain and distress, probably associated with suffocation.

Birds Raised for Meat

It takes a lot of chickens to meet Americans' appetite for wings, nuggets, and fried drumsticks. Modern agriculture meets that demand by growing chickens as fast as they can. Unlike laying hens, who just need to produce as many eggs as possible, "broilers" need to pack on pounds. They grow four times faster than birds raised in the 1950s.[5] And while that is good for the farmer's bottom line, it's awful for the chicken. The excess weight leads to severe leg problems, sometimes even the inability to walk, which means that a chicken may not be able to access food and water. We know that these chickens feel pain because studies have found that birds with deformed legs are more likely than those with normal legs to eat feed that is laced with painkillers.[6]

Pigs

"Forget the pig is an animal. Treat him just like a machine in a factory," an issue of *Hog Management* trade magazine advised back in 1976.[7] On today's hog farms, breeding sows are in fact treated as piglet-producing machines with no consideration for their natural needs. These mother pigs are confined for nearly all of their four-month pregnancy in gestation crates. The crates are so small that for this entire time, they can take a step forward or backward but can't turn around. To give birth, they are moved to farrowing crates which allow them to lie on their sides so they can nurse their piglets through bars.

Under natural conditions, piglets nurse for twelve weeks or more as they gradually wean themselves. On hog farms the weaning period has gotten shorter and shorter in an effort to squeeze more and more pregnancies out of the sow. Piglets are typically weaned at about three weeks and sent to a weanling facility, where they are housed in pens with bare, slatted flooring. Or they go directly to the finishing barn where they are crowded into pens.

Because of ammonia levels, respiratory problems are the leading killer of pigs grown for meat.[8] Like birds, they are bred to grow faster than their bodies can handle, and many develop painful leg conditions and eventually are unable to walk. If piglets fail to grow properly, they are killed on the farm. According to the American Association of Swine Veterinarians and the Pork Checkoff, appropriate ways to kill young piglets include blunt trauma with a "quick, firm blow to the top of the head." Although the idea is to kill the piglets quickly, this doesn't always happen and videos show injured piglets writhing in pain. Older pigs who aren't growing quickly enough to be economically viable may be killed through carbon dioxide, gunshot, or electrocution.[9]

Pigs are surprisingly social, intelligent, and playful. Under natural circumstances, they engage in nesting behavior and have a strong tendency to root and live in small social groups. With no opportunity to engage in any of their natural behaviors, crated pigs develop repetitive behaviors like banging their heads against the cages and biting the metal rails. Pigs who are crammed together in pens can develop aggressive behavior, so farmers often cut off their tails without anesthesia to prevent tail-biting. The male piglets are also castrated without any treatment for pain.

But the natural personalities of pigs aren't reflected in the unnatural environment of a farm. Former hog farmer Bob Comis said it best: "During 10 years as a pig farmer I came to know pigs as well as I know my own dog. That's why I quit."[10]

Dairy Cows

Bucolic scenes of black-and-white cows grazing on a hillside create a sense of the happy and safe farm. But many dairy cows spend their lives enclosed in barns or they are kept on large feedlots, where they live on a layer of mud and feces and among swarms of flies.

Again, it's efficiency at all costs, which means cows are bred to produce as much milk as possible. According to USDA statistics, the average dairy cow produces five times more milk today than in 1940.[11,12] They are also constantly impregnated to produce more milk. Being pushed to such limits means they develop painful diseases, such as udder inflammation, and they often become unable to walk comfortably or at all.

On most farms, both male and female calves are taken from their mothers shortly after birth. This allows the mother cow to return to producing milk for human consumption. Farmers say that the cows don't mind, but cows have a strong maternal instinct that makes the separation traumatic. In 2013 the *Newburyport News* in Newbury, Massachusetts, reported on strange noises coming from a local dairy farm. The reporter shared that "According to Newbury police Sergeant Patty Fisher, the noises are coming from mother cows who are lamenting the separation from their calves." The separation of mother cows from their calves is a yearly occurrence and is a normal function of a working dairy farm, Fisher said. "It happens every year at the same time."[13]

Calves on Dairy Farms

Like any mammal, cows produce milk only after they've given birth. In the early days of dairy farming, male calves were kept or sold as breeding stock. As farms got bigger and the number of male calves outnumbered the need for breeders, farmers needed a new solution. That solution was veal. A direct outgrowth of dairy farming, veal farming is a way to turn unneeded calves into meat and money.

While female calves are sent to live in individual huts until they are ready to be bred and milked, the newborn males are sold and transported to a veal farm. They, too, are housed in individual pens for about eight weeks and then transitioned to small group pens. The calves are sent to slaughter at about five months of age.

Cows Raised for Beef

A common thread in animal food production is that most of these animals never see the outdoors until they are loaded onto a truck bound for the slaughterhouse. Cattle raised for beef are the exception since most graze outdoors for the first part of their lives. Of all farmed animals, beef cattle probably have it the best for these first few months. They graze and socialize as nature intended. They aren't free from abuse though, since they are often branded with a hot iron and the males are tied down and castrated without any type of pain relief. Eventually, the cattle are moved to a facility where they will put on weight at a much faster rate. Even "grass fed" cattle may be sent to a barn to live the rest of their lives indoors where they are fed a mix of legumes and hay. (Grass-fed refers only to what cows eat; not where they eat it.)

Most beef cattle are loaded onto trucks and shipped to crowded feedlots. After the relatively peaceful four to six months on the ranch, the feedlot is most likely an unpleasant adjustment for cattle. They are often crammed into these barren facilities where their diet is switched from grass and forage to grains and soy. Harris Ranch in Coalinga, California, is a feedlot that holds more than 100,000 beef cows for fattening. They live on a layer of dirt mixed with feces, and the stench can be smelled from miles away.

Because of the stress of their new environment and the switch to an unnatural diet, cattle in feedlots are prone to illness including respiratory disease. It is a common practice to lace their feed with antibiotics, which also help the cattle grow faster.[14] One estimate is that as much as 80 percent of all antibiotics sold in the United States are used on farmed animals, and this may contribute to antibiotic resistant bacteria. In fact the very air around feedlots has been found to contain DNA that codes for antibiotic resistance.[15]

ALL FARMED ANIMALS ARE SENT TO SLAUGHTER

Some farmed animals, like cows on small dairy farms or cattle grazing on the range, may live in relative comfort for at least the first part of their lives. But all farmed animals, unless they die from starvation, thirst, infections, or injury on the farm, are eventually sent to the slaughterhouse. For many, it is the first time they ever see the outdoors as they are packed onto trucks. Some are healthy animals who have been raised specifically for slaughter. Others are tired and worn-down dairy cows, breeding pigs, and laying hens who have outlived their economic value. All of these animals are killed well before they achieve their natural lifespan.

As slaughterhouses have consolidated, animals are trucked long distances to their deaths. They are typically not fed for many hours at a time and are subject to extreme heat and freezing cold, as well as highway accidents. It is legal to transport cows and pigs for up to twenty-eight hours without providing food or water. For chickens and turkeys, there is no limit on how long they can be held on trucks. Dairy cows may be so weak and tired that these gentle animals are unable to walk from the truck to the slaughterhouse. Animal science experts note that many of these cows are far too sick to be transported

long distances, but are loaded onto trucks anyway. In a journal of veterinary medicine, one group noted that these practices are common
and that they mean considerable suffering for the cows.[16] Once she
arrives at the slaughterhouse, a cow who can't walk can't legally be
slaughtered so she may be repeatedly shocked to get her to stand up.

Some of these stumbling, confused animals are the youngest of
calves. About 15 percent of calves are slaughtered when they are just
a few days or weeks old for "bob veal."[17] One investigation showed
workers kicking and electrically prodding newborn calves who strug-
gled to walk to slaughter.

With the exception of kosher and halal slaughter, mammals must
be rendered unconscious before they are killed according to the federal
Humane Slaughter Act. This is often done with a shot from a captive
bolt pistol. With the fast pace of the slaughter line, it's a given that
some animals won't be properly stunned on the first try. The American
Meat Institute considers a 95-percent stun rate acceptable, and research suggests that between 95 and 99 percent of animals are stunned
with the first shot.[18] But the fact that "only" 1 to 5 percent of cows are
insufficiently stunned on the first try means that as many 345,000 to
1.7 million cows per year must be stunned more than once—or they
remain conscious during at least part of the slaughter process.[19]

Fast line speeds at the slaughterhouse are typically to blame for
the fact that animals are often conscious as they move down the line.
Workers are under too much pressure to keep the line moving and
cannot take the time to worry about a still-conscious animal who has
slipped by.

And as weak as the federal Humane Slaughter Act is, it doesn't
even cover chickens and turkeys (or rabbits). There is no federal requirement for these animals to be stunned or unconscious when they
are slaughtered. Hung upside down, their heads are dragged through
an electric stunning bath before a blade cuts their throats. Then they
are dunked into a scalding tank for easier feather removal. Although
standard practices in slaughterhouses are aimed at ensuring that they
are dead by this time, USDA data shows that as many as a half-million

chickens and turkeys each year are still alive as they drown in near boiling water.[20]

NATURAL DISASTERS AND ACCIDENTS AFFECT FARMED ANIMALS, TOO

When the flood waters swept over eastern North Carolina during Hurricane Florence in 2018, tens of thousands of chickens and pigs had no way to escape. Estimates are that more than 5,000 hogs and 3.4 million chickens and turkeys drowned, many of them presumably imprisoned in their crates. There was nothing the farmers could do. Because huge numbers of farmed animals are confined in massive sheds on today's farms, when catastrophes strike, there is no escape. In 2010, for instance, 60,000 chickens died from heat exhaustion on a North Carolina farm when the fans stopped working following a power outage. A year earlier, nearly 4,000 pigs met the same fate when a vandal turned off the fans on an Iowa farm. And on a single farm in Texas, 800,000 hens died in a fire.

FISH AND OTHER SEA CREATURES

It may seem difficult to warm up to a fish, but these animals are more complex than once thought. There is evidence that some types of fish are capable of planning and using tools and some even have the capacity for facial recognition.[21] Research suggests that fish can feel pain and experience suffering as well. They react to pain by changing their behavior, which suggests a consciousness of discomfort. We don't know what pain feels like to a fish, but it seems fair to give them the benefit of the doubt, especially since the ways in which they are farmed, caught, and killed are particularly inhumane.

Bottom-trawling nets pull hundreds of tons of animals from the ocean, squeezing them together in the nets sometimes for hours as they are dragged along the ocean floor. When hauled out of the water, the surviving fish undergo decompression and suffer agonizing deaths.

Other animals suffer and die as a result of commercial fishing since drift nets kill tens of thousands of sea mammals such as dolphins, whales, otters, seals, and sea lions per year.

FACTORY FARMS HURT HUMANS, TOO

In 1906 Upton Sinclair's famous book *The Jungle* was published, detailing the lives of Lithuanian immigrants working in filthy and inhumane conditions in Chicago's stockyards and slaughterhouses. His book led to landmark changes in the meat industry as well the establishment of the forerunner of the US Food and Drug Administration. But, more than a century later, slaughterhouse workers, many of whom are immigrants, still work under incredibly dangerous conditions. The fast pace of line speeds in the slaughterhouse mean that workers make thousands of repetitive movements per day giving rise to muscle and nerve injuries. Witnessing the pain and fear of the animals being killed can also give rise to psychological trauma.

Most slaughterhouse workers are people of color living in low-income communities or are immigrants from Latin America. Some are undocumented and are unable to report injuries or seek medical care or report harassment and violations in the workplace for fear of being deported or losing their job. Like exploitation and inhumane treatment of animals, the exploitation of slaughterhouse workers helps keep the cost of animal foods low and production high.

Alternatives to Factory Farms

Learning about the lives and deaths of farmed animals can be disheartening, but there is good news, too. There have been small changes in factory farming practices at the state level, nearly all in response to the efforts of animal protection activists. Voters in some states have passed measures to do away with some of the cruelest confinement systems. But given the extensive and routine cruelty associated with factory farming and the strength of an industry that resists even the smallest improvements, meaningful change for all farm animals is a long way off. Animal cruelty is an inherent part of factory farming.

For many people, the answer is to seek meat, milk, and eggs from animals who were well treated. A number of different labels are meant to identify food from these animals. Three labels that suggest better treatment of animals on farms, and sometimes during transport, are "GAP-Certified" (which is associated with Whole Foods Markets), "Certified Humane," and "Animal Welfare Approved," but none of these labels cover all animals and/or all aspects of production. It's also easy to get confused. For example, the "American Humane Certi-fied" label is not associated with better welfare for animals. You'll see this label on pork that may have come from a farm that uses gesta-tion crates and on cartons of eggs from caged hens.[22] Terms like "all-natural," "free range," "humanely-produced," and "pasture-raised," have no legal definitions.

The organic label mandates some basic welfare standards for ani-mals since it requires access to the outdoors and conditions that allow some freedom of movement. But there are no specific definitions for these space requirements or the quality of the outdoor environment. In 2010, the Cornucopia Institute, an organic farm watchdog group, released a report that was based on visits to more than 15 percent of USDA-certified organic egg farms and surveys of all name-brand and private-label industry egg companies. They found that most of the industrial-scale producers were confining tens of thousands of hens inside henhouses, commonly only offering tiny concrete or wooden porches as "outdoor access."[23] Whether or not organic farms comply with standards, animals raised on these farms are not protected from the same types of mutilation as animals on nonorganic farms and they are subject to the same suffering during transport and slaughter.

For most products touted as "humanely produced," cruelty lurks behind the cheerful label. Even if free-range dairy farms provide better treatment for cows, their male calves are still taken from their mothers within hours of birth and sold for veal production. Chickens in cage-free facilities can spread their wings, but they still spend their entire lives packed by the tens of thousands into windowless warehouses. The male chicks are still killed at birth and the females are debeaked. They go to the same slaughterhouses as caged chickens.

Seeking out these labels can be valuable while you are making a transition to a vegan diet. But there is no way to ensure that any milk, eggs, or meat you consume were produced with no animal suffering. And they always come from animals who died within years of their natural lifespan.

ANIMAL RIGHTS

People dress their dogs in fuzzy coats for a brief walk in the snow, adopt kittens from shelters, and flock to national parks to photograph grizzly bears and moose. Most humans love animals and are sometimes in awe of them. How then can people sanction the practices of keeping pigs in gestation crates and hens in cages before sending them to an early death?

British psychologist Richard Ryder answered that question in 1970 when he coined the term "speciesism," which was later popularized by Princeton University philosopher Dr. Peter Singer in his 1975 book *Animal Liberation*.[25] Singer wrote that just as "racists violate the principle of equality by giving greater weight to the interests of members of their own race, speciesists allow the interests of their own species to override the greater interests of members of other species."

Not only do we consider the interests of humans to be paramount, we also believe that certain animals matter more than others. Or that they have different purposes. That's a judgment that varies among cultures, but in the United States, we've largely determined that dogs and cats are beloved companions while pigs, chickens, and cows are food. Yet, there is no logical or moral reason to distinguish among these animals.

An animal rights ethic asks us to put aside the issue of species and to consider only whether an animal is sentient and capable of suffering. It doesn't mean we treat all species the same in every situation.

TUNING IN TO ANIMALS

At just three weeks of age, a little female piglet from a farm in Iowa was loaded onto a truck with hundreds of other pigs. The weanlings were headed to a facility where they would be held in pens for several months to be fattened up for slaughter. When the truck arrived and the piglets were unloaded, this one little animal somehow managed to hide. The truck headed to a truck wash where it was flooded with water to clean out the excrement. As the water swooshed out, an employee saw the half-drowned piglet float by. He grabbed her and with nowhere to take the piglet, called the Iowa Farm Sanctuary. The sanctuary staff took the piglet in, named her Unsinkable Molly Brown, and gave her a safe home for the rest of her life. At the sanctuary, Molly loves being around people, especially if she can convince someone to give her a belly rub. She enjoys being outdoors during the day, but evenings usually find her in the cozy barn, snuggled up with her best friend, a potbelly pig named Stella.

Molly is among a handful of lucky animals who escaped a factory farm and eventual slaughter. Every year, 10 billion animals are killed to feed the demand for beef, pork, chicken, eggs, milk, and cheese in the United States. It's impossible to wrap your brain around those numbers and most of us don't even want to try to imagine all of that suffering. When we talk about the conditions on factory farms, what sometimes gets lost in the discussion is that each of these billions of animals is a feeling individual. If the massive numbers and unimaginable suffering make you feel tempted to tune out, it can be helpful to focus on just one of these animals and to realize that your choices make a difference. Every single time you pass up a hotdog or omelet or glass of milk, you are taking a stand against the abuse of an animal like Molly.

If you are able, we highly recommend visiting a farm animal sanctuary to have the opportunity to know these animals. There are close to 100 of them in the United States and many more throughout the world.[24] If an in-person visit isn't possible, read about the animals on the sanctuary websites or follow their accounts on Instagram for inspiring stories and photos. Seeing what is possible for these animals when they are rescued and safe is a good way to stay committed on your vegan journey.

And it doesn't mean that animals have the exact same rights as humans. It simply means that we don't decide whether an individual deserves protection based on their species alone. Since a chicken or a cow or a pig all experience fear and pain, and wish to avoid death, we really have no compelling reason to believe they deserve less protection than a dog.

VEGAN DIETS AND CLIMATE CHANGE

Shifting your diet away from meat, dairy, and eggs does more than protect animals—it helps to shrink your carbon footprint as well. Animal agriculture takes a toll on planetary resources and helps propel global warming.

Global warming is perhaps the most pressing issue of our time. It drives climate change, which includes extreme weather patterns, changes in precipitation, rising oceans, flooding, droughts, wildfires, and hurricanes. Climate change threatens not just public safely, but also public health and food security. For example, rising temperatures and increasing concentrations of carbon dioxide in the atmosphere increase pollen production and make the allergy season longer. These same conditions help invasive weeds and insects thrive, which threatens food crops. Rising sea levels and flooding create conditions for the spread of infectious diseases.

And, of course, climate change has devastating effects on wild animals, too. In the Arctic, polar bears are losing the sea ice they require for survival as it melts into the ocean. At the other end of the globe, seabirds and marine mammals of the Antarctic are also seeing their food supplies dwindle with the shrinking ice. Warmer, more acidic oceans are killing parts of Australia's Great Barrier Reef, which has been described by UNESCO as one of the richest and most complex natural ecosystems on earth. It's where humpback whales give birth, sea turtles breed, and more than two hundred species of birds come to roost and nest. Higher temperatures, melting ice, acidic oceans, and habitat losses are a threat to the remarkable biodiversity of the planet, to human health, and to our food and water supplies.[26]

Animal Agriculture and Climate Change

Scientists agree that global warming is a problem caused by human activity. It's due to increases in greenhouse gases (GHGs), particularly carbon dioxide, in the atmosphere. These gases trap heat, preventing it from escaping into the outer atmosphere. Two human activities that contribute significantly to global warming are the burning of fossil fuels and agriculture.

While all agriculture contributes to global warming, eating plant foods instead of animal products is one important way to shrink your carbon footprint. Growing animals to produce meat, eggs, and dairy takes a disproportionate amount of resources like land, water, fertilizer, and fossil fuels and that translates to higher GHG emissions.

It's not a new concept. Back in 1971, author Frances Moore Lappé calculated the true cost of meat production in her seminal book *Diet for a Small Planet*.[27] She coined the phrase "protein factory in reverse" to describe the wasteful process of meat production and its toll on land, fuel, and water. Specifically, she showed that there is more protein and energy in the grains and beans fed to farmed animals than in the meat, eggs, and milk that they produce. The excess protein and calories that the animals ingest ends up supporting their energy needs and contributing to growth of body parts that humans don't consume.

This inefficiency means that we get far too little return on the substantial resources—land, water, and fuel—that is poured into growing animal feed. For example, the Amazon rainforest is being cleared in part to expose land to grow soybeans. As the single largest tropical rainforest in the world, the Amazon is home to at least 10 percent of the world's known species. It's been called the "lungs of the planet" because of its valuable role in removing carbon dioxide from the air and converting it to oxygen. As the rainforest shrinks, so does its carbon-reducing capacity.

A common misconception is that eating soyfoods like tofu and veggie burgers is the reason the Amazon is disappearing. But it's not humans who are eating those soybeans from the rainforest—the beans are processed into animal feed and shipped off to dairy, hog, and chicken farms and to cattle feedlots. If we ate these beans directly instead of funneling them through the "protein factory in reverse" of animal agriculture, we'd be able to grow enough on far less land.[28] Eating soyfoods doesn't destroy the Amazon, it helps save it.

Eating beans and grains directly instead of feeding them to farmed animals conserves land, water, fertilizer, and fossil fuel. By one estimate, it takes almost three times as much water and thirteen times as much fertilizer to produce food for a meat-eater compared to a vegetarian.[29]

Clearing forests, processing massive amounts of animal feed, housing and transporting animals, and generating fertilizer all produce GHGs. The manure produced by farmed animals also releases GHGs and so do the digestive systems of cows, through burps and flatulence. When British researchers measured average greenhouse gas emissions from people eating all different types of diets including vegan, vegetarian, and varying amounts of meat, they found that the less animal food a group ate, the lower the GHG emissions associated with their diet. Emissions associated with meat-eaters were twice as high as those in vegans.[30]

Animal agriculture not only requires vast amounts of water, a precious and dwindling resource on our planet, but manure from these farms is also a source of water pollution.[31] On hog farms, waste is stored in outdoor pits called manure lagoons. When hurricanes strike the low-lying areas of coastal North Carolina where many of these hog farms are located, some of the manure lagoons are breached, pouring contents into the surrounding landscape.

Even in the best of times, these hog farms are a public health nuisance. Manure is routinely removed from the lagoons and sprayed on surrounding fields as fertilizer, creating a mist and a stench that impacts nearby communities. In North Carolina, hog farms produce nearly ten billion gallons of feces and urine per year. The farms are often located near low-income communities of color who don't have the financial clout to mobilize against the farms, making this a case of environmental racism and an important social justice issue. Exposure to the manure that permeates the air is linked to birth defects, asthma, and foodborne illness.

Locavore vs. Veggie Burger

Since fossil fuel is a major contributor to global warming, it might seem like eating locally is the best approach to dietary choice. But most carbon emissions related to food are due to production, not transportation.

Some plant foods are better than others, though, when it comes to resource use and global warming. Protein-rich beans are one of the most sustainable foods (they also improve soil health by fixing nitrogen). One group of researchers suggests that a simple change, replacing beef in American diets with beans, could help the United States meet up to 75 percent of its GHG reduction goals.[32] And even though food processing takes energy, even processed foods like soymilk, tofu, and veggie burgers produce far fewer greenhouse gases than comparable animal foods. Enjoying veggie burgers in place of burgers made from beef has considerable benefits for the environment.[33]

ANIMAL RIGHTS, HUMAN RIGHTS, CLIMATE CHANGE, AND VEGAN DIETS

With every step you take toward a vegan diet, you're reducing your contribution to some of the worst animal cruelty in the world and to the destruction of the planet. It's a powerful choice especially for those in industrialized countries like the United States. We consume almost twice the amount of meat as people living in developing countries. The impacts of our dietary habits are felt by those around the globe who have few choices about what they will eat, are the most vulnerable to food and water shortages, and who also have the fewest resources to respond to climate change. It means that those of us who do have a choice about what we will eat are in a uniquely privileged position— we have the opportunity, with every bite of food we take, to make a difference for farmed animals and for the rest of the people living on this planet.

CHAPTER 2

Making the Transition

When you go meatless and dairy-free, what on earth do you eat? Some of the best food you've ever tasted!

It would seem that dropping entire food categories from your menus would leave a diet that feels restricted. But upon going vegan, many people find that their food horizons actually expand as they explore new menu items like crusty barbecued Indonesian tempeh, Moroccan chickpea stew, Thai peanut sauce, and cashew cream cheesecake. Dining at a vegan table is anything but dull!

But what if exotic fare isn't your thing? What if you have neither the patience nor time to follow a recipe? That's fine. You can build healthful and appealing vegan meals around convenience foods and easily prepared dishes—old standbys that have been a part of your diet all of your life, like spaghetti with marinara sauce.

There are plenty of wonderful cookbooks and recipe websites for vegans who like to experiment in the kitchen. But you can be a happy, healthy vegan without ever cracking open a cookbook. After all, it doesn't take much instruction to bake a potato, flavor beans with onions and salsa, and round out the meal with steamed spinach. Much of the cooking that people do—whether or not they are vegan—is just this type of casual, unstructured preparation.

GETTING STARTED

It's not hard to create great vegan meals and find substitutes for the foods you've always enjoyed. Yes, there is a learning curve as you switch from the diet you've always known to one that is based on plant foods. But if you take it one step at a time, going vegan is a fun adventure.

Some people dive into a vegan diet and lifestyle overnight while others need to test the waters and make a gradual transition. The transition can occur in any number of ways, and it's up to you to decide what feels logical and practical. Don't assume that you have to go vegetarian—omitting meat while still eating eggs and dairy—as the first step toward veganism. Some people do, and that's fine, but it's not the only, or necessarily best, way to begin reducing your intake of animal products.

The tips in this chapter cover a broad range of big and small changes and offer options for different cooking and eating styles. Choose the ones that seem most realistic to begin with and then keep making changes at the pace that feels right for you.

KEYS TO SUCCESS

You may know someone who tried a vegan diet but went back to eating animal foods because they found it too difficult or didn't get what they expected from a vegan diet or didn't feel well. It's unfortunate because with some basic knowledge of food choices, sensible expectations, and a bit of support, staying vegan for life becomes much more realistic. Whether you are just taking steps toward a vegan diet or have been eating this way for a while, these tips can help ensure your success.

BE SMART ABOUT NUTRITION. It's true that you won't feel well on your vegan diet if you're falling short of vitamin D or vitamin B_{12} or not getting enough protein or fat. It's easy enough to get everything you need, but you do need to know how. In this book,

---

continues

we've provided everything that we believe you need to know to stay healthy on your vegan diet. For a quick primer, all of this information is condensed into a handful of guidelines in Chapter 10. If you follow those guidelines, you don't need to worry about whether your vegan diet is providing what you need.

CELEBRATE THE BENEFITS OF A VEGAN ETHIC. As you explore vegan choices, you might see some welcome changes in your health. Vegan diets are associated with lower blood pressure and cholesterol levels. Some people shed weight when they go vegan. But if you don't achieve health benefits or if those benefits are smaller than you expected, it doesn't mean your vegan diet "doesn't work." A vegan diet always works because it always reduces your contribution to animal exploitation and shrinks your carbon footprint. There is no other diet that can make those promises. Focusing on these guaranteed benefits of veganism makes it easy to embrace it as a long-term commitment.

DON'T WORRY ABOUT HOW YOU'LL FEEL WHEN YOU STOP EATING ANIMAL FOODS. You won't experience "detox" symptoms and won't feel any type of physical withdrawal. Foods like cheese and ice cream might be tempting at times, but we don't have actual physical addictions to these foods. And you will find plenty of satisfying vegan alternatives to them.

ENJOY A VARIETY OF VEGAN FOODS. Throughout this book, we're going to encourage you to make generous use of whole plant foods. But that doesn't mean that other foods are off limits. You don't need to go fat-free or raw to be a healthy vegan. It's okay to enjoy some refined grains and more processed foods. It won't make or break your health and it's likely to make your vegan diet more fun and pleasurable.

DON'T SWEAT THE SMALL STUFF. Even foods like white sugar and maple syrup—seemingly vegan—can be processed with animal ingredients. Some food additives and food colors can be either animal- or plant-derived—and you'd have no way of knowing which is

continues

in your food. Some vegans prefer to avoid such foods, but we see no need to do so. Avoiding these minute animal ingredients won't make your diet any healthier. Nor will it lessen animal suffering or help protect the environment in any meaningful way. The only thing it will do is make your vegan diet more restrictive, time-consuming, and difficult to follow. It's possible to get so bogged down in these details that you will simply find a vegan diet too laborious to follow. And the people around you may be less inspired to explore veganism if they believe that this meticulous attention to detail is required.

HONOR YOUR PROGRESS; DON'T WORRY ABOUT PERFECTION. No matter how devoted you are to being vegan, you may stumble sometimes in your commitment. For many people these stumbles occur around social situations or travel. If you lapse in your food choices now and then, don't let that derail all your efforts. Instead, celebrate the changes you've already made and are continuing to make and keep moving forward. Vegan choices get easier over time.

FIND SUPPORT. For some, it can feel isolating to be vegan. Local vegan organizations or meet-ups can be a good source of support. If you don't have any local resources, join the mentorship program at Vegan Outreach: https://veganoutreach.org/vmp/. The program will connect you with an experienced vegan mentor who will help you with everything from figuring out what to bring to a work potluck, to talking to your children's teachers about their diet, to answering questions from friends and family.

Make Small, Easy Substitutions Right Away

There are many changes you can make that don't require any real knowledge about cooking or meal planning. They won't make much difference in your meal preparation, but they will reduce your intake of animal foods immediately. First, make a few ingredient swaps by replacing mayonnaise with a commercial vegan choice (you'll find these right in the mayo aisle at the grocery store) and choosing vegan salad dressings. You'll also find cubes of vegetable bouillon next to the ones made from chicken—another easy exchange in recipes. Look for reduced-sodium versions of Worcestershire sauce. They're better for you and they usually don't contain anchovies.

One of the easiest changes you can make is to replace cow's milk with some type of plant milk. Because plant milks are used in the exact same ways as cow's milk, you don't need to learn anything new. It's just as easy to pour almond or oat milk over your morning cereal as it is to use cow's milk. You can use these milks in baking and in sauces, too. And given the variety of plant milks on the market, you will have no trouble finding one you like. Try milks made from soy, rice, hemp, oats, walnuts, flaxseeds, hempseeds, pea protein, or almonds on cereal, in baking, to make chocolate pudding, or to wash down a cookie. Look for choices that are fortified with calcium. If you don't like one, try another.

Explore Vegan Meats

When you want something "meaty," the selection of vegan choices is amazing. Check the frozen and refrigerated sections of specialty foods stores as well as your regular grocery store. You'll find vegan burgers, sausages, hotdogs, sandwich slices, pepperoni, Canadian bacon, pulled pork, chicken nuggets, corn dogs, ground beef, and much more. Different options appeal to different palates, so keep tasting until you find the items that you and your family enjoy. Look for products made by Gardein, Field Roast, Tofurky, Lightlife, Beyond Meat, Impossible Foods, and Yves, among others.

Vegans can also look to Asian cuisine for tofu and tempeh, two traditional meat substitutes. Read more about these staples of Asian diets in the Soyfoods Primer on pages 38–42. Both can be cubed, marinated in a simple sauce (try any barbecue, Thai peanut, or teriyaki sauce), and then baked or sautéed. Serve them over rice or tossed with cooked vegetables.

REDUCING MEAT: WHERE TO START

If you are taking first steps toward a vegan diet by reducing your meat intake, it might seem logical to start by eliminating red meat. We humans tend to relate more to other mammals like cows and pigs, and sometimes feel less unease about eating birds and fishes. And of course, concerns about health and the environment have many people cutting back on steak and pork chops. But in some ways, it makes more sense to eliminate the flesh of smaller animals like chickens first. It takes as many as 200 chickens to provide the same number of meals as one cow, so eliminating chicken meat from your diet impacts more animals. And what we know about chicken farms tells us that treatment of these animals is especially cruel.

This is not to say that there is any single best way to transition to a vegan diet. Every step you take toward reducing and eliminating animal products from your diet makes a difference and is a way of voicing your support for animals. But if you'd like to start with changes that have an especially valuable impact, consider removing chicken meat from your menus.

Get to Know the New Vegan Dairy

Vegan cheeses of the past sometimes left something to be desired in terms of their flavor, texture, and meltability. That has all changed. A wide selection of cheeses made to mimic cheddar, Parmesan, ricotta, mozzarella, Camembert, and more have made their way into both specialty and mainstream grocery stores and they keep getting better every day. Some are aged and cultured products that are at home at the fanciest wine and cheese party. Others are kid-friendly choices for an old-fashioned grilled cheese sandwich.

While a handful of these products contain small amounts of the milk protein casein, most are reliably vegan. Look for products made by Follow Your Heart, Violife, Vegan Gourmet, Daiya, Field Roast, and cultured cheeses made by Miyoko's Creamery, Kite Hill, and Treeline.

Here are additional ideas for phasing dairy out of your meals:

- Spread your morning bagel with nondairy cream cheese made by Tofutti, Daiya, Kite Hill, or Follow Your Heart. Most larger grocery stores carry one of these brands in the natural foods section. Even Trader Joe's has a vegan cream cheese!
- Spoon a few dollops of vegan sour cream into soup or on top of burritos.
- Try a nondairy creamer made from coconut or soy. Or make a soymilk foam for cappuccino.
- Have fun exploring the vast array of nondairy frozen desserts. Who needs ice cream when there is Coconut Bliss in the world?
- Everything that replaces dairy in your diet doesn't have to be an analogue. Spread almond butter or mashed avocado on toast instead of butter for a more healthful choice and a nice change of pace. Soaked cashews blended in a food processor or blender with lemon juice, salt, and olive oil makes a fast cheese spread.

Identify Ten Great Vegan Dinners

Start with what you know. What's on family menus that is already vegan or could be vegan with just a tweak or two? How about pasta with marinara sauce? Or tomato soup? (Prepare it with soymilk instead of cow's milk.) Make Sloppy Joes using a canned sauce and meatless "ground beef."

Next, spend some time with cookbooks, the internet, and your own recipe collection to identify seven to ten easy vegan dinners that you like and can prepare without much fuss (unless you like to fuss, of course). That's as much variety as most omnivores enjoy, and families are usually very happy with a ten-day cycle of their favorite meals. Over time, you'll probably grow tired of some and replace them with others, but for starters, this short list of meals will get you through your first months as a vegan.

Take Advantage of Convenience Foods

You don't have to be a sophisticated or creative cook in order to follow
a vegan diet. It's nice to know a few basics—how to bake a potato,
cook brown rice, and steam vegetables—but that's no more or less
than anyone, eating any type of diet, needs to know.

Anyone can make these ten vegan dinners:

- Baked potato topped with vegan baked beans and shredded soy
  cheese and accompanied by frozen spinach sautéed in olive oil.
- Veggie burger on a roll with salad and prepared salad dressing.
- Pasta salad: Toss cooked pasta with canned chickpeas, onions,
  chopped raw vegetables, and vegan mayonnaise.
- Burritos: Use leftover beans or canned vegan refried beans.
  Spoon onto warm tortillas, roll them up, and top with chopped
  tomatoes and guacamole.
- Pasta with sauce from a jar (add sautéed veggies or soy sausage
  for your own "homemade" touch).
- Chili beans with veggie burger crumbles served over rice with
  steamed carrots.
- Soup and salad: Progresso makes vegan lentil soup. Campbell's
  Tomato Soup—very possibly the most famous soup in America—
  is vegan. Just add any plain nondairy milk. Make it go a little farther with a healthful addition like pasta, rice, or beans.
- Taco salad: Toss together greens, chopped tomato, chopped onion, rinsed canned black beans, defrosted corn, and cubes of avocado. Dress with olive oil and lime or lemon juice and top with
  a handful of crushed tortilla chips.
- Tofu and vegetable stir-fry: Marinate chunks of firm tofu in prepared peanut or teriyaki sauce and stir-fry with frozen vegetables. Serve over rice or noodles.
- Whole-grain main-dish salad: This is a great way to use up
  leftover cooked grains. Toss brown rice, couscous, barley, or

whatever you have on hand with chopped onion, defrosted frozen peas and corn, sunflower seeds, and rinsed canned beans. Top with your favorite dressing or with olive oil and lemon juice.

Look to Global Cuisine

Some of the best eating patterns in the world—from both a culinary and health standpoint—are based on plant foods. When you start exploring meals from Italy, India, Mexico, China, Thailand, and other locales, it can open your world to exciting new vegan dishes. Look in cookbooks and online for recipes for pasta or Asian noodle dishes, curries, stir-fries, and pilafs (made with grains, nuts, and dried fruits). And look for restaurants that serve traditional cuisines from around the world when eating out since they are likely to have a good choice of vegan dishes.

Experiment with Beans

Most Americans didn't grow up eating beans, which is too bad. They are super nutritious foods and among the world's cheapest and most abundant sources of protein. That's why beans have played a role in the diets of nearly every culture. If you can't get organized enough to cook beans from scratch, it's fine to use canned. Try bean dishes that are familiar, like baked beans (you can buy the canned vegan variety), bean burritos, and lentil and split pea soups.

One way to update your attitude about this group of foods is to become familiar with their uses around the world. Chickpeas slow-baked in rich tomato sauce, along with pasta and a glass of Chianti is a meal featuring the traditional flavors of Sicily. Other wonderful bean-based delicacies are garlic-infused Cuban black beans, spicy Indian lentil curry, and lemony chickpea hummus from the Middle East. Truly, beans are anything but boring!

WHAT TO DO WITH BEANS

It's a simple matter to turn cooked beans into a tasty dish. Here are some super-fast ideas for ways to flavor beans. Most of these dishes can be served over rice or other grains—or spooned over a baked potato.

BLACK, PINTO, AND KIDNEY BEANS

- **Mexican-style beans:** For each cup of cooked beans, stir in ¼ cup salsa and ¼ cup corn kernels. Heat and serve over rice topped with shredded nut or soy cheese or chopped avocado and tomatoes.
- **Mediterranean beans:** Sauté ½ cup chopped onion and two stalks celery in 3 tablespoons olive oil until tender. Stir in two cans beans (rinsed) or 3 cups cooked beans, 4 ounces sliced pimiento-stuffed green olives, and a 4-ounce can chopped chile peppers.

WHITE BEANS (GREAT NORTHERN, BABY LIMA, OR CANNELLINI)

- **Beans with mushrooms:** Sauté 1½ cups sliced mushrooms in 2 tablespoons olive oil. Add 3 cups cooked beans and season with black pepper and fresh lemon juice. You might also add canned or chopped tomatoes.
- **Barbecued beans:** Mix 3 tablespoons prepared barbecue sauce into each cup of cooked beans.
- **Zesty beans with tomato sauce:** Mix 3 tablespoons prepared spaghetti sauce (try a spicy one) into each cup of cooked beans.
- **Italian-style beans with figs:** Sauté ¼ cup chopped onion and a clove of minced garlic in 1 tablespoon olive oil. Add 3 cups cooked beans and ½ cup chopped dried figs. Season with 1 teaspoon each dried basil and rosemary.
- **Hoppin' John:** Sauté 1 cup chopped onion and 2 minced garlic cloves in 3 tablespoons olive oil. Add 4 cups of beans and ¼ teaspoon ground cayenne pepper (more if you like your food very

spicy). Add ¼ cup chopped veggie bacon (or a sprinkle of bacon bits) if you like. Prepare this dish with black-eyed peas for a traditional southern New Year's Day supper. It's supposed to bring good luck for the coming year.

- **Beans with apples and sausage:** Sauté ½ cup chopped onions in 2 tablespoons olive oil. Add 3 cups cooked beans, 1 diced apple, and 4 ounces vegan sausage, crumbled. Simmer until everything is heated through and apples are tender.

ALL BEAN TYPES

- **Sloppy Joes:** Add a 15-ounce can of Sloppy Joe sauce to 2 cups cooked beans. Heat and serve over whole wheat hamburger rolls.
- **Bean and potato soup:** Sauté 1 cup chopped onions and two cloves minced garlic in 2 tablespoons olive oil. Add 2 cups diced potatoes, 2 cups cooked beans, and 8 cups vegetable broth. Simmer for 20 minutes until potatoes are tender. Season with basil and oregano.
- **Bean and grain salad:** Toss 3 cups of any cooked grain with 1 cup cooked beans. Season with bottled or homemade salad dressing. Add ¼ cup each of minced onion, chopped celery, dried cranberries or raisins, and/or shredded carrots for added flavor and crunch.

Add What's Missing: The Power of Umami

If you find it difficult to eliminate certain animal products from meals, it's possible that what you're really struggling with is umami. This flavor/essence of foods has been described as the fifth taste (in addition to salt, sweet, bitter, and sour), and certain foods like aged cheese are packed with it. It was discovered more than one hundred years ago, but scientists are still learning about what makes umami so satisfying. We may have an innate penchant for it since breast milk is high in umami.

Fortunately, it's easy to add umami to vegan meals. Ingredients that are high in umami include ripe tomatoes and concentrated tomato products like tomato paste, ketchup, and sun-dried tomatoes; wine; fermented soy products such as miso and tamari; concentrated yeast products such as Marmite and nutritional yeast; umeboshi plums and umeboshi vinegar; sauerkraut; balsamic vinegar; olives; dried mushrooms; and dried sea vegetables. In fact, the scientist who discovered umami first identified it in kombu, a sea vegetable.

Certain cooking practices like roasting, grilling, and caramelizing also bring out the umami aspect of foods. Here are some tips for adding umami to your menus:

- Add nutritional yeast to scrambled tofu, beans, vegetables, or pasta. Nutritional yeast blended with nuts and a little salt makes a delicious umami-rich substitute for Parmesan cheese.
- Toss vegetables with balsamic vinegar before roasting them.
- Blend sun-dried tomatoes with any type of cooked beans for a sandwich spread.
- Add a dash of red wine, miso, balsamic vinegar, or a sprinkle of dried sea vegetables, like nori or kombu to soups.
- Stir tomato paste into bean dishes or soups.
- Toss pasta with tapenade made from olives. Or spread the tapenade on sandwiches.

Take Advantage of Familiar Favorites for Breakfast

Many people eat the same breakfast every single day, perhaps with a slight variation on the weekends. Hot or cold cereal with nondairy milk, toast with nut butter, juice, and fruit make a very hearty and healthy vegan breakfast that will suit the needs of most family members. Overnight oatmeal is a popular breakfast-to-go choice. Look for recipes on the internet and substitute nondairy yogurt or any plant milk. Pancakes, vegan French toast, or scrambled tofu are good choices for more leisurely weekend breakfasts. Don't be afraid to think beyond traditional breakfast foods. A veggie burger or soup is just as good for breakfast as for dinner.

Identify Snacks, Treats, and Desserts That Are Vegan

You might want to experiment with egg-free baking (see next section on this page) but you'll also find a growing number of vegan baked goods and frozen desserts in stores. Old-fashioned, all-purpose cookbooks have recipes for fruit crumbles and crisps that are vegan—or that can be "veganized" by replacing butter with margarine or coconut oil.

Many snack chips are vegan and so are several brands of commercial cookies, including Oreos. Take a peek in the freezer section of your natural foods store, too, for frozen desserts such as Coconut Bliss, hempseed-based Tempt, and So Delicious products. Well-known traditional ice cream manufacturers like Ben and Jerry's, Häagen Dazs, and Breyers have jumped into the dairy-free market with their own vegan flavors.

Learn to Bake Without Eggs

The egg's main claim to fame is its role as a functional participant in cooking. In baking, it helps with leavening, and in savory foods, like veggie burgers, it's a binding agent. But other ingredients have those same properties, and there are plenty of effective ways to replace eggs in cooking.

To keep vegan loaves, burgers, and croquettes from falling apart, add a little bit of flour, bread crumbs, or rolled oats.

For egg-free baking, you are likely to get better results by using refined flours since they are lighter and more easily leavened. (It's fine to use whole grains, though, just as long as you know to expect a somewhat heavier product.)

Look for recipes that call for just one or two eggs since it is easy to replicate them with a vegan version. Most cake mixes lend themselves well to vegan baking. For foods that don't require a great deal of leavening, like pancakes, you can simply eliminate the eggs and add an extra two tablespoons of water or soymilk.

Try one of the following to replace eggs in baked goods.
For each egg:

- Combine 1 tablespoon ground flaxseeds with 3 tablespoons cold water and blend until thick and viscous. The consistency is just like raw egg.
- Mix 1 tablespoon full-fat soy flour with 3 tablespoons water.
- Mix together 1 tablespoon white vinegar and 1 teaspoon baking soda to make an instant, light foam.

DISCOVER AQUAFABA

Chances are, you already have a remarkable egg substitute sitting in your pantry. Aquafaba is the liquid from canned chickpeas. With a similar consistency to raw egg whites, this liquid can be whipped to create meringues, toppings for pies, and even homemade marshmallows and can be used as a substitute in baking. Replace one egg with 3 tablespoons of aquafaba. If you want to learn more about how to use aquafaba, head over to Facebook and join the Aquafaba (Vegan Meringue—Hits and Misses) group. Finally, two cookbooks provide extensive information on using aquafaba. One is *Vegan for Everybody* by America's Test Kitchen and the other is *Aquafaba* by Zsu Dever.

Go Egg-Free for Breakfast and Lunch

When it comes to replacing eggs on the menu, there is nothing like tofu. Mash tofu and sauté it in vegan margarine with mushrooms and a sprinkle of nutritional yeast for "scrambled tofu." Or chop firm tofu and mix with onion, celery, and vegan mayonnaise for vegan egg salad. You may want to track down some black salt (called *kala namak*), which can be found in Indian groceries or ordered online. It smells and tastes exactly like egg yolks. Try it in scrambled tofu or in recipes for vegan omelets. The Just, Inc. food company sells Just Eggs, a liquid product that can be scrambled or used to make omelets.

Pack Up Vegan Food to Go

There are thousands and thousands of vegan recipes for dinner and at-home meals. But you can brown-bag it vegan-style, too. If your workplace has a microwave oven, you can enjoy instant soups packaged as individual servings (the kind in cardboard cups) or prepared burritos. Use the weekend to prepare a big pot of soup or beans and then freeze individual portions for grab-and-go meals to heat at work. If you don't have access to a microwave, take leftover beans, soups, or stews to work in a good-quality thermos.

If you prefer a sandwich or wrap for lunch, there are plenty of vegan options beyond PB&J. Here are a dozen ideas to get you started:

- Almond butter with sliced bananas
- Chopped chickpeas, onions, and celery mixed with vegan mayo and a dash of lemon juice
- Baked tofu strips with tomatoes, lettuce, and vegan mayo
- Cashew cheese with sliced olives and red onions
- Vegan bologna and cheese slices with mustard
- Vegan tofu "egg" salad
- Tahini with shredded carrot and raisin salad
- Walnut-basil pesto with lettuce and sliced tomatoes
- Curried tofu spread
- White beans pureed with sun-dried tomatoes with lettuce, tomatoes, and avocado
- Lentil spread made with onions, nutritional yeast, and sunflower seeds, topped with shredded cabbage and tahini
- White beans and avocado (smash them together with a fork or potato masher) with sprouts and pickles

Keep Learning

The variety of vegan products is growing like wildfire. In particular, meats made from plants are appearing on restaurant menus across the country—including fast-food restaurants—and in both the natural foods sections and the meat case in grocery stores. They make it easier than ever for vegans to dine out and create fast meals at home. As you explore, experiment, and taste, your menus will evolve, and you'll find solutions to menu-planning problems. Even longtime vegans find that their menus and diets develop over time based on new products and changing lives. Maybe you need to identify a list of restaurants where you can meet friends or take business clients or host a child's birthday party. Local vegan societies are often the best resource for these kinds of questions. Phone apps like HappyCow and Vanilla Bean are useful guides to finding vegan restaurants. And the internet offers a wealth of ideas for vegans who entertain and need ideas for a vegan cocktail party or for family get-togethers.

VEGAN ON A BUDGET

Making the change to a vegan diet won't automatically save you money, but it's easy enough to plan healthy and enjoyable meals with a budget in mind. There's a balance, though: the best way to cut back on food expenses is to eat out less frequently and limit pricey convenience foods. But that usually translates to more time spent cooking, and not everyone has the time or ability to cook most of their meals. Here are a few ideas that will help you save money without spending hours in the kitchen.

- Cook beans and grains from scratch but in large enough quantities to have on hand for several meals. Leftovers don't have to be the same old thing. Serve black beans over rice the first night and then mixed with corn and salsa and wrapped in a corn tortilla the next. If you still have beans left over, you can add a can of tomatoes for a third dinner. Or cook up a pot of chickpeas and use half to make hummus for sandwiches and half in a pasta and bean soup. The versatility of beans means that they can appear in meals throughout the week without getting boring. You can also batch cook and freeze beans in smaller portions to have on hand for lunches.

- Get the most from higher-cost ingredients. Nuts, in particular, tend to be expensive, but a small amount goes a long way. One tablespoon of ground nuts mixed into a serving of cooked grains can add substantial flavor for very little cost. The same is true of more deluxe foods like sun-dried tomatoes, olives, and curry paste.

- No amount of leftovers is too small to save. If you have just a quarter cup of rice left, toss in some shredded carrots and a little bit of tahini and roll it up in a whole wheat tortilla for a wrap sandwich. Little odds and ends in the refrigerator can often be pulled together into a salad or soup.

- Keep frozen vegetables on hand. They are just as nutritious as fresh and often cost less. And they make it so easy to create fast dinners without having to make an extra trip to the store. If you have fresh vegetables that you can't use before they go bad, cut them up and freeze them to use later.

- Many bakeries sell day-old bread and baked goods at a discount. Stock up there or at a bakery outlet nearby. Freeze loaves so you won't run out.

- Freeze bits of leftover canned ingredients like tomato paste and coconut milk. Keep a couple of ice cube trays in the freezer just for small amounts of these ingredients.

- If you have Asian, Middle Eastern, or Indian grocery stores in your area, you may find "specialty" foods at much lower prices. This can be your ticket to saving on some of the more expensive vegan staples like soymilk, tahini, and tempeh.

- Visit www.localharvest.org/csa to find a community-supported agriculture group in your area, and talk to them to see if it would be a good fit for you. These programs allow you to buy shares in local farms—a good way to support small vegetable farmers and get quality produce—but depending on the specifics, they may or may not be a bargain.

- If you can't make everything from scratch, choose a few items that will save you real money and that you enjoy (or at least don't mind) doing. Homemade cakes and cookies can save lots of money. Making your own seitan from gluten flour is also a huge money saver and it is far easier than most people think; you can make a big batch every few months and freeze it. Other ways to save include homemade salad dressings, peanut sauce, and hummus.

- If you have even a small sunny spot in your yard or on a patio or balcony, you can grow your own vegetables. Tomatoes, lettuce, and greens can all be grown in pots. Leafy greens like kale and Swiss chard will give you a harvest throughout the summer and well into the fall. If you like cooking with fresh herbs, a small herb garden—in the ground or in a pot or on the windowsill—is a must since these foods are expensive at the grocery store.

All the standard advice that works for budget-minded omnivores applies to vegan grocery shopping: make a list and stick to it; buy in season; look for specials; avoid impulse purchases; and take advantage of bulk-food warehouse stores.

SOYFOODS PRIMER

You don't have to include soyfoods in your vegan diet, but they are so versatile and nutritious that many vegans make them a staple of their menu. This group of foods has a long history of use in Asian countries, and they've been the focus of much research over the past couple of decades. We'll talk about nutrition, health, and safety issues related to soy in Chapter 9. Here is a quick rundown of the most commonly consumed soyfoods.

Soybeans. Soybeans are generally tan in color, but they can also be black or brown. They're a good source of protein, fiber, calcium, iron, and folate. Cooked soybeans have a flavor often described as "beany." It's a flavor that marries well with tomato sauces and spicy foods.

Edamame. These are soybeans that are harvested at about 75 percent maturity, while they are still green and have the nutrition of the whole soybean but with a milder flavor. In Japanese cuisine, they are boiled in the pod and then served as a popular bar food (with beer). You can find edamame already shelled in either the produce or frozen food section. Boil them for fifteen minutes and eat as a vegetable, add them to grain salads, or use them to make a delicious variation on hummus. They're a good source of protein, fiber, and calcium.

Soynuts. Made from dry soybeans that have been soaked and then roasted, these are a good snack and a crunchy addition to salads. They are relatively high in fat and calories and are a good source of both protein and calcium.

Soymilk. This is the liquid expressed from soaked, pureed soybeans. It's a good source of protein and usually fortified with calcium, vitamin D, vitamin B_{12}, and sometimes riboflavin. (Soymilk sold in Asian markets is often not fortified, so be certain to check labels.) Plain, unsweetened soymilk can stand in for cow's milk in just about any circumstance. Vanilla or chocolate soymilk can be used in smoothies or desserts.

Tofu. Made in the same way that cheese is made from cow's milk, tofu is produced by adding a curdling agent to soymilk. Though it is the source of many jokes in the Western world, tofu has a long and sacred history in the East. It's believed that the first tofu shops were located within the walls of Buddhist temples and the first tofu makers were monks. There is still a sense of the sacred attached to tofu and tofu making in many parts of Asia today. It has been used for nearly two thousand years in China and is a daily staple in most Asian households. Throughout Asia tofu is made fresh daily from soybeans in small shops and sold on the street by vendors.

If calcium sulfate is used in the manufacturing process, tofu is a good source of calcium. The protein content varies depending on processing, but some types, especially those that are more firm, are very high in protein.

Two properties give tofu great culinary versatility. First, its flavor is relatively bland. Second, it is a porous food that takes on the flavor of other foods and ingredients with ease. This explains why tofu is at home in spicy entrees or in creamy sweet desserts.

The key to success with tofu is to choose the right type for the job. If you are stir-frying chunks of tofu with veggies to serve over rice, choose firm tofu. Soft tofu is perfect to mash or puree as a filling for sandwiches or lasagna. And the tofu that is traditional to Japanese cooking, silken tofu, is a soft, custard-like food that can be blended or pureed for sauces, smoothies, or desserts. It is a great replacement for the cream in creamed soup recipes.

Frozen tofu takes on a chewy, spongy texture that makes it a useful meat substitute. Freeze it right in the unopened package. Then defrost, squeeze out the liquid, and chop or shred it.

Okara. The word "kara" refers to the hull of the soybean, and the addition of "o" turns it into "honorable hull." This is the portion left behind when liquid is squeezed from the soaked soybean to make soymilk. It's high in protein and fiber and is sometimes used to give a protein boost to baked goods like muffins or cookies. In Japan, okara is sometimes sautéed with vegetables and served with rice. You may be able to find okara in natural foods stores, but the best place to track it down is in an Asian market.

Fermented Soyfoods

Tempeh. In Indonesia, it's spelled *tempe*, and it is an ancient cultural staple of cooking in that part of the world. Today, tempeh making is still a home-based art in which whole soybeans are treated with a "starter" and wrapped in banana leaves to ferment. Tempeh can be made from soybeans only or soybeans in combination with grains. The texture is tender and chewy, and the savory flavor is sometimes described as "nutty," "yeasty," or "mushroom-like"—or just indescribably delicious. In traditional meals, it's sautéed with vegetables and served over rice, sometimes with peanut sauce. Tempeh baked in barbecue sauce is a favorite with many vegans. Like tofu, tempeh takes to marinades and flavorings very well. Tempeh is a good source of protein, fiber, iron, and calcium. Contrary to popular opinion, however, it is not a good source of active vitamin B_{12} (for more on B_{12}, see pages 85–94).

Miso. You may be familiar with miso soup, the common starter in many Japanese restaurants. With a full-bodied flavor that is unmatched by any Western condiment, miso captures the essence of Japanese cooking. This salty, fermented soybean paste (usually with the addition of other beans or grains) comes in different colors—white, red, and brown—and the flavor varies greatly among types, with some being more fruity or wine-like than others. In fact, in Japan, miso production is regarded in a similar fashion to winemaking in other parts of the world. Miso is very high in sodium and a little goes a long way. Use it to make broths and sauces.

Natto. Made from whole soybeans fermented with a bacterial culture, natto has a distinctive aroma, flavor, and texture, which is often described as "gooey." It is a popular breakfast food in Japan, served with rice, but has not made its way onto many American menus. It may be the only known plant food that is high in vitamin K_2.

Western Soyfoods

Soy Curls. Made from the whole soybean, once these are dehydrated in hot water or broth, they can be marinated and then sautéed to produce a chewy and flavorful meat substitute. They are a favorite for making vegan bacon with the addition of liquid smoke and tamari.

Textured Vegetable Protein (TVP™). Made from defatted soy flour, TVP is a dried granular product that can be rehydrated with boiling water and used in place of ground beef. Plain TVP tastes best when cooked in tomato sauce and is good for pasta dishes or chili. In her cookbook *Vegan Comfort Food*, Alicia Simpson recommends rehydrating 1 cup dry TVP with 1 cup of dark vegetable stock and 1 tablespoon of hickory liquid smoke. TVP is a very inexpensive source of protein with a long shelf life, and it's a good source of protein, fiber, and calcium.

Isolated Soy Protein. Many veggie meats use soy protein as a base. For those who are just making the transition to veganism, are too busy to cook, or crave protein-rich foods, veggie meats made from soy protein isolate can be life-savers.

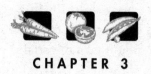

CHAPTER 3

Understanding Vegan
Nutrient Needs

Nutrition science was born in the early 1800s with the discovery of protein, carbohydrates, and fats. But long before that, humans knew a lot—strictly through trial and error—about food and health without actually understanding what the protective factors in foods were.

The first documented nutrition experiment was performed in 1747 by Dr. James Lind, a ship's doctor with the British Royal Navy. At the time, being a sailor was a dangerous occupation, not just because of storms and piracy, but because as many as half of all sailors who set out on long voyages died from scurvy. Theorizing that it had something to do with the lack of fruits and vegetables on board, Lind fed different diets to a small group of sailors and noted that those who consumed lemons and limes didn't get scurvy.

While the navy made good use of the information, ordering all British ships to carry limes, the reason that these foods were protective wasn't known for another two hundred years when researchers discovered vitamin C. (And while Lind got all the credit for discovering the cure for scurvy, Chinese sailors had been growing greens on their ships to ward off scurvy since at least the fifth century.)

As early as 1916, well before the discovery of many vitamins, nutritionists were recommending intake of certain "protective foods." The first recommended daily allowances (RDAs) were read over the radio to Americans in 1941 and have been updated and expanded a number of times since then.

Today, recommendations for individual nutrients are overseen by the National Academies of Sciences, Engineering, and Medicine (referred to in this book as the National Academies). While these are official recommendations, the science behind them is sometimes still not entirely settled. In some cases, there isn't enough research for anything more than an educated guess. And actual individual requirements are affected by lifestyle, overall diet, and genetics, which means that it's impossible to pin down the exact nutrient requirements of any one person.

The recommendations are set at levels that are believed to meet the needs of the majority of Americans. Therefore, for any given nutrient, many Americans will need less than the recommended amount while others might need more.

VEGANS AND THE RDAS

The dietary recommendations are aimed at omnivores and, in a few cases, nutrient needs might be higher for vegetarians and vegans. Protein requirements are believed to be slightly higher because plant protein isn't digested quite as well as protein from animals. It's a small difference and it's easily satisfied with vegan diets as long as calorie needs are met and your diet includes high-protein plant foods. Zinc needs may also be higher, and it's possible that some vegans have intakes that are less than optimal.

The situation for iron is a little more controversial. We'll see that vegans have higher requirements but how much higher is a subject of some debate. We've included the National Academies recommendations for iron in the chart on page 46, but we don't think that vegans should worry too much about getting this much iron. We'll talk much more about this issue in Chapter 8.

NUTRIENT INTAKE OF VEGANS: HOW DOES IT COMPARE TO RECOMMENDATIONS?

Studies show that vegans are likely to consume more of certain nutrients—vitamin C, thiamin, riboflavin, niacin, folate, and sometimes iron—than omnivores.[1] In contrast, many vegans have intakes of calcium and zinc that are lower than the recommendations. In the chart on page 46, we've compared recommendations for selected nutrients to actual intakes of groups of British vegans and North American vegans. The study in North American vegans included supplements and fortified foods, while the ones among British vegans didn't. It's also important to note that the type of dietary surveys used in these studies are not ideal for comparing intakes to recommendations. So we use them to look for trends and problems, but not for drawing absolute conclusions about the adequacy of any particular diet.

We also made a notation about recommended intakes of protein, iron, and zinc since they may be higher for vegans. We'll talk more about these issues later.

GOOD DIETS ARE GOOD ADVOCACY

Whether you are already vegan or just starting to take steps in that direction, eliminating animal products from your lifestyle is an effective way to make a difference. It reduces animal suffering, removes your financial support for factory farming, and represents a stance against the use of animals. And most of us who care about animals would like to see those around us explore a vegan diet, as well.

The meat, dairy, and egg industries would like to portray vegan diets as inadequate. So the last thing we want to do is give them any ammunition. Some vegans balk at the idea of taking vitamin B_{12} supplements, because they think it makes vegan diets appear inadequate.

NUTRIENT INTAKES OF VEGANS

	Recommended Nutrient Intakes for Adults (*adjusted recommendations for vegans)		Intakes of British Vegans 2003[2]		Intakes of North American Vegans 2013[3]	Intakes of British Vegans 2016[4]	
	Men	Women	Men	Women	Men and Women	Men	Women
Protein, grams	54 (*60)	46 (*51)	62	56	71		
Vitamin A, retinol activity equivalents	900	700			1,108 (calculated from beta-carotene intakes)	623	623
Vitamin C, milligrams	90	75	155	169	293		
Vitamin E, milligrams	15	15	16.1	14	18.5		
Vitamin B6, milligrams	1.3	1.3	2.2	2.1	3.2		
Folate, micrograms	400	400	431	412	723		
Calcium, milligrams	1,000	1,000	610	582	933	862	839
Iron, milligrams	8 (*14)	18 (*33)	15.3	14.1	22.2	20	18
Magnesium, milligrams	420	320	440	391	591		
Zinc, milligrams	11 (*16)	8 (*12)	7.9	7.2	11.3	9	8
Potassium, milligrams	4,700	4,700	3,937	3,817	4,120		

But taking a chance with nutrient deficiencies is the worst thing we can do for our own health and it also may affect how others view vegan diets.

It's tempting to believe that vegans will meet all their nutrient needs as long as they eat a variety of whole foods. After all, people were eating long before anyone knew what a nutrient was. But our forebears learned what to eat through many generations of trial and error. People who ate foods that sustained them and kept them healthy survived to pass those habits onto their offspring. Vegan diets don't have that history or that cultural context. While many populations have thrived on plant-based diets, those diets have always included some animal foods. We can't look to culture to guide us, but fortunately we can look to science.

And it's not just vegans who need to take advantage of modern nutrition knowledge. Despite a history of healthful eating practices, nutrient deficiencies have cropped up in many populations over the centuries. In the early twentieth century, iodine deficiency was widespread in parts of the United States. The response was to add iodine to salt, which has proven highly effective in preventing the scourge of iodine deficiency. In this case, not just science but food processing came to the rescue.

Promoting veganism as a lifestyle that is practical, easy, and realistic is important, too. Time, convenience, and taste are primary factors in people's food choices. That's why overly restrictive diets can create the wrong kind of image for veganism. Trends among some vegans to give up more and more foods—added fats, cooked foods, and plant-based meats and cheeses—are counterproductive, especially because these dietary restrictions have few health benefits for most people.

For example, the idea behind a raw foods diet is based on a few scientific principles that are shaky at best. There is really no good evidence to suggest that eating primarily raw food is any better for you than eating mostly cooked whole plant foods. In fact, some of the beneficial compounds in foods, such as lycopene (an antioxidant in tomatoes that protects against prostate cancer), are available only when foods are cooked. The vitamin A precursor beta-carotene is more readily available from cooked foods as well and is also better absorbed in the presence of some fat. A raw foods diet can be helpful for weight control, since it has a lower caloric density, but this also means that it isn't appropriate for children.

A gluten-free diet is an absolute necessity for those who have celiac disease, a permanent intolerance to gluten. But this autoimmune disease affects only 1 percent of the population. The percentage of people who have an intolerance to gluten (but don't have celiac disease) is also relatively small. That means that most vegans have no reason to eliminate gluten from their diets. In fact, some research suggests that gluten-free diets are associated with reductions in levels of beneficial gut bacteria and increased levels of harmful microbes. For those who don't have celiac disease, it may be beneficial to include some gluten in their diet. (Of course, those who have allergies, including nonceliac wheat allergy, need to adjust their diets accordingly.)

Promoting these additional restrictions that have no known health advantage for most people doesn't do anything to help animals or promote vegan diets. To the contrary, it creates an image of vegan diets that makes them look more difficult and less appealing. If we want others to follow our lead in adopting more compassionate food choices, it makes sense to avoid unnecessary restrictions and make vegan diets as accessible as possible.

The nutrition recommendations in this book, which are based on solid, current science, are aimed at making your vegan diet healthful and realistic. You'll see that it's easy to meet nutrient needs by eating a variety of cooked and raw plant foods, and it's also reasonable to plan some family meals using convenience products without compromising your health.

SUPPLEMENTS IN VEGAN DIETS

With the exception of vitamin B_{12}, it's possible to get all of the vitamins and minerals you need from plant foods and sunshine (for vitamin D). Depending on individual circumstances, though, vitamin supplements can provide an important way to meet nutrient needs, especially for vitamin D, iodine, calcium, and omega-3 fats.

While it's possible to purchase vitamin supplements that are food concentrates, many are synthetic—that is, they are synthesized in a laboratory. As long as they are well digested, synthetic vitamins and minerals will do their job. In fact, in some cases they are a better source of nutrition than the food concentrates. For example, some "natural" vitamin B$_{12}$ supplements are produced by companies that have not used proper testing standards and, therefore, the B$_{12}$ is not a reliable source of that nutrient. And for many people, especially with aging, the vitamin B$_{12}$ in supplements is much more available for absorption than vitamin B$_{12}$ that occurs naturally in animal foods.

The US Pharmacopeia (USP) verifies the quality, purity, and potency of dietary supplements for companies that take part in their certification program. Supplements that display the "Dietary Supplement USP Verified" mark on labels have been tested to verify that they dissolve properly. (Vitamin and mineral supplements that don't carry the USP symbol may still be of high quality; it just means they haven't been certified.) Other independent organizations that offer similar guarantees are ConsumerLab.com and NSF International.

The supplements we recommend throughout this book and that are summarized in Chapter 10 are for nutrients that can be low enough in vegan diets to lead to a deficiency. While a multivitamin can provide a number of these nutrients all at once, taking them as separate supplements will allow you to take only the supplements you need. A few things to keep in mind regarding supplements: First, most of us have sufficient stomach acid to dissolve supplements for thorough absorption. But if you have reason to believe that your stomach acid isn't strong, it's a good idea to crush or chew vitamin and mineral supplements. Also, supplements sometimes require a bit of attention to balance. For example, high doses of zinc can inhibit copper absorption. Taking 50 milligrams of zinc per day (the RDA for vegans is 12 to 16 milligrams) can cause a copper deficiency in just a few short weeks. This is one reason to rely on a well-balanced diet to provide enough nutrients, using supplements to make up for any shortfall.

KEEPING NUTRITION SIMPLE

Humans require more than forty essential nutrients. Most people know that they need nutrients like vitamin C, protein, and calcium. But they may never have heard of the B vitamin biotin or the mineral vanadium and have no idea that they need to consume foods that

NUTRIENT RECOMMENDATIONS:
SOME TERMINOLOGY

Depending on the available research, determining precise needs is easier for some nutrients than for others. If researchers don't have enough data, or the findings are conflicting, it can be difficult to reach conclusions about optimal intakes. Therefore, current recommendations fall into several different categories, which are collectively known as the DRI (Dietary Reference Intakes):

RECOMMENDED DIETARY ALLOWANCE (RDA): The amount of a nutrient that is believed to be sufficient to meet the needs of 97 to 98 percent of the population. It varies for different age groups and between men and women.

ADEQUATE INTAKE (AI): When there isn't enough data to establish an RDA, the National Academies sets an AI, which is based on both studies and observations of what healthy populations consume.

TOLERABLE UPPER INTAKE LEVEL (UL): This is the maximum daily intake of a nutrient that is likely to be safe. Some nutrients can be extremely toxic at higher than normal levels, although excessive intakes are almost always associated with supplements.

The RDAs and AIs are also used to generate **Daily Values** (DV), which are used strictly for food labeling purposes. The amounts of vitamins and minerals in a food are listed as a percent of the DV. For example, the DV for calcium is 1,300 milligrams, so if a food contains 10 percent of the DV for calcium per serving, it provides 130 milligrams of calcium. The DVs serve as a general guide to help you determine which foods are good sources of certain nutrients. A food that provides at least 20 percent of the DV for any nutrient can be considered a good source. These food labels can also guide you toward limiting foods that are high in things you want to avoid. A good rule of thumb is to aim for foods that provide 5 percent or less of the DV for saturated fat and sodium.

provide these nutrients. And it's definitely not something you need to worry about. Most nutrients are so readily available in all different types of diets that we don't need to think about how to get them.

In this book, we're going to focus on just nine nutrients—protein, calcium, iron, zinc, iodine, alpha-linolenic acid, and vitamins B_{12}, A, and D. We'll briefly mention a handful of others and talk about DHA, an omega-3 fat that doesn't have essential nutrient status (meaning that, while a growing body of evidence suggests that it's important, it hasn't been established as a dietary essential). These are the nutrients that are of special interest to vegans and are the center of vegan nutrition. Getting enough of them isn't difficult. You just have to know how to do it.

UNDERSTANDING NUTRITION RESEARCH

The amount of nutrition information in the media and on the internet is staggering. Much of it is conflicting and often studies looking at the same question come up with completely different answers.

In fact, for essentially all heavily researched areas, you can build a case for just about anything by picking and choosing the studies that support your point. Some advocates do this to make vegan diets look more beneficial. And some vegan detractors pick a completely different set of studies to make vegan diets look bad.

The key to understanding nutrition research is to look at the *entire body of evidence* and see what *most studies* say. Rarely can a single study provide a definitive answer to a question. There are always inconsistencies and there are always study flaws. In addition, different types of studies carry different weight. So the strengths and weaknesses of certain types of studies have to be balanced against the strengths and weaknesses of others.

We're going to get into the weeds just a little bit here as we look at the different types of studies. You can learn everything you need to know about being healthy on a vegan diet without diving into this information about nutrition research, so feel free to skip this section if you prefer. But for those who want to know how we've arrived at the recommendations we make in this book, this information provides some background.

Types of Studies

WEAKEST EVIDENCE

These types of studies don't provide conclusive evidence but are conducted primarily to determine if further research is warranted.

- Neither *in vitro* (studies conducted in test tubes or cell culture often using single cells) nor *animal studies* can serve as the basis for conclusions about diet and disease. Aside from any ethical considerations and despite their widespread use, findings about nutrition from animal studies often can't predict what is going to happen in humans.
- A *case study* is an observation about one or perhaps several patient histories and their treatment and disease outcomes that is published in a scientific journal. Often these types of reports can be used as the basis for generating a hypothesis, but they don't provide definitive answers. In contrast, if a report isn't published in a peer-reviewed journal, it is merely an anecdote and has little or no value in contributing to nutrition knowledge. A great deal of nutrition information on the internet and in books— including books by doctors and other health professionals—is based on anecdotes rather than actual science.

BETTER EVIDENCE: EPIDEMIOLOGIC RESEARCH

Epidemiologic studies look at health conditions in populations and try to determine whether those conditions are paired with other factors. For example, they might try to determine whether people who get cancer tend to eat fewer fruits. These studies can establish that two factors have occurred together but not that one causes the other. They are prone to *confounding variables*, which means that there might be unidentified issues that cause two factors to be associated. For example, if researchers find that people with low fruit intakes are more likely to get cancer, it seems logical that fruit is protective against this disease. But what if those who don't eat fruit also don't exercise? It's difficult to establish whether it is lack of fruit or lack of exercise or a combination of both that raises the risk.

There are several types of epidemiological studies and some provide stronger evidence than others.

- *Ecological studies* (also called correlational studies) compare food habits and disease rates among different groups of people. One ecological study that is familiar to many vegans is the China Study, which compared the types of food consumed and average disease rates in different counties in China, mostly during the 1980s. Although the China Study didn't look at vegan diets, it did find that the more plant foods and less animal foods consumed in a given county, the lower the rates of chronic diseases like heart disease and certain cancers. It's not possible to draw firm conclusions about diet and health from ecological studies like the China Study because this type of research doesn't control for other factors. But the studies do give rise to hypotheses about diet that stimulate further research that is designed in a way to give us better answers.

    Another ecological study that many vegans are familiar with looked at rates of hip fracture and protein consumption in different countries. The results showed that as protein intake increases, so does the rate of hip fracture. But contrary to popular opinion, that study didn't show that high protein intake causes weak bones and in fact, it may have misled us about the relationship of protein to bone health. (We talk more about why that is in Chapter 5.) It did set the stage for clinical studies on how protein might impact calcium metabolism.

    One interesting type of ecological study is the migration study. It looks at changes in health of people when they relocate and acquire the food and lifestyle habits of their adopted home-land. These kinds of studies can help show whether risk for certain diseases is related more to genetics or lifestyle.

Ecological studies are limited by the fact that there are many factors that affect health outcomes and these can't be completely controlled for in the analysis of the data. Additionally, individual food intakes can only be roughly estimated.

- *Retrospective studies* compare past eating habits between people with and without a particular disease. For example, if people with heart disease are more likely to have eaten a diet high in saturated fat, it would suggest that saturated fat might be a factor in heart disease. Some of the most interesting findings about soyfood consumption and breast cancer risk come from retrospective studies that look at breast cancer rates in women who consumed soyfoods in childhood and adolescence. The main drawback of these studies for nutrition research is that people's memories of their previous diet can be faulty, especially if their food choices have changed over the years.

- *Cross-sectional studies* compare eating habits and disease rates in groups of people at one moment in time. One problem is that people who have similar diets might have other lifestyle factors in common that could impact their disease rates. Another is that people who have become ill may have recently changed their diet.

- *Prospective studies* (also called cohort studies) follow large numbers of people who are (usually) healthy when the study begins. As the population is followed, eating patterns of those who eventually get a disease are compared to those who do not. These studies require a lot of subjects—numbering in the tens of thousands—and take place over a long period of time, but they carry the most weight of any epidemiologic studies. Much of what we know about the health of vegans comes from two large prospective studies, the Adventist Health Study in North America and the EPIC-Oxford Study in the United Kingdom. We describe these studies in more detail in Chapter 15.

BEST EVIDENCE: CLINICAL TRIALS

The *randomized clinical trial* (RCT) is the gold standard in nutrition research. It's the most credible type of study because it randomly assigns people to different groups and then controls what they eat. Ideally, the study is double-blinded, which means neither the subjects nor the researchers know who is in the experimental or control group until the study is completed. These studies can be very powerful, and ideally, everything we want to know about nutrition would be tested through RCTs. They are useful for testing the effects of a particular supplement or food on disease markers, like cholesterol or bone density. But, unfortunately, they are expensive and difficult to conduct for long periods of time. So they tend to be used for short-term studies that might test the effect of saturated fat on blood cholesterol levels, for example, but are rarely used for determining whether saturated fat causes people to die from heart disease.

We'll look at a number of RCTs in Chapter 15 where we consider the ways in which diet impacts chronic disease. For example, the Ornish study, which explored the impacts of eating a vegetarian diet along with other lifestyle changes on atherosclerosis, is a well-known RCT.

Other Considerations

A WORD ABOUT STATISTICS

Statistical analyses are always performed to eliminate the probability that different outcomes occurred by random chance. Generally, a finding is *statistically significant* if there is less than a 5 percent chance that it occurred by chance. When studies are small in size, it becomes difficult to show statistical significance. Even if there are measurement differences between different foods, supplements, or diets, if they aren't statistically significant, researchers conclude that there was no effect.

One way to make good use of the data from smaller studies is to do a *meta-analysis*. This is a statistical analysis of a large number of studies for the purpose of integrating the findings. It is often done to compensate for the small size of individual studies.

FUNDING AND OTHER TYPES OF BIAS IN RESEARCH

Scientific journals make sure that studies are credible and worth publishing by having them reviewed by other researchers qualified to do so. The reviewers can recommend that the study be published or not, based on what they think of the study design and other factors. However, the phenomenon known as publication bias means that journals are more likely to publish studies with positive findings—that is, studies where something "worked"—than a study with a negative finding. For example, a study that finds that vitamin C helps prevent colds will have a better chance of getting published than one that finds no effect of vitamin C. Researchers have developed methods to test for publication bias for well-researched subjects, but it remains an influence on contemporary nutrition science.

There is also a great deal of concern about the impact of funding on research. Most nutrition research is funded by the government, but some is paid for by the food industry. Although data is rarely fabricated, funding may affect the way a study is designed or the way the findings are reported. So, knowing about funding sources is important.

Industry funding is not the only source of bias. Many researchers have a vested interest in a particular theory and may have built their careers or even written books based on a particular belief about nutrition and health.

In conclusion, we can make educated statements about vegan nutrition only by looking at what most of the studies say (rather than drawing conclusions from individual studies) and by focusing on the studies that are likely to yield the most reliable information. The information in this book draws from that approach.

CHAPTER 4

Plant Protein

Nutrition researchers declared more than thirty years ago that plant foods can provide adequate protein.[1] But "where do you get your protein?" is a question that most vegans have heard more times than they can count. Many of the questions about protein in plant-based diets stem from confusion over what it means for proteins to be "complete."

COMPLETE AND INCOMPLETE PROTEINS

Proteins are made of chains of twenty different amino acids. Some amino acids can be made by the body (generally from other amino acids) and therefore we don't need a dietary source of them. Others—the *essential amino acids* (EAAs)—must be supplied by the diet.

Proteins in the human body tend to have a consistent percentage of the different EAAs. Because the percentage of EAAs in animal products and soybeans are a close match to those in the human body, proteins from these foods are considered "complete." Plant foods like grains, beans, and nuts have a lower percentage of at least one essential amino acid, making them "incomplete." For example, beans (other than soybeans) are low in the EAA methionine, and grains are low in lysine. But when grains and beans are consumed together, their amino acid profiles complement each other and produce a mix that is "complete" and therefore a good match to the body's needs.

In the early 1970s, the idea that vegetarian meals should contain complementary proteins was popularized in *Diet for a Small Planet* by Frances Moore Lappé.[2] Soon after that, research showed that it's not necessary to eat complementary proteins at each meal because the body maintains a storage of the essential amino acids.[3] We need to keep replenishing that storage with all the amino acids, which we can get by eating a variety of plant foods. But the old idea that certain combinations of plant foods—the complementary pairings—must be consumed together isn't true.

While fruit is extremely low in protein, and oils don't provide any, all other plant foods contain protein. One common misconception is that plant foods are completely lacking in one or more amino acids. That's not true—all plant sources of protein contain at least some of every essential amino acid. In fact, you could get enough protein and all the essential amino acids by eating just one type of food like pinto beans. You'd need to eat a lot of them, though—about four cups per day. That's not practical, partly because it would be boring, but also because all those beans are likely to displace foods that are needed to satisfy other nutrient requirements. So eating a variety of protein sources makes better nutritional sense.

PROTEIN RDA FOR VEGANS

Protein needs are calculated on the basis of body weight. Scientists use the metric system, so US protein needs are determined using your weight in kilograms.

The protein RDA for adults is 0.8 grams of protein per kilogram of body weight. The World Health Organization recommends a very slightly higher intake at 0.83 grams per kilogram of body weight.[4] Since protein needs vary considerably among individuals, the RDA is designed to cover the needs of 97 percent of the population and is presumably more than what many people need. Without any way of knowing where you fall on the protein-needs spectrum, and because some protein experts believe that current protein recommendations are too low, it's a good idea to play it safe and aim for the RDA.[5]

But along with most other vegan dietitians, we recommend a somewhat higher protein intake for vegans. This is because plant proteins are not digested as well as animal proteins.[6] Since both cooking and processing often improve protein digestibility, this may be less of an issue for vegans who consume some processed foods. Veggie meats, energy bars, and protein powders that are made with soy protein isolate, for example, provide very well digested protein. For those who are depending on whole foods like legumes, nuts, and grains for most of their protein, the digestibility factor comes into play.

It's not a big difference, but vegans should strive for a protein intake of 0.9 grams per kilogram of body weight. This translates to around 0.4 grams of protein per pound of body weight. So a vegan who weighs 150 pounds would need 60 grams of protein (150 × 0.4) per day. Although the RDA for protein is based on total body weight, nutritionists often calculate protein needs based on "ideal" body weight. That's because fat tissue maintenance requires very little protein. You can find a number of calculators online to determine your ideal body weight. (Note that while these tools are useful for estimating your protein needs, they may not be the best approach to setting weight-loss goals. We talk more about concerns with the concept of "ideal" weight in Chapter 17.) Since calculating protein needs is not an exact science, we encourage you to err on the side of a bit more protein (10 to 15 percent more) than your ideal body weight would require.

PROTEIN RECOMMENDATIONS FOR YOUNG VEGANS

Age (years)	Females (grams/day)	Males (grams/day)
1–2	18–19	18–19
2–3	18–21	18–21
4–6	26–28	26–28
7–10	31–34	31–34
11–14	51–55	50–54
15–18	50–55	66–73

For children and teens, we base our recommendations on the RDA aimed at the needs of different age groups with an added amount for vegans. (We address protein needs of athletes in Chapter 14.)

MEETING PROTEIN NEEDS ON A VEGAN DIET: THE IMPORTANCE OF LEGUMES

While the chart on pages 61–62 shows that many plant foods are good protein sources, legumes are especially rich in protein. Legumes include beans, peas, lentils, soyfoods (like tofu, soymilk, and veggie meats), and peanuts. (Most people think of peanuts as nuts, but they are botanically legumes and, from a nutritional standpoint, they have more in common with pinto beans and lentils than walnuts and pecans.) Our food guide specifies at least three to four servings per day of these foods. A serving is pretty modest: ½ cup of cooked beans, ½ cup of tofu or tempeh, a three-ounce veggie burger, 1 cup of soymilk, or 2 tablespoons of peanut butter.

In addition to being protein-rich, these foods are the only good plant sources—with a few exceptions—of the essential amino acid lysine. A diet that gets most of its protein from grains, nuts, and vegetables is likely to be too low in lysine.

You can get a rough idea of how much lysine you need by multiplying your weight (in pounds) by 19. This calculation includes a small factor that makes up for the slightly lower digestibility of protein from whole plant foods. For example, a person weighing 140 pounds would need 2,660 milligrams of lysine per day. The chart on pages 61–62 shows that the best sources of lysine are legumes, quinoa, and pistachios.

If you follow our recommendations to consume at least three to four servings of legumes per day, you'll meet lysine needs with ease. That doesn't mean that beans, peanuts, and soyfoods are absolutely essential in vegan diets. While it is difficult to meet protein and lysine needs without them, it's possible, and we provide guidance on how in Chapter 10, when we look at meal planning guidelines for vegans.

PROTEIN AND LYSINE CONTENT OF SELECTED VEGAN FOODS

Recommended Intakes	Multiply your body weight in pounds by 0.4	Multiply your body weight in pounds by 19
Food	Protein in grams	Lysine in milligrams
Legumes, Peanuts, and Soyfoods ½ cup cooked unless otherwise noted		
Black beans	7.6	523
Garbanzo beans	7.5	486
Kidney beans	8.1	526
Lentils	8.9	623
Navy beans	8.7	598
Pinto beans	7.7	488
Seitan*, 3 ounces	22.5	656
Edamame	11	665
Soy protein powder, 1 scoop	25	1,598
Pea protein powder	22	1,634
Rice protein powder	25	741
Tempeh	15.5	754
Textured vegetable protein	11	657
Tofu	10–20**	582**
Tofu, soft	8–10**	534**
Vegetarian baked beans	6	378
Veggie meats, 3 ounces	6–18	***
Peanuts ¼ cup	9	330
Peanut butter, 2 tablespoons	8	290
Pasta made from chickpeas, lentils, or black beans	11	n/a
Pasta made from edamame	12	n/a
Plant Milks, 1 cup		
Almond milk	1	n/a
Hempseed milk	2	n/a
Oat milk	3–4	n/a
Pea milk	8	n/a
Rice milk	1	n/a
Soymilk	7–10***	439
Nuts and Seeds		
Almonds, ¼ cup	7.3	205
Almond butter, 2 tablespoons	7	196
Brazil nuts, ¼ cup	4.7	139
Cashews, ¼ cup	5.2	280
Flaxseeds, 1 teaspoon ground	0.5	22
Pecans, ½ cup	2.5	78

continues

PROTEIN AND LYSINE CONTENT OF SELECTED VEGAN FOODS *continued*

Recommended Intakes	Multiply your body weight in pounds by 0.4	Multiply your body weight in pounds by 19
Food	Protein in grams	Lysine in milligrams
Nuts and Seeds *continued*		
Pistachios, ¼ cup	6.4	367
Sesame seeds, 2 tablespoons	3.2	102
Sunflower seeds, 2 tablespoons	3.6	164
Tahini, 2 tablespoons	5.3	172
Walnuts, ¼ cup	4.4	124
Grains and Starchy Vegetables ½ cup cooked unless otherwise noted		
Barley	1.7	66
Oatmeal	3	158
Pasta	3.5	162
Potato, 1 baked	4.5	131
Quinoa	4.0	221
Rice, brown	2.5	86
Rice, white	2.0	80
Sweet potato, 1 medium	2.2	88
Taco shell, 1 medium 5-inch	1.0	26
Whole wheat bread	2–6	85
Vegetables, ½ cup cooked or 1 cup raw		
Broccoli	2.3	117
Carrots	0.6	62
Collards	2.6	96
Corn	2.3	116
Eggplant	0.4	19
Green beans	1.2	57
Kale	1.75	104
Spinach	2.6	164
Turnips	0.5	22
Turnip greens	0.8	54

*Seitan is wheat protein. It is not a legume, but because of its high protein content, it is usually grouped with legumes and soyfoods for meal-planning purposes.

**Firm tofu is usually higher in protein than soft tofu, but the protein content of different brands and types of tofu varies widely.

***Amount varies by brand.

Protein and Calories

In addition to overseeing minimum requirements for nutrients, the National Academies specifies an Acceptable Macronutrient Distribution Range (AMDR) for protein, carbohydrates, and fat. According to these recommendations, an acceptable protein intake is anywhere from 10 to 35 percent of total calories.

We sometimes hear questions from vegans about how we could possibly need to get as much as 10 percent of our calories from protein. After all, human breast milk is only 6 percent protein and it supports health during early infancy, which is the fastest period of growth of the entire life cycle. How could adults—who aren't growing at all—need a more protein-dense diet than a baby?

Infants actually have extremely high protein needs based on their body weight. They require almost 0.7 grams of protein per pound of body weight, compared to around 0.4 grams for vegan adults. But infants have a distinct advantage when it comes to meeting protein needs: They are little eating machines. A 13-pound baby can consume as much as 500 calories per day. Although their food has low protein density, babies get plenty of protein simply because they eat so much food. And an additional advantage is that the protein in breast milk has high bioavailability.

Unless you're on a mission to gain weight, you can't eat quite as enthusiastically as the average one-month-old. A young infant needs around 9 grams of protein per day and 500 calories. Compare that to the needs of a 135-pound vegan woman—she needs at least six times more protein but is likely to need only about four times more calories. Obviously, she needs to pack more protein into those calories and requires a more protein-dense diet.

People who are very physically active can often get away with a diet that is less protein dense, because, like babies, they end up eating a lot of calories. On the flip side, those who are cutting calories need to pack enough protein into fewer calories and need a more protein-dense diet.

You don't need to worry about the math, though—just make sure you follow our recommendations for including legumes in your diet. That's all it takes for most vegans to get at least 10 percent of their calories from protein.

PROTEIN: MEALS THAT DELIVER

It's easy to build vegan meals that pack a substantial protein punch. Each of these meals provides at least 20 grams of protein.

EASY OATMEAL BREAKFAST

- 1 cup of oatmeal with ½ cup soymilk
- 1 slice whole wheat bread with 2 tablespoons almond butter

Total protein: 20.5 grams

INDONESIAN TEMPEH WITH PEANUT SAUCE

- 1 cup of rice
- ½ cup tempeh
- ¼ cup peanut sauce
- 1½ cups steamed broccoli

Total protein: 35 grams

BEAN AND "BEEF" TACO DINNER

- 2 taco shells
- ½ cup refried beans
- ¼ cup veggie "ground beef" cooked in tomato sauce
- Chopped tomatoes and lettuce
- 1 cup steamed spinach

Total protein: 20 grams

PASTA PRIMAVERA

- 1 cup pasta
- ½ cup garbanzo beans

continues

```
┌─────────────────────────────────────────────────────────┐
│                                                           │
│  PROTEIN: MEALS THAT DELIVER  continued                   │
│  ─────────────────────────────────────────────           │
│                                                           │
│    •  2 tablespoons pine nuts                             │
│    •  1 cup chopped broccoli                              │
│    •  ½ cup roasted red pepper strips                     │
│    Total protein: 23 grams                                │
│                                                           │
│                                                           │
│                    LUNCH ON THE GO                        │
│                                                           │
│    •  Instant lentil soup with 2 tablespoons pumpkin seeds│
│    •  1 slice whole wheat bread with mashed avocado       │
│    Total protein: 21 grams                                │
│                                                           │
└─────────────────────────────────────────────────────────┘
```

INADEQUATE INTAKES

Overt protein deficiency is rare among Americans and occurs in other parts of the world where people don't have enough food. Many vegan advocates point out that people don't end up in hospitals because of a protein deficiency. It's true that in countries where food is abundant, acute deficiency of protein doesn't occur. But diets that are marginal in protein—not quite deficient, but not quite optimal—can result in loss of muscle mass, poor bone health, and compromised immunity. And those kinds of problems do occur in the United States.

We'd like to say that vegans never need to worry about protein, but that isn't entirely true. There are a few situations where vegans may fall short on meeting their protein needs.

Vegan diets that are low in protein-rich foods like legumes are likely to be too low in protein. And because low-calorie diets raise protein requirements, people who are dieting or simply not eating enough for other reasons (like chronic illness) may need to boost their intake of protein-rich foods like legumes or soyfoods.

Although we rarely see this among vegans, someone who relies heavily on foods that are high in refined carbohydrates like potato chips, French fries, and soft drinks is likely to fall short of meeting needs for protein—and just about all other nutrients.

And extreme versions of vegan diets, such as raw foods or fruitarian regimens, are often low (or completely lacking) in the higher-protein plant foods like legumes and soyfoods and can lead to a marginal protein intake. That's one reason these types of diets are not recommended for children. As we noted, the science on protein needs is still evolving and some experts believe that getting a little bit more of this nutrient has its advantages. Higher protein intakes may help manage appetite,[7] improve blood pressure control,[8] and can also protect bone and muscle mass.[9] In particular, there are concerns that older people may need more protein to avoid muscle and bone loss.[10-12] Although high-protein diets are sometimes associated with high cholesterol and greater risk of cardiovascular disease, cancer, and kidney disease, for most Americans, a high-protein diet results from a high intake of meat and dairy foods. Getting a little extra protein on your plant-based diet doesn't carry those same risks.[13]

Our recommendations for food choices are aimed at ensuring that you'll meet protein needs, and since the protein is coming from healthful plant foods, we're not concerned if you get a little extra. We talk more about the benefits of protein for older people, for weight loss, and for athletes in subsequent chapters.

DO VEGANS GET ADEQUATE TRYPTOPHAN?

One common belief, often voiced by critics of vegan diets, is that plant foods don't provide adequate tryptophan. This essential amino acid is needed to make the neurotransmitter serotonin, and low levels of serotonin are linked to depression. Meat is higher in tryptophan than plants, but a well-balanced vegan diet is almost guaranteed to provide more than enough of this amino acid. The recommendation for tryptophan is 5 milligrams for every kilogram of body weight. Adding in a factor for plant protein digestion, this translates to a vegan RDA of 5.5 milligrams per kilogram of body weight or 2.5 milligrams of tryptophan per pound.

For example, a vegan who weighs 130 pounds would need 325 milligrams of tryptophan, which is easily provided on a vegan diet. A diet that includes one cup of black beans, ½ cup of tofu, and one cup of brown rice would provide nearly 400 milligrams of tryptophan.

In fact, eating foods that are very high in protein, like meat, doesn't necessarily increase the amount of tryptophan in the brain. That's because high levels of other amino acids in these foods block absorption of tryptophan from the blood into the brain. Eating foods like legumes that provide both protein and carbohydrates can actually enhance the passage of tryptophan into the brain.[14]

TRYPTOPHAN CONTENT OF SELECTED VEGAN FOODS

Recommended intake: Multiply your weight in pounds by 2.5	
	Tryptophan (in milligrams)
Tofu, ½ cup	155
Oatmeal, ½ cup	118
Soymilk, 1 cup	105
Black beans, ½ cup cooked	90
Peanut butter, 2 tablespoons	78
Garbanzo beans, ½ cup cooked	70
Quinoa, ½ cup cooked	48
Brown rice, ½ cup cooked	29
Broccoli, ½ cup cooked	24

TIPS FOR MEETING VEGAN PROTEIN NEEDS

- Consume adequate calories. If your calorie intake is low because you are trying to lose weight or for any other reason, you may need to add a few additional protein-rich foods to your menus.
- Eat a variety of plant foods every day.
- Follow the guidelines in the Food Guide in Chapter 10 and aim for at least three to four servings of legumes in your daily menu. A serving is ½ cup cooked beans, ½ cup tofu or tempeh, ¼ cup peanuts, 1 cup soymilk, or 2 tablespoons peanut butter.
- If beans give you discomfort from gas production, see our tips on page 265 for ways to manage this.
- If you include plant milks in your diet, choose soymilk or pea milk at least some of the time. Milks made from almonds, hempseeds, and rice are usually low in protein.

CHAPTER 5

Eating for Healthy Bones
Calcium and Vitamin D

C alcium in vegan diets can be a confusing issue, especially since there is so much conflicting information about its impact on bone health. In this chapter, we sort through the evidence about calcium and vitamin D and bone health. We also look at other ways in which nutrition impacts bone health.

CALCIUM

For most of human history, people got their calcium from plants, primarily wild, leafy greens. Dairy foods didn't become part of the human diet until around ten thousand years ago and even then they were consumed only in some parts of the world. Calcium-rich greens were so abundant in early diets that some nutritional anthropologists speculate that people consumed at least 1,000 and possibly as much as 3,000 milligrams per day of calcium from these foods, or about three times our current recommended intakes.[1,2] The cultivated greens that are available to vegans today are lower in calcium than the wild vegetables available to our ancestors, but they can still make a significant contribution to calcium intake. Vegans can also get calcium from some legumes and nuts, and from fortified foods.

There is no question about whether vegan diets can provide enough calcium. They can. But that doesn't mean that they always do. In studies of vegans, average calcium intakes have often fallen well below recommendations.[3] More recent research suggests that vegans may be doing better in regard to calcium intake, however.[4,5] This may be because more foods are fortified with this nutrient or perhaps because better information about calcium content of plant foods is available.

Calcium and Bones

While bones might seem solid and static, they are actually quite dynamic. The skeleton acts as calcium storage, providing a steady supply of calcium to the blood where it is needed for muscle relaxation, nerve cell transmission, and a host of other functions. Some of this calcium is regularly lost in the urine and must be replaced by dietary sources. As a result, bones are in motion—breaking down to release calcium to the blood and then taking up new calcium and rebuilding. Getting enough calcium is important for bone health, but reducing the amount that is lost through the urine could be important, too.

Bones grow through the first three decades of life, becoming longer, heavier, and denser. By their late twenties or early thirties, most people have achieved *peak bone mass*, and their skeleton is as heavy and dense as it is going to get. There is some evidence that peak bone mass determines bone health and risk for osteoporosis in later years.

Beginning at age forty-five or so, there is a shift in metabolism and bone mass begins to decline. Efforts to slow calcium losses from the body and provide enough calcium to keep bones strong are important for preventing osteoporosis, especially for women, who can begin to lose bone rapidly after menopause.

Good bone health depends on a complex interplay of factors that affect both absorption of calcium and calcium losses from the body. Diet, lifestyle, and genetics all play a part in calcium balance. Figuring out how these factors interact and affect calcium needs has been an ongoing subject of debate among researchers, and some of the issues may be especially important for vegans.

Calcium is different from other nutrients in that it isn't associated with an acute deficiency disease. With most nutrients, if your intake is too low, you'll get sick. That's not true for calcium because levels in the blood are very tightly controlled. Even a small change in those levels can be life-threatening, so the body utilizes stored calcium in the bone plus the filtering system of the kidneys to keep calcium concentrations within strict boundaries. You can't ascertain calcium status by measuring blood levels of this mineral because those levels are always the same. But while a low calcium diet doesn't cause an acute nutritional deficiency, a chronically low intake can raise the risk for osteoporosis later in life.

Osteoporosis is a crippling and debilitating disease of severe bone loss—as much as 30 to 40 percent of total bone—that affects an estimated 10 million Americans. Eighty percent of Americans with osteoporosis are women.

When nutrition scientists look at the relationship of diet to bone health, they look at both bone density and fracture rates. And the findings are anything but clear. How much calcium humans need and the extent to which varying intakes affect bone health are topics of intense research. Many large epidemiologic studies fail to show that high calcium intakes protect against bone fractures.[6,7]

Protein and Calcium

A couple of decades ago, studies of bone health among people in different countries revealed an interesting pattern. Rates of hip fracture (which is often used as a marker for bone health) were highest in countries with the highest intakes of animal protein, even though calcium intake was also high.[8] The findings suggested that too much protein was worse for bones than too little calcium. And, in fact, there is a biological explanation to back this.

High doses of certain proteins increase the blood's acidity, kicking off a chain of reactions to bring blood back to a more neutral pH. A release of calcium from the bones is one part of the process. The theory has been that the more acidic the blood, the greater the loss of calcium from bones. Meat proteins are among the most acid-producing foods, followed by proteins from grains and dairy. Diets high in fruits and vegetables are the least acidic.

Based on this, it seems to make sense that people who eat animal protein should need more calcium to replace what is constantly being leached from their bones. Conversely, wouldn't vegans, whose diets contain no animal proteins, have lower calcium needs? This sounds like an obvious conclusion, but it's not quite that straightforward.

First, the studies comparing different populations have limited usefulness. These are ecological studies, and we saw in Chapter 3 that they provide only weak evidence. There are just too many cultural and genetic variations among people of Asian, African, and Caucasian backgrounds for us to make direct comparisons about their protein intakes and bone health. For example, people of African descent have a genetic predisposition toward stronger, heavier bones[9] while a slight genetic advantage in hip anatomy among Asians protects against fracture.[10,11]

There are cultural differences too. Older Asians appear to be less likely to fall, which lowers risk for a bone fracture.[12] In fact, while Asian populations fare well in comparisons of hip-fracture rates, their spinal bone health is similar to Westerners.[13,14] This suggests that there is something in their genes or lifestyle that is specifically protective against hip fracture but doesn't affect other parts of the skeleton. If diet were the protective factor, the benefits would likely show up in all parts of the skeleton.

As a result, these cross-cultural studies might tell us more about culture and genetics than about diet, which means these comparisons don't tell us a whole lot about how much calcium Western vegans might need. It's better to look at clinical research, where the effects of protein are directly observed and measured. Findings from clinical studies show the following:

- Consuming isolated protein—that is, just the pure protein portion of a food—has a direct and significant effect on calcium losses, but that effect is often lost when subjects are fed whole, high-protein foods. The reason may be that other factors in foods, like phosphorus, counteract the urinary losses.[15]

- While protein can increase calcium losses, it also enhances calcium absorption from foods. There is evidence that these positive effects on absorption may outweigh or at least compensate for the negative effects of calcium loss.[16,17] In fact, it appears that the calcium that shows up in the urine when people eat more protein is not actually coming from the bones, which means it might simply be due to the higher absorption of calcium from the diet.[18,19]

- In some studies, higher protein intake is actually associated with better bone health, and protein supplements can help bone fractures heal more quickly.[20–23]

In addition to the positive effects of protein on calcium absorption, high-protein diets improve muscle mass, which is associated with better bone health. And protein also boosts levels of compounds that may stimulate bone formation.[24]

Studies of vegetarians suggest that emphasizing protein-rich foods is good for bones. Among Seventh-Day Adventists, women who had the highest intakes of legumes and veggie meats were less likely to suffer a wrist fracture, and in both men and women, eating more of these foods was linked to lower risk for breaking a hip.[25,26] The best overall approach for bone health appears to be a diet that provides plenty of calcium and protein as well as a generous intake of fruits and vegetables, which can help neutralize any potential acidic effect of protein-rich foods.[27]

This is an example of how the research has evolved over the decades in ways that allow us to make better, health-supporting recommendations for vegans. Where we once thought that vegans could get away with lower calcium intakes due to their more modest consumption of protein, we now know that getting plenty of both protein and calcium is important for strong bones.

Vegan Diets and Bone Health

While we don't have much information about bone health in vegans, the few available studies suggest that some vegans have lower bone density.[28] In a study in the United Kingdom, fracture rates were higher in vegans only when their calcium intake was low.[29] In Taiwan, a greater likelihood of having a spinal fracture may have been due to low protein intake.[30] These studies tell us that many vegans need to give more attention to both calcium and protein to protect their bone health.

Calcium Without Milk?

Recommendations for daily calcium intake for Western populations range from 700 milligrams in the United Kingdom to 1,000 milligrams in the United States. There is evidence to suggest that 700 milligrams may meet the needs of most people, but it also may not be enough for everyone. Calcium needs can vary considerably among individuals, primarily because there is a big genetic variation in absorption rates. Aiming for the US recommendation of 1,000 milligrams for adults and 1,200 for those over fifty can provide good insurance. At this point, we see no reason why vegans would need any less calcium than people eating other types of diets.

Getting calcium from plants might seem a little strange in a society that is so focused on dairy foods as a source of calcium. While a strong dairy lobby has convinced many consumers that milk and other dairy foods are essential for a healthy diet, the ability to drink milk into adulthood is not the norm throughout the world.

Normal development throughout most of the world involves a gradual loss of the enzyme needed to digest milk sugar after children are weaned from breast milk. Indications are that a mutation occurred some ten centuries ago among northern Europeans that resulted in the continued production of this enzyme, allowing that population to drink milk into adulthood. In the United States, we refer to the lack of this enzyme as "lactose intolerance." But that's definitely a Western bias since this "intolerance" is not a lack or an abnormality; it's part of normal human development in most people.

Meeting Calcium Needs on a Vegan Diet

The amount of any nutrient in a food is not equal to the amount that actually makes its way from the intestines into the bloodstream. The bioavailability of a nutrient from a particular food refers to the amount of that nutrient that is likely to be absorbed and used, and it's affected by a number of factors.

A few leafy green vegetables that are rich in calcium—spinach, beet greens, Swiss chard, and rhubarb—are also high in naturally occurring compounds called oxalates that bind calcium and make it essentially unavailable to the body. But the availability of calcium from low-oxalate vegetables—kale, collards, broccoli, and turnip greens—can be as high as 50 percent. That is, we absorb as much as half of the calcium from these foods. While that might not sound like a lot, it's a very good absorption rate compared to other foods. Calcium absorption from soyfoods, like calcium-set tofu (tofu that is processed with calcium-sulfate) and fortified soymilk, is also good at around 25 to 30 percent, which is about the same as from cow's milk. Calcium absorption from nuts and legumes is somewhat lower, around 20 percent.[31-34]

The recommended intake of 1,000 milligrams of calcium is based on the assumption that most people absorb around 30 percent of the calcium in their diet. If you're eating a varied diet that includes several different types of calcium sources, including low-oxalate leafy greens and soy products, you don't need to worry that some of the calcium from other foods is absorbed less efficiently.

It's possible to get plenty of calcium just from eating foods that are naturally rich in this mineral, but it does take some effort. (This is equally true for people who consume dairy foods, since many people who drink milk don't meet calcium requirements. That's why so many products on the market—from cereals to juices to protein bars—are fortified with calcium.) Using fortified foods like juices and nondairy milks can make it easier to meet calcium recommendations on a vegan diet.

It's also helpful to pay attention to the effects of processing. For example, frozen leafy greens are higher in calcium than fresh, although this is simply because their volume tends to be more concentrated. Processing also affects the amount of calcium in different types of tofu. Tofu production involves ingredients that cause soymilk to curdle. The two most common—often used together—are magnesium-chloride (*nigari* in Japanese) and calcium-sulfate. When calcium-sulfate is used, tofu is often an excellent source of calcium. Also, firm tofu tends to have a higher calcium content than soft. It's important to read package labels, though, since the amount of calcium in different brands and different types of tofu varies widely.

Aim to eat at least 3 cups per day of some combination of foods that are good sources of well-absorbed calcium. These include fortified plant milks, fortified juices, calcium-set tofu, oranges, and low-oxalate leafy green vegetables like kale, mustard greens, turnip greens, bok choy, and collard greens.

TIPS FOR GETTING ENOUGH CALCIUM

- Choose plant milks that are fortified with calcium, and give the carton a good shake before pouring since the calcium can settle to the bottom.
- Look for calcium-set tofu, which is tofu that includes calcium-sulfate as an ingredient.
- Learn to love greens! The ones that are low in oxalates—kale, turnip, mustard, and collard greens—are good sources of well-absorbed calcium as well as other nutrients that are important for bone health.
- Make your own trail mix using soynuts, almonds, and chopped figs and keep it on hand for snacks.
- Choose calcium-fortified brands if you drink fruit juices.

- If your intake falls short, make up the difference with a small supplement. (Although high-dose supplements of calcium have been linked to risk for heart disease, a small daily supplement of 500 milligrams or less is safe.)[35]

VITAMIN D

Adequate vitamin D is every bit as important as calcium for maintaining bone health. It improves calcium absorption and limits losses of calcium in the urine. But is vitamin D a nutrient? Not exactly, since we can make all we need when our skin is exposed to ultraviolet rays from sunlight. In fact, for most of human history, this is where people got their vitamin D since it occurs naturally in very few foods. But as people moved away from the equatorial zones and began to spend more time indoors, vitamin D deficiency became a problem. In the early 1900s, rickets (soft bones that don't develop well in children) was a significant public health problem that led to fortification of cow's milk with vitamin D.

While the focus has long been on bone health, more recent research suggests that suboptimal vitamin D levels are linked to fibromyalgia, rheumatoid arthritis, multiple sclerosis, depression, muscle weakness, diabetes, hypertension, and cancer.[36] This has led to some controversy over how much vitamin D we actually need. According to the National Academies, we need enough to maintain blood levels that are at least 20 ng/ml. To maintain those levels, the current RDA for vitamin D in adults is 600 International Units or 15 micrograms (vitamin D can be measured either way; 1 microgram equals 40 International Units). But many experts believe that blood levels should be much higher and that levels above 30 ng/ml are preferable for optimal health.[37] Until the issue is resolved, taking a supplement providing between 600 and 1,000 International Units of vitamin D is a reasonable choice. It's always a good idea to include an assessment of vitamin D levels when your doctor orders routine blood tests.

Vitamin D$_2$ vs Vitamin D$_3$

There are two types of vitamin D used in fortified foods and supplements. Vitamin D$_3$ or *cholecalciferol*, is derived from animals, usually from sheep's wool or fish oil. Vitamin D$_2$, or *ergocalciferol*, is usually obtained from yeast and is vegan. The evidence suggests that the two types are absorbed equally as well but that blood levels of vitamin D$_2$ decline more quickly when megadoses of the vitamin are consumed.[38,39]

In a study in Germany, people who took supplements of vitamin D$_3$ had higher blood levels of vitamin D at the end of eight weeks compared to the group that was taking supplements of D$_2$. But both types of supplements resulted in blood levels that were well within the healthy range established by the National Academies.[40]

For vegans who do not have a vitamin D deficiency, taking a daily supplement of 600 to 1,000 International Units of vitamin D$_2$ appears to be as effective as vitamin D$_3$ for maintaining healthy blood levels of vitamin D. If you are deficient in vitamin D and have had trouble raising your levels, then it's possible that vitamin D$_3$ is the best choice. There is currently one brand of vitamin D available that has been verified to be vegan vitamin D$_3$. Called *Vitashine*, it is sourced from lichen.

Getting Enough Vitamin D for Optimal Health

Concern about skin cancer has people using powerful sunscreen or shying away from sun exposure altogether. However, in addition to blocking the harmful effects of the UV light on the skin, sunscreen blocks vitamin D synthesis. And there are plenty of other factors that affect vitamin D synthesis in the skin. Older people need longer exposure and so do people with dark skin. Smog can interfere with vitamin D synthesis and the farther away you are from the equator, the more sun exposure you need to make vitamin D. Some research suggests that Americans living in the northern part of the country do not make any vitamin D during the winter months.[41]

To make adequate vitamin D for one day, a light-skinned person needs ten to fifteen minutes of midday (10 a.m. to 2 p.m.) sun exposure, without sunscreen, on a day when sunburn is possible.[42] Dark-skinned people need twenty minutes and older people need thirty minutes.[43,44]

If your sun exposure doesn't match these guidelines, then you need to take a supplement or use fortified foods.

The only significant, natural sources of vitamin D in foods are fatty fish, eggs from chickens who have been fed vitamin D, and mushrooms treated with ultraviolet rays. Many people think that milk is a good natural source of vitamin D, but it isn't. Milk contains no vitamin D unless it has been fortified and is no more natural a source of this vitamin than any other fortified food.

Many foods, including most breakfast cereals, are fortified with vitamin D. Almost all use vitamin D_3, which is derived from animals. Most brands of fortified soymilk and other nondairy milks use vitamin D_2, which comes from yeast exposed to UV rays.

For food labeling purposes, the Daily Value for vitamin D is 10 micrograms (400 International Units). So if a food provides 25 percent of the Daily Value for vitamin D, it contains 2.5 micrograms (100 International Units) of vitamin D per serving. Vitamin D–fortified plant milks normally have 2 to 3 micrograms (80 to 120 International Units) per cup. You can see from these numbers that it's not that easy to meet the recommended 600 International Units per day from fortified foods. If your sun exposure isn't adequate, you will probably need to use a vitamin D supplement. Most natural foods stores carry supplements of plant-derived vitamin D_2.

FRUITS AND VEGETABLES FOR HEALTHY BONES

Calcium and vitamin D have well-deserved reputations as bone-strengthening nutrients, but they don't act alone. Diets that emphasize fruits and vegetables are linked to strong bones, possibly because they are good sources of potassium and magnesium, two minerals that are involved in bone metabolism.[45] Recommendations for potassium are 2,600 milligrams per day for women and 3,400 for men. Many Americans fall short of meeting potassium needs. Also, much higher potassium intakes have been used in studies aimed at reducing hypertension so it's possible that increasing intake of this mineral beyond current recommendations could be best for overall health. We talk more about this in Chapter 15. In addition to eating plenty of fruits and vegetables, replacing meat with beans is an effective way to consume more potassium, since legumes are excellent sources of this mineral. The best sources of potassium are spinach, Swiss chard, cooked and canned tomato products and tomato juice, orange juice, bananas, and legumes.

Many of the same foods that provide potassium are also good sources of magnesium. In addition, this mineral is abundant in whole grains and some nuts and seeds. Recommendations for magnesium intake are 320 milligrams for women and 420 milligrams for men. But again, higher intakes might have some benefits for managing blood pressure. Intakes of both potassium and magnesium above the RDAs are safe when these minerals come from foods rather than supplements. The table on pages 81–83 shows the amounts of calcium, potassium, and magnesium in vegan foods.

Fruits and vegetables also provide vitamin C, which is needed for synthesis of the connective tissue in bones and helps prevent bone loss, and vitamin K which is essential for activation of a protein needed for healthy bones.[46,47] Inadequate intake of this vitamin, which is found in many leafy green vegetables, is linked to poorer bone density and greater likelihood of fracture.[47,48] We talk more about vitamin C and vitamin K in Chapter 8.

A HEALTHY LIFESTYLE TO PROTECT BONES

Making sure you meet needs for protein, calcium, and vitamin D, and striving to eat plenty of fruits and vegetables are important habits for protecting bone health. Limiting sodium intake and being moderate with alcohol consumption are helpful as well since both are linked to risk for bone loss.

But exercise may be the most important factor of all in preventing bone loss. Staying active is crucial to bone density and strength. Choose weight-bearing and high-impact exercise to get the greatest benefit, such as strength-training, jogging, and step aerobics. Biking and swimming don't do much to strengthen bones.

Finally, maintaining a healthy weight can protect your bones, and by this, we mean don't let your weight get too low. When it comes to bone health, being a few pounds above your ideal weight is better than being a few pounds below it. Rapid weight loss is associated with bone loss, so if you have some pounds to shed, aim for a slow reduction while building more muscle and protecting bones through exercise.

CALCIUM, POTASSIUM, AND MAGNESIUM CONTENT OF FOODS

Recommended Adult Intake	Calcium 1,000 milligrams	Potassium Women: 2,600 milligrams Men: 3,400 milligrams	Magnesium Women: 320 milligrams Men: 420 milligrams
Legumes (½ cup unless otherwise noted)			
Baked beans	63	379	40
Black beans	51	400	45
Chickpeas	40	239	39
Edamame	130	485	54
Great northern beans	60	346	44
Lentils	19	365	36
Navy beans	62	415	61
Refried beans	40	397	44
Bean pasta, black bean	57	550	n/a
Bean pasta, chickpea	22	480	n/a
Bean pasta, edamame	70	630	71
Hummus, homemade	56	208	32
Peanut butter, 2 tablespoons	17	189	57
Soymilk, fortified, 1 cup	300	284	36
Soynuts, ¼ cup	59	632	62
Tofu, firm, made with calcium sulfate	434	150	37
Tofu, firm, made with calcium sulfate plus nigari	253	186	47
Tofu, soft, prepared with calcium sulfate and nigari	138	149	33
Soy yogurt, 1 cup	300	n/a	n/a

continues

CALCIUM, POTASSIUM, AND MAGNESIUM CONTENT OF FOODS   *continued*

Recommended Adult Intake	Calcium 1,000 milligrams	Potassium Women: 2,600 milligrams Men: 3,400 milligrams	Magnesium Women: 320 milligrams Men: 420 milligrams
Tempeh	92	342	67
TVP	80	594	n/a
Vegetables (½ cup cooked or 1 cup raw unless otherwise noted)			
Beet greens	***	654	49
Bok choy	80	315	10
Broccoli, fresh	31	229	16
Broccoli, frozen	30	142	12
Butternut squash	42	291	30
Cabbage	36	147	11
Carrot juice, 1 cup	60	683	33
Collard greens cooked from fresh	134	111	20
Collard greens cooked from frozen	178	213	25
Corn, 1 cup	2	416	57
Kale, cooked from fresh or frozen	88	85	15
Mustard greens, cooked from fresh	82	113	9
Mustard greens, cooked from frozen	76	104	10
Okra, 1 cup	81	303	57
Parsnips, 1 cup	48	499	39
Baked potato	26	926	48
Potato, ½ cup	3	256	16
Rutabaga, 1 cup	66	472	32
Spinach, ½ cup cooked	***	420	80
Swiss chard	***	480	75
Winter squash, 1 cup	32	406	16
Sweet potato, 1 cup cubes	40	448	33
Tomato, 1 large	18	431	20
Tomatoes, canned	43	264	15
Turnip greens, 1 cup	104	163	17
Yam, 1 cup cubes	26	1,224	32
Fruits			
Banana	6	422	32
Dates, 3 Medjool	46	696	39
Figs, 4 dried	54	228	23
Figs, 2 fresh	35	232	17
Orange	61	238	14
Orange juice, fortified, ½ cup	349	443	27

continues

CALCIUM, POTASSIUM, AND MAGNESIUM CONTENT OF FOODS   *continued*

Recommended Adult Intake	Calcium 1,000 milligrams	Potassium Women: 2,600 milligrams Men: 3,400 milligrams	Magnesium Women: 320 milligrams Men: 420 milligrams
Nuts and Seeds			
Almond butter, 2 tablespoons	86	243	97
Almonds, ¼ cup	88	259	97
Brazil nuts, 3 nuts	24	99	56
Tahini, 2 tablespoons	39	129	99
Grains (cooked)			
Barley, ½ cup	9	73	17
Kamut, ½ cup	8	170	48
Oatmeal, ½ cup	11	82	31
Spaghetti, 1 cup	10	55	25
Whole wheat spaghetti, 1 cup	26	395	42

*** Calcium from these foods is poorly absorbed.
n/a not available

TIPS FOR BUILDING HEALTHY BONES ON A VEGAN DIET

Building and keeping strong bones depends on a number of lifestyle factors. They are all important.

- Aim for a diet that is rich in calcium, using the tips for meeting calcium needs on pages 75–77.
- Eat a protein-rich diet by eating at least three to four servings of legumes per day.
- Include plenty of vegetables and fruits in your diet, especially ones that are rich in potassium and magnesium.
- Get adequate vitamin D through daily sun exposure during the warm months or by using fortified foods and/or a supplement providing 25 micrograms (1,000 International Units) per day.
- Stay active and include weight-bearing exercise in your fitness routine.
- Avoid excess sodium and alcohol.

CHAPTER 6

Vitamin B$_{12}$

Y ou may have heard that vitamin B$_{12}$ is a controversial topic among vegans. But among nutrition professionals (including those of us who specialize in vegan diets), there is no controversy at all: All vegans need to take a vitamin B$_{12}$ supplement or consume foods that are fortified with this nutrient.

Vitamin B$_{12}$ is needed for cell division and formation of healthy red blood cells. Overt B$_{12}$ deficiency can produce a condition called macrocytic or megaloblastic anemia, in which blood cells don't divide and reproduce normally. It's also needed to produce myelin, the protective sheath around nerve fibers. As a result, deficiency can also result in nerve damage. But even if your B$_{12}$ levels aren't low enough to produce these acute deficiency symptoms, a marginal intake may increase the risk for certain chronic conditions like dementia.

The scientific name for vitamin B$_{12}$ is cobalamin because the B$_{12}$ molecule contains the mineral cobalt at the center of its structure. Commercial preparations of vitamin B$_{12}$ used in supplements and fortified foods are called cyanocobalamin. This supplemental form is converted in the body to vitamin B$_{12}$ coenzymes, which are the compounds needed for B$_{12}$ activity.

VEGAN SOURCES OF VITAMIN B$_{12}$

All of the vitamin B$_{12}$ in the world is made by bacteria, and that includes bacteria living in the digestive tracts of animals and humans. It seems like we could just use what these bacteria produce, but they are too far down in the intestines to be of any use to us. We absorb vitamin B$_{12}$ in our small intestine; the bacteria producing it live in our large intestine.

There are also molecules that are very similar to vitamin B$_{12}$ but that have no true vitamin activity for humans. These are inactive B$_{12}$ analogues. Most methods for measuring vitamin B$_{12}$ in foods don't differentiate between true vitamin B$_{12}$ and the inactive analogues. That's been a source of confusion for a long time. Foods like fermented soy products, sourdough bread, and some sea vegetables have all been credited at one time or another as good sources of vitamin B$_{12}$. But studies show that what they really contain are primarily inactive analogues.[1] There is a double risk associated with depending on these foods for vitamin B$_{12}$, because the inactive analogues can actually block the activity of true vitamin B$_{12}$.[2]

Some companies may claim that a food contains active vitamin B$_{12}$ even though the testing methods they use can't discern between active B$_{12}$ and inactive analogues. Currently, the only way to know if a food contains active vitamin B$_{12}$ is to feed it to humans and look for vitamin B$_{12}$ activity. The standard way to do this is to see how different foods affect levels of a compound called methylmalonic acid (MMA). MMA levels increase in B$_{12}$ deficiency, and consuming foods that contain active vitamin B$_{12}$ causes those levels to drop. Many foods that are commonly believed to be good sources of vitamin B$_{12}$ actually have no effect on MMA levels, which means that they contain primarily inactive analogues.

Plants have no need for B$_{12}$, which is why they usually don't contain any. Occasionally, a plant food might be "contaminated" with vitamin B$_{12}$. That is, it contains vitamin B$_{12}$ by accident. For example, the "starter" used to make tempeh, which is a fermented soyfood, might accidentally contain B$_{12}$-producing bacteria. Seaweed might pick up bacteria that produce B$_{12}$-analogues. There is some evidence that sea vegetables such as chlorella, dulse, and nori contain vitamin B$_{12}$, but again, these haven't been shown to be reliable and significant sources of the active vitamin.

Although one study found that supplements of chlorella led to a drop in MMA levels in vegans who were B$_{12}$ deficient, their MMA levels were still higher than ideal. And they had to take forty-five tablets per day to achieve this. What studies like this tell us is that some sea vegetables may be contaminated with vitamin B$_{12}$ but that this doesn't present a practical or reliable way to meet needs.[3]

In cases where vitamin B$_{12}$ shows up unexpectedly in plant foods, we don't know how it got there. That is, we don't know if the plant made it (which is unlikely) or if it came from fecal or insect contamination. This means we can't know how reliable other batches of the same food might be as a source of B$_{12}$.

Most humans get vitamin B$_{12}$ by eating animal products. Cows and other true herbivores are able to absorb the vitamin B$_{12}$ produced in their intestines by bacteria. Others, including many primate species, eat at least small amounts of animal products (including insects or even feces), which can be a good source of B$_{12}$.

It would follow that soil and water that are contaminated with human or animal waste should contain vitamin B$_{12}$, and they might. But while there is speculation about this among research scientists, there is no direct evidence for it. One paper that has gained support among some vegan groups was actually just an abstract in *Science* magazine from 1950 by researchers with the New York Botanical Gardens. The methods used didn't determine whether the B$_{12}$ was active. A more recent finding that plants could take up vitamin B$_{12}$ from manure-treated soil didn't show whether the B$_{12}$ was active vitamin or inactive analogue. And it doesn't really matter because the amounts were so tiny that they didn't have any nutritional significance.[4] A few studies have found that when vitamin B$_{12}$ is injected into the growing medium of plants, some of these plants can take up enough of the vitamin to provide reasonable amounts in the diet. This may supply us with new B$_{12}$ sources for vegans in the future, but for now is not of any practical significance.[5] And supplements are probably more economically effi-cient than running the vitamin B_{12} through plants.

Humans definitely evolved to get by on pretty low intakes of vita-min B_{12}. We have a rather complex physiological way of recycling it, and we also can store relatively large amounts in our livers—sometimes enough to prevent overt deficiency for as long as three years. As a re-sult, some vegan advocates insist that no one needs to worry about vitamin B_{12} until they have been a vegan for several years and that we can get by with taking supplements just "once in a while." We think this approach is a mistake for a couple of reasons.

First, not everyone has a three-year B_{12} supply. It depends on what your diet has been like over time. Building up generous B_{12} stores can take many years of consuming the vitamin in quantities that exceed daily needs. If you have been eating a mostly plant-based or lacto-ovo vegetarian diet before becoming vegan—that is, a diet that is more moderate in animal foods than what most Americans eat—your vita-min B_{12} stores may be relatively low. Some people may find themselves running through their B_{12} supply in just a few months. In addition, vitamin B_{12} stores may not be sufficient to prevent mild, marginal-type deficiencies, as we'll see below.

VITAMIN B_{12} DEFICIENCY

Overt deficiency occurs when vitamin B_{12} stores drop to near zero. Often, the first sign is megaloblastic anemia, which is reversible with vitamin B_{12} therapy.

But sometimes B_{12} deficiency anemia is "masked" by the vitamin folic acid (also called folate), which can step in and do part of vitamin B_{12}'s job. So you can be deficient in vitamin B_{12} but not have anemia if your diet is high in folate. This may sound like a good thing, but it's not since folic acid won't prevent the nerve damage that can occur with B_{12} deficiency. If B_{12} intake is low and folate intake is high, B_{12} deficiency can go unnoticed until it progresses to a more advanced stage. It's an important issue for vegans since we typically have a high intake of folate, which is found in leafy greens, oranges, and beans.

The neurological damage that can result from a B$_{12}$ deficiency typically begins with tingling in the hands and feet and can progress to far more serious symptoms. Often the symptoms can be reversed, but some neurological damage can be permanent. This is especially true in babies born to mothers who don't have adequate vitamin B$_{12}$ intake during pregnancy.

The anemia and neurological symptoms associated with overt B$_{12}$ deficiency are fairly obvious. But a second type of "mild" deficiency doesn't have acute symptoms. It does its damage over time—often decades—and is only detected through medical tests. When B$_{12}$ levels in the blood start to drop, levels of an amino acid called homocysteine begin to rise. Elevated homocysteine is linked with cognitive decline[6,7] and brain atrophy,[8] but there is also evidence for increased risk of birth defects,[9] low bone mineral density,[10,11] and possibly stroke.[12]

Research shows that vegetarians and vegans who supplement with vitamin B$_{12}$ have healthy levels of homocysteine, while those who don't take supplements have high homocysteine levels.[13] Folate and vitamin B$_6$ also affect the vitamin homocysteine, but most vegans get plenty of those.

Studies that have looked at both blood levels of vitamin B$_{12}$ and at levels of MMA suggest that not just vegans, but vegetarians who include dairy and eggs in their diets, are at high risk for vitamin B$_{12}$ deficiency if they don't supplement.[14,15] In vegetarians who had low blood levels of vitamin B$_{12}$, taking supplements improved their artery function, which could lower their risk for cardiovascular disease.[16] These findings present strong evidence that vegans who don't use supplements—and who insist that they feel fine—may be damaging their health over the long term.

While this might sound like vitamin B$_{12}$ is a big problem for vegans, it's an issue that's so easily resolved it shouldn't be a concern. In fact, it's a concern only when vegans don't get good advice about vitamin B$_{12}$ or don't want to use supplements or fortified foods.

We think that vegans actually have the advantage when it comes to vitamin B$_{12}$. Here is why: as people age, no matter what type of diet they follow, their ability to absorb vitamin B$_{12}$ found naturally in foods begins to decline.[17] Vitamin B_{12} in animal foods is bound to protein, and the decrease in stomach acid that tends to occur in older people makes it harder to release B_{12} from the protein so it can be absorbed. Because the vitamin B_{12} in supplements and fortified foods is not bound to protein, it is more easily absorbed by older people. For this reason, the National Academies recommends that all people over age fifty get at least half of the RDA for B_{12} from some combination of supplements and fortified foods. Many older people may not know this, but vegans who are paying attention to good nutrition advice are already using vitamin B_{12} supplements or fortified foods.

SUPPLEMENTING VS. MONITORING

It has been suggested that anyone who is worried about whether or not they should take supplements should simply get their B_{12} levels tested. But that doesn't make any sense. You don't want to wait until your levels are low to start supplementing. And if your levels are normal, you should supplement in order to maintain them. There is no reason not to take supplements. They are inexpensive and safe. So you can have your B_{12} levels tested if you want, but regardless of the results, you should follow the advice about vitamin B_{12} supplements and fortified foods we've outlined next.

MEETING VITAMIN B_{12} NEEDS

The recommendations we make in this chapter are based on supplements and fortified foods that utilize the form of vitamin B_{12} called cyanocobalamin. It may seem like this doesn't make sense since cyanocobalamin has to be converted to the active form of vitamin B_{12}, called methylcobalamin, before it can do its job. So why not just take the methyl version directly? It's not because cyanocobalamin is "better." It's because it's been very well studied and we have more reliable information about appropriate doses for protecting B_{12} status. There is some evidence that methylcobalamin is less stable in supplements and it seems that it takes very high doses to maintain B_{12} levels. Since there is extensive research showing that cyanocobalamin is effective in maintaining good vitamin B$_{12}$ status, and since your body easily converts it to the active form of the vitamin, it's the best choice for supplements. And while there is a small amount of cyanide in cyanocobalamin supplements, the amount is inconsequential compared to what occurs naturally in the diet. A twice weekly supplement of 1,000 micrograms of cyanocobalamin would provide an average of 6 micrograms of cyanide per day which is well below the minimum risk level of 3,175 micrograms per day.[18]

There are a couple of important things to keep in mind about supplementing with B$_{12}$. First, it's a good idea to choose supplements that are chewable (or in liquid form) to maximize vitamin B$_{12}$ absorption.

Also, the body is used to getting little bits of vitamin B$_{12}$ here and there throughout the day. When confronted with a big dose of B$_{12}$, it absorbs just a tiny fraction of the whole amount. So when you take vitamin B$_{12}$ infrequently, you need rather large amounts in order to get enough. The RDA for vitamin B$_{12}$ is just 2.4 micrograms for adults. But if you are getting your daily dose from a supplement, you may need as much as 25 to 100 micrograms. And if you supplement just two or three times a week, you may need 1,000 micrograms each time.

To meet your vitamin B$_{12}$ requirements on a vegan diet, do any *one* of the following:

- Consume two servings per day of fortified foods providing 2 to 3.5 micrograms of vitamin B$_{12}$ each.
- Take a daily vitamin B$_{12}$ supplement of at least 25 micrograms (25 to 100 micrograms is a good range).
- Take a supplement of 1,000 micrograms of vitamin B$_{12}$ two times a week.

Getting B$_{12}$ from Fortified Foods

Plant foods are reliable sources of active vitamin B$_{12}$ only if they are fortified with the vitamin. On food labels, the Daily Value for vitamin

B_{12} is 6 micrograms. So if a food provides 25 percent of the Daily Value, it contains 1.5 micrograms.

Nutritional yeast is a popular choice with many vegans. Its cheesy-yeasty flavor is especially appealing mixed into bean and grain dishes or sprinkled over popcorn. Nutritional yeast is grown on a nutrient-rich culture and contains only the nutrients that are in that culture. So don't assume that every type of nutritional yeast is a good source of vitamin B_{12}. Some Red Star brand nutritional yeast contains vitamin B_{12} and is widely available, often in the bulk food section of natural foods markets. It's usually labeled VSF, which stands for Vegetarian Support Formula. (Don't confuse nutritional yeast with brewer's yeast, which is a byproduct of beer making and is not a good source of vitamin B_{12}. Neither brewer's yeast nor nutritional yeast is the active yeast used in bread making.)

A growing number of plant milks are fortified with vitamin B_{12} and you may also find it added to some brands of tofu, although this is less usual. In Canada, vitamin B_{12} is added to veggie meats by law, but it's far less common for these products to be fortified in the United States.

VITAMIN B_{12} CONTENT OF FORTIFIED VEGAN FOODS

Food	Vitamin B_{12} Content (micrograms)
Nutritional yeast, VSF, 1 tablespoon	4.0
Soymilk, fortified, 1 cup	1.2–2.9*
Protein bar, fortified	1.0–2.0*
Marmite yeast extract, 1 teaspoon	0.9

*Amount varies by brand.

VITAMIN B_{12} FACTS

- The vitamin B_{12} in supplements comes from bacterial cultures—it's never isolated from animal products.
- B_{12} pills should be chewed or allowed to dissolve under the tongue.
- Seaweed (e.g., algae, nori, spirulina), brewer's yeast, tempeh, or "living" vitamin supplements that use plants as a source of B_{12} cannot be relied upon to protect vitamin B_{12} status.

- Neither rainwater nor organically grown, unwashed vegetables are a reliable source of vitamin B$_{12}$.
- About 2 percent of people can't absorb B$_{12}$. This disease is called *pernicious anemia*. Being vegan has nothing to do with this condition, but if you are supplementing regularly with vitamin B$_{12}$ and still suspect that you have symptoms of vitamin B$_{12}$ deficiency, such as extreme fatigue or neurological problems, then by all means get your B$_{12}$ levels tested. Pernicious anemia is treated with vitamin B$_{12}$ injections or large doses of oral supplements.

IS A VEGAN DIET NATURAL?

It wouldn't be right to ignore the four-hundred-pound gorilla in the room, so let's ask the obvious question: Since vitamin B$_{12}$ is not found in plant foods and vegans must take supplements, doesn't that make a vegan diet unnatural?

Many vegans have bent over backward to convince themselves that humans evolved as vegans and that supplemental vitamin B$_{12}$ is only needed because we have moved so far away from our natural environment. But there is a tremendous amount of evidence that humans evolved eating some animal products. While B$_{12}$ is not needed in large amounts, it may take more than can be picked up from unwashed produce to sustain optimal levels. That's especially true during pregnancy and lactation, when a woman needs to consume enough B$_{12}$ for her own needs and to pass on to her baby.

In fact, adding small amounts of animal products to the diet has been shown *not* to cure B$_{12}$ deficiency. At least one study showed that some lacto-ovo vegetarians may have vitamin B$_{12}$ status that is similar to that of vegans when neither group supplemented.[19] If consuming small amounts of animal foods doesn't improve vitamin B$_{12}$ status, then it is unlikely that inadvertently ingesting B$_{12}$ from unwashed produce would be enough to sustain vegans through the life cycle in a pre-vitamin-supplement culture.

On the (now defunct) PaleoVeganology website, paleontologist Robert Mason said this about the evolution of human diets: "This touches on the issue of how vegans should handle the caveman argument. Many of us are tempted to strain credulity and torture the evidence to 'prove' humans are 'naturally' vegan. This is a trap, and one into which carnists (especially paleo-dieters) would love us to fall; the evidence isn't on our side. There's no doubt that hominids ate meat. . . . The argument for veganism has always been primarily ethical, and ought to remain that way. It's based on a concern for the future, not an obsession about the past."[20]

And Tom Billings, who wrote the Beyond Veg website, says, "Further, if the motivation for your diet is moral and/or spiritual, then you will want the basis of your diet to be honest as well as compassionate. In that case, ditching the false myths of naturalness presents no problems; indeed, ditching false myths means that you are ditching a burden."[21]

We agree that it just doesn't matter whether a vegan diet is our historical way of eating or not. The fact is, it makes sense *now* to choose a vegan diet. And whose diet is really natural, anyway? The assumption that there is one natural prehistoric diet, which can be approximated today and would be optimal for modern humans, is dubious at best.

Today's commercial plant foods and meats are different from the foods available in prehistoric times. We eat hybrids of plants and we feed foods to animals that they would not normally eat. Additionally, the US food supply is routinely fortified with a host of vitamins and minerals. Even those people who strive to eat a more "natural" diet as adults have normally benefited from fortified foods as children. It is quite unlikely that anyone is eating a natural diet in today's world.

Taking a daily vitamin B_{12} supplement is a small thing that can make all the difference in your health as a vegan. Based on our current knowledge of vitamin B_{12} requirements and sources, supplementation is not a subject for debate—vitamin B_{12} supplements or fortified foods are an essential part of a well-balanced and responsible vegan diet at all stages of the life cycle.

CHAPTER 7

Fats

Making the Best Choices

S tudies show that, on average, vegans consume a little less than 30 percent of their calories from fat.[1] That's a bit lower than the average for nonvegan Americans, but not by much. The big difference is in the type of fat that vegans consume since plant foods are much lower in saturated fat than meat, dairy, and eggs.

The term "fat" is a big category that includes a number of different fatty acids, two of which are essential to our diet. Actual requirements for essential fats are low, but there may be advantages to eating some fat-rich foods overall. In this chapter, we'll look at ways to ensure you are meeting essential fatty acid needs. First, though, we want to answer the question of how much total fat vegans can safely consume.

HOW MUCH FAT SHOULD VEGANS CONSUME?

Despite the popularity of vegan diets that eliminate all high-fat foods, the evidence for the benefits of this approach is limited. It's true that compared to usual Western eating habits, low-fat vegan diets offer advantages for health. But there is no evidence that they provide benefits compared to higher-fat plant-based diets.

In the famous Seven Countries Study, Ancel Keys and his colleagues sought to answer questions about the impacts of traditional eating patterns and lifestyles in different countries on risk for cardiovascular disease. They found the lowest risk was among people living on the island of Crete, who also happened to have the highest fat intake of all the populations studied.[2] Importantly, their diet was built around healthful plant foods and included foods rich in health-promoting fats. Since then research has continued to show the benefits of fat-rich plant foods. For example, some types of fat have beneficial effects on blood cholesterol levels. There is a large body of research showing that nuts, which are among the highest-fat foods in vegan diets, protect against heart disease and may even be beneficial for weight management.

Fat is also essential for the absorption of vitamins D, E, and K as well as beta-carotene, the plant compound that is converted to vitamin A. Very low fat diets can result in poor absorption of these nutrients and also of a number of health-promoting phytochemicals.

This does not suggest that you should eat unlimited amounts of high-fat foods. Very high fat diets can raise risk for chronic diseases and can also push calorie intake too high. But the range of healthful fat intakes is fairly wide. According to the National Academies, the Acceptable Macronutrient Distribution Range for fat intake is between 20 and 35 percent of calories. This translates to about 45 to 78 total grams of fat per day for a person consuming 2,000 calories.

Very low fat diets are never appropriate for vegan children, who need higher fat foods to meet calorie and nutrient needs. The acceptable range of fat intakes for toddlers (ages one to three years) is 30 to 40 percent of calories. For children ages four to eighteen, it is 25 to 35 percent.

While some vegans prefer and thrive on lower fat intakes, these diets are not the right choice for everyone. Eating diets that are very low in fat could be the reason that some people abandon vegan diets and return to eating meat. Many people think of meat as "protein," forgetting that meat is also typically high in fat. Those who don't feel well on vegan diets sometimes add meat back to their diet because they're convinced that they aren't getting adequate protein—when, in fact, they might have felt better by simply adding more fat to their menu.

Plant foods that provide healthy fats can make vegan diets more interesting and easier to plan. For many, this provides an easier transition to a vegan diet and makes this way of eating a more realistic choice for the long term. From both a practical and a health point of view, it doesn't make sense to ban all high-fat foods from your diet. We do need to choose fats wisely, though, and in particular need to make sure that we're meeting needs for the essential fatty acids.

MEETING ESSENTIAL FATTY ACID NEEDS

Two fatty acids, both of which are polyunsaturated, are considered essential nutrients for humans. **Linoleic acid** (LA) is an essential omega-6 fat and **alpha-linolenic acid** (ALA) is the essential omega-3 fat. Even vegan diets that are relatively low in fat almost always provide enough linoleic acid. Recommended amounts are 12 grams for women and 17 grams for men. Walnuts, seeds, soyfoods, and many vegetable oils are especially rich in linoleic acid. Vegans tend to have adequate intakes of this nutrient, often consuming more than nonvegetarians.[3,4]

Some vegans may not meet needs for the omega-3 essential fatty acid, ALA, however, since this fat is found in only a handful of plant foods. Recommended intakes of ALA for adults are 1.1 grams per day for women and 1.6 grams for men. Meeting those needs isn't difficult, but it requires a little bit of attention to food choices.

LONG-CHAIN OMEGA-3 FATS

In addition to the essential fat ALA, the omega-3 family includes a couple of other fatty acids that are of considerable interest in nutrition. These are EPA and DHA, which are the "long-chain" omega-3 fatty acids. These fats have been thought to be important for lowering risk

ALA CONTENT OF VEGAN FOODS

Recommended intake is 1.1 grams for women and 1.6 grams for men	
	ALA in grams
Nuts and Seeds	
Flaxseeds, ground,* 1 tablespoon	1.6
Hempseeds, 1 tablespoon	0.8
Chia seeds, 1 tablespoon	2.5
Walnuts, 6 halves	1.0
Walnuts, chopped, ¼ cup	2.6
Oils, 1 tablespoon	
Flax oil	7.3
Hempseed oil	2.5
Walnut oil	1.4
Canola oil	1.3
Soy oil	0.9
Soyfoods, ½ cup cooked	
Firm tofu	0.2
Tempeh	0.2
Soybeans	0.5

*Flaxseeds should always be ground to enhance ALA absorption.

for cardiovascular disease, and possibly also for protecting cognitive function and eye health.

Since the long-chain omega-3 fats are found primarily in cold-water fish and to a much smaller extent in eggs, lacto-ovo vegetarians consume very little, and vegans generally have none in their diets (although some vegans may consume very small amounts of EPA from sea vegetables).[5] Whether or not this matters is a big question in vegan nutrition.

Potential Benefits of DHA and EPA: The Science Behind the Claims

The relationship of DHA and EPA to heart disease risk is a topic of much debate among nutrition experts. A number of studies (and large reviews of studies) have suggested that consuming these fats reduces the risk of heart disease but others have found no benefit.[6–11]

DIETARY FATS: TERMS YOU NEED TO KNOW

THE ESSENTIAL FATTY ACIDS

LINOLEIC ACID (LA): An omega-6 fatty acid found in grains, seeds, nuts, and oils, especially safflower, sunflower, corn, and soy oil.

ALPHA-LINOLENIC ACID (ALA): A short-chain omega-3 fatty acid found in flaxseeds, chia seeds, hempseeds, walnuts, canola oil, and some soyfoods.

LONG-CHAIN OMEGA-3 FATS

DHA (DOCOSAHEXANOIC ACID): Found in fatty fish, some eggs, and algae. It can be manufactured in the body from ALA, but optimal conditions for conversion are not well known.

EPA (EICOSAPENTAENOIC ACID): Found in fatty fish, sea vegetables, and algae. It can be manufactured in the body from ALA, and small amounts can be made from DHA.

Although the omega-3 blood levels of vegetarians have been measured often enough to show that they are clearly lower than in fish-eaters, the actual effects of these lower levels aren't clear.[4,5,12–16] For example, two studies of the effects of DHA and EPA on blood clotting in vegetarians came up with conflicting findings. DHA and EPA consumption can slow blood clotting, which is one way they might help reduce heart disease risk.

A 1999 study in Chile found that vegetarians had significantly more platelets (which are involved in blood clotting) and a shorter bleeding time than nonvegetarians, which suggests greater blood-clotting activity. But when the vegetarians took supplements of EPA and DHA for eight weeks, it didn't affect clotting activity (although other factors changed).[17,18]

In contrast, an earlier study in the United Kingdom found only small differences between vegetarians and nonvegetarians in factors that affect blood clotting. Bleeding times were similar between the two groups.[13] So, of two studies looking at these effects, vegetarians fared worse than meat-eaters in one but were largely the same in the other.

The findings are also conflicting when we look at heart disease risk in vegans compared to pescovegetarians—vegetarians who eat fish. In the United Kingdom, vegans had a somewhat higher risk of death from heart disease compared to pescovegetarians.[19] But among North American vegetarians (including both lacto-ovo vegetarians and vegans), vegetarians had a much lower risk for heart disease than pescovegetarians. In fact, the fish-eaters had about the same risk as subjects who consumed all types of meat.[20] While that's encouraging, findings on heart disease risk in vegans haven't been as impressive as we'd expect, especially given their lower blood cholesterol and blood pressure levels. It's possible that omega-3 fat status is part of the explanation for this but we just don't know.

DHA is also found in high concentrations in the retina of the eye and in the brain's gray matter. It might help protect against depression and cognitive decline, although again, the findings are conflicting, and we don't have any studies on this in vegans.

DHA and EPA in Vegan Diets

While vegans don't have direct sources of DHA and EPA in their diets, the body can synthesize them from the essential fatty acid ALA under the right conditions. Conversion of ALA to these long-chain fats varies considerably based on genetics and lifestyle factors, but on average, 5 percent of ALA is converted to EPA and 0.5 percent is converted to DHA.[21,22] Synthesis of EPA and DHA is enhanced by estrogen and seems to be best in women during childbearing years.[21] But at any stage of life, poor nutrition and chronic disease like diabetes can reduce production of these fats.

Some evidence suggests that high intakes of the omega-6 fatty acid LA suppress conversion of ALA to DHA and EPA.[23,24] This is because metabolism of LA and ALA compete in the body for the same enzyme. It's possible that consuming less LA frees up the enzyme allowing ALA to convert to the long-chain fats more efficiently. A common recommendation is to reduce LA intake to achieve a ratio of LA to ALA that is no greater than 4 to 1. But the ratio in vegan diets is more typically around 15 to 1 due to relatively high intakes of LA.[1] As a result, dietary strategies to boost ALA intake and lower LA intake have become popular among some vegans. But do they work?

Studies in vegans have shown conflicting results.[25-27] In general it seems that for the ratio to have an effect, levels of LA may need to be extremely low—as low as 2.5 percent of total calories—to maximize synthesis of the long-chain omega-3 fats.[28] This is not a practical goal for most people.

Another strategy is to simply consume more of the essential omega-3 fat ALA. Some research has found this to be effective in raising blood levels of DHA and EPA in vegans, particularly in women.[29,30]

Adding another layer of complexity to the issue is that some experts warn that restricting LA too much might raise the risk for heart disease since these fats help lower blood cholesterol levels. The World Health Organization and Food and Agriculture Organization recommend an LA intake between 2.5 and 9 percent of calories, saying that the higher end of the range reduces risk for heart disease.[31] The National Academies also doesn't recommend a specific ratio of LA to ALA, but rather recommends consuming diets that provide between 5 and 10 percent of calories from LA and 0.6 and 1.2 percent of calories from ALA. Vegan intakes of LA in recent studies have ranged from 5.1 to 9.3 percent of calories, putting them within the recommended range.[4,32-34]

Right now, the research leaves us with many unanswered questions about how to maximize DHA and EPA status. The optimal ratio of LA to ALA for maximizing synthesis of the long-chain omega-3 fats isn't known and it's possible that the most effective ratio is too low in LA and too high in ALA to be realistic or healthful. It is easy enough to modify the ratio of these fats in your diet by limiting foods that are very high in LA such as safflower, sunflower, corn, and soybean oil, and getting more fat from nuts, avocado, olives, and olive and canola oils. But beyond those choices, we don't recommend efforts to achieve a specific ratio.

Our recommendations focus on ensuring adequate intakes of both essential fatty acids rather than on specific ratios. But where does all of this leave us in terms of DHA and EPA in vegans? One last option for enhancing status is to take direct supplements of these fats.

DHA Supplements

Fish get their DHA from algae, and vegans can go to the same source. Preliminary research suggests that a supplement providing 200 milligrams of DHA from microalgae per day for three months can raise blood DHA levels in vegans by as much as 50 percent.[35] Other studies of vegetarians (not necessarily vegans) have also shown the positive effects of taking DHA supplements.[36]

But because the research on the overall benefits of omega-3s is so conflicting, it's hard to know whether these supplements are necessary for vegans. While we are not convinced that they are, we're also not convinced that the lower blood levels of DHA and EPA in vegans is unimportant. Until we know more, supplementing with very small amounts, around 200 to 300 milligrams of DHA every two or three days is a reasonable approach for those vegans who wish to err on the side of caution. Because ALA converts more efficiently to EPA than DHA, and because some DHA can convert back to EPA, it's likely that taking supplements of DHA alone is enough provided you are meeting needs for ALA. There is some evidence, although again it's conflicting, that omega-3 supplements could help with symptoms of depression. In this case, EPA might be more effective than DHA. If you've been diagnosed with depression, talk to your health-care provider about EPA and whether supplements would be a good choice for you.

The main problem with these supplements is that they are expensive. Our recommendation to take a small dose just every few days makes them a little more affordable, but, whether or not you include them in your diet remains a personal decision.

A few vegan foods such as soymilk, energy bars, and olive oil are sometimes fortified with algae-derived DHA, providing what may be a more reasonable option for some vegans.

VEGETABLE OILS IN VEGAN DIETS

Vegetable oils aren't essential in vegan diets, but for those who enjoy them, they can fit into healthy menus. While frying meat and peeled potatoes in hot oil doesn't result in the most health-promoting meal, there's a world of difference between that and drizzling a little extra-virgin olive oil over a platter of roasted red peppers.

Oils are part of some of the healthiest cuisine in the world, and when they are used judiciously in diets that emphasize plant foods, there is no reason to believe that they are harmful. (We look at the research on fats and heart disease in Chapter 15.) Just a little bit of oil can make flavors pop and also enhance nutrient absorption.

The way in which oils are processed affects their nutrient content and also guidelines for using and storing them. Cold pressed or expeller-pressed oils are extracted through mechanical crushing and pressing. They are higher in phytochemicals, including antioxidants, than refined oils but are more susceptible to rancidity. Keep these oils in the refrigerator. You can even freeze them if a bottle is going to last you for a long time. (Freeze them in an ice cube tray so you can defrost a little at a time.)

These oils also have a low smoke point, which means that, compared to refined oils, they begin to break down at lower temperatures, producing potentially toxic compounds. It's best to use them in dressings rather than for cooking. Smoke point is affected by the type of fatty acids in the oil as well as processing and you may want to keep several different oils on hand for different culinary purposes.

Here are general guidelines for choosing the right oil in your food preparation:

- For high-temperature cooking (400 to 450 degrees): refined soy oil, peanut oil, avocado oil, olive oil (not extra-virgin)
- For moderate-temperature cooking (400 degrees and lower): canola oil (either refined or expeller-pressed); expeller-pressed avocado oil, grapeseed oil
- For low-temperature cooking (350 degrees or lower): cold-pressed sesame oil; extra-virgin olive oil
- For flavoring and drizzling after food is cooked or for salad dressings or to heat at very low temperatures (below 320 degrees): expeller-pressed nut oils like walnut and almond; toasted sesame oil
- For use in small quantities as a source of ALA: hempseed and flaxseed oils. These oils are fragile, so always keep them in the refrigerator and never heat them.

What About Coconut Oil?

Packed with saturated fat—it has more than either butter or lard—coconut oil has developed a surprising reputation as a health food. This is partly because some research has shown coconut oil to have antimicrobial properties. Virgin coconut oil contains a number of protective phytochemicals as well and, in populations where people eat healthy diets containing plenty of fiber-rich plant foods, coconut oil consumption isn't associated with heart disease.[37] One reason may be that the main fat in coconut oil raises blood levels of HDL-cholesterol (the "good" cholesterol) more than it raises the more harmful LDL-cholesterol.[38] Whether or not this matters is something we don't know since the impact of HDL-cholesterol is a subject of some debate.

Adding coconut oil to your diet is unlikely to have any particular benefit and, as with all added fats, we advise keeping intakes low. But for those eating a heart-healthy vegan diet, it's fine to use occasional coconut oil in your meals when you need a solid fat for cooking. While refined coconut oil has a higher smoke point, it's stripped of its health-promoting phytochemicals. Be sure to choose virgin coconut oil and use it only at temperatures below 350 degrees.

FAT IN VEGAN DIETS: PRACTICAL GUIDELINES

Keep total fat intake in the moderate range. The consensus among experts is that fat intakes across a wide range are compatible with good health. Excessive fat intake is not healthy, but that doesn't mean that all fat is bad. The World Health Organization cautions against consuming a diet that is less than 15 percent fat for adults or less than 20 percent for premenopausal women.[31] We recommend that vegans strive for a fat intake somewhere between 20 and 30 percent of calories. That means between 22 and 33 grams of fat for every 1,000 calories you consume. Here is a quick guide to approximate amounts of fat in plant foods.

AVERAGE AMOUNT OF FAT IN VEGAN FOODS

	Average Amount of Fat (in grams)
Avocado, ¼ cup cubes	5.5
Leafy green vegetables, ½ cup cooked	0.2–0.35
Nuts, ¼ cup	17–20
Seeds, 2 tablespoons	8
Soybeans, ½ cup cooked	7
Tempeh, ½ cup	9
Tofu, firm, ½ cup	11
Tofu, soft, ½ cup	4.5
Vegetable oils, 1 teaspoon	5

Avoid fats that are associated with chronic disease. We'll talk more about these in Chapter 15, but both saturated fat and trans fats may raise the risk for heart disease and diabetes and could be associated with cancer risk as well. Generally speaking, vegans don't need to worry since saturated fats tend to be low in plant-based diets and in the United States, trans fats have been banned.

Be sure to meet your needs for the essential omega-3 fatty acid ALA. Use the table on page 98 to make sure you're getting enough of this fat.

Consider taking a DHA supplement. While we don't know whether low levels of DHA are of any significance to the health of vegans, if you want to err on the side of caution, a DHA supplement will ensure that you are getting the same fatty acids in your diet that people get from eating fish. For those vegans who suffer from depression, a supplement that provides both DHA and EPA may be preferable. For those who prefer not to take these supplements, an alternative is to consume an additional 2 grams of ALA per day since this may enhance synthesis of DHA and EPA.

CHAPTER 8

Vitamins and Minerals
Maximizing Vegan Sources

Protein, calcium, and vitamins B_{12} and D get most of the attention in vegan diets. But there are a few other nutrients that deserve consideration, namely iron, zinc, iodine, and vitamin A. We'll touch briefly on vitamin K, riboflavin, and selenium, too.

MINERAL ABSORPTION ON VEGAN DIETS

Minerals like iron and zinc are absorbed less well from plant foods than from animal products. There are a number of reasons for this, but the most important is the presence of phytate in the diet. This phosphorus-containing compound is found in whole grains, legumes, seeds, and nuts. (Smaller amounts are found in vegetables, too.) Phytate binds minerals, making them less absorbable. Refining grains reduces their phytate content, but it also reduces the mineral content of a food, so it isn't much of a solution.

A number of food preparation techniques help liberate minerals from phytate and can greatly increase absorption. Fermentation, which includes the activity of both yeast and sourdough starters in bread making, as well as the production of fermented foods like tempeh and miso, greatly increases mineral availability. This makes leavened bread a better source of well-absorbed iron and zinc than crackers and flatbreads.

Toasting nuts and seeds, and sprouting beans and grains, reduces the effects of phytate. So does soaking these foods and discarding the water before using them in a recipe. Foods that contain vitamin C are especially effective for increasing iron absorption.

Phytate isn't all bad, though. It's an antioxidant that acts in ways that could reduce cancer risk. This suggests a benefit to getting minerals from plant foods. If you use food preparation techniques to break the bond between phytate and iron or zinc, you'll improve mineral absorption while getting the potential health benefits of phytate.

IRON

Iron is a part of hemoglobin, the component of red blood cells that carries oxygen to the cells. It's also a part of many enzymes involved in energy production and immune function. Even among Americans who eat meat, iron deficiency is the most common nutrient deficiency. Poor iron status is seen most often in toddlers and premenopausal women and is especially common in pregnant women.[1-3]

We need a constant supply of iron in our diets because we lose it through daily sloughing off of intestinal and other cells. Premenopausal women lose more iron than men because of menstrual losses. Their iron needs are more than twice what men require, which explains why iron deficiency is so much more common among younger women. With menopause, iron needs decrease. The recommended daily iron intake is 18 milligrams for premenopausal women and 8 milligrams for men and postmenopausal women.

Iron Deficiency

There are two stages of iron deficiency. In the first, iron stores become depleted and there may be a decrease in hemoglobin levels and mild symptoms like tiredness and difficulty concentrating. In the next stage—overt iron deficiency anemia—hemoglobin drops to subnormal levels, which can cause symptoms such as pale skin, fatigue, weakness, shortness of breath, an inability to maintain body temperature, loss of appetite, and hair loss. But these symptoms can also be due to other nutritional deficiencies or conditions, and true iron-deficiency anemia can be diagnosed only through a blood test. A blood test can also help your physician differentiate between anemia due to iron deficiency and anemia due to vitamin B_{12} deficiency.

Meat Iron vs. Plant Iron

You might be surprised to know that vegans typically consume more iron than either lacto-ovo vegetarians or meat-eaters.[4-7] The issue for vegans is how well that iron is absorbed.

Foods contain two forms of iron, called heme and nonheme iron. Heme iron is much more readily absorbed by the body and is not much affected by other factors in the diet. Nonheme iron is absorbed at a much lower level, and its absorption can be inhibited or enhanced by other dietary components, including phytate. Meat contains both types of iron, but plant foods contain only nonheme iron. So strategies to boost absorption are important for people who get all their iron from plant foods.

Because phytate reduces iron absorption, all the food preparation methods we mentioned earlier—fermentation, leavening breads, soaking, sprouting, and cooking—can boost iron absorption. But the most effective way by far to release iron from phytate is to add vitamin C-rich foods to meals. Vitamin C changes the iron into a form that is more easily absorbed. The effects of vitamin C on iron absorption are rather dramatic. Just 5 ounces of orange juice, providing 75 milligrams of vitamin C, can quadruple the amount of iron you absorb from a meal.[8] In one study in India, children with iron-deficiency anemia (who probably did not have high vitamin C intakes) were given 100 milligrams of vitamin C at lunch and dinner for sixty days. Most made a full recovery with a significant improvement in their anemia.[9]

But simply taking a daily vitamin C supplement won't improve your iron status, since the iron and vitamin C must be consumed at the same time. The key to optimizing iron status for vegans is to include iron-rich and vitamin C–rich foods in the same meal. Vitamin C is found in oranges, grapefruits, strawberries, many green leafy vegetables (broccoli, kale, collards, Swiss chard, Brussels sprouts), bell peppers (yellow, red, and green), and cauliflower. You should know, however, that certain dietary factors like tannins in coffee and tea and high doses of calcium reduce absorption of nonheme iron. It's important to take calcium supplements between meals, and if you are trying to maximize iron absorption, to avoid drinking coffee and tea with meals.

Vegans have a definite advantage over lacto-ovo vegetarians when it comes to iron because milk is a poor source of this mineral. In addition to displacing iron-rich foods from the diet, it interferes with iron absorption. Excessive consumption of milk can increase the risk for iron deficiency, especially in young children.[10]

Vegan and Vegetarian DRI for Iron

Vegetarians typically have iron stores that are at the lower end of the normal range—that is, lower than the stores of meat-eaters, but still adequate.[11,12] It's important to maintain these stores by eating plenty of iron-rich foods. And since nonheme iron is absorbed at a lower rate, vegetarians and vegans need more dietary iron than meat-eaters. But how much more is controversial. The National Academies established a vegetarian recommendation that is 1.8 times higher for vegetarians than omnivores. But this was based on a (completely unrealistic) test diet that was low in vitamin C and high in factors (like tannins from tea) that reduce iron absorption.[13] In other words, it represents a worst-case scenario rather than the way most vegetarians and vegans actually eat.

Based on these recommendations, a premenopausal vegan woman would require 33 milligrams of iron per day. While it's possible to plan a diet that provides this much iron, it would be extremely difficult to consume this much without supplements.

IRON CONTENT OF VEGAN FOODS

*Recommended intakes are 18 milligrams for women and 8 milligrams for men.**	
	Iron (in milligrams)
Breads, Cereals, and Grains	
Barley, pearled, ½ cup cooked	1.5
Bran flakes, 1 cup	12
Bread, white, 1 slice	1.4
Bread, whole wheat, 1 slice	0.8
Cream of Wheat, ½ cup cooked	6
Oatmeal cooked from rolled oats, ½ cup	1
Oatmeal, instant, 1 packet	3.6
Pasta, enriched, ½ cup cooked	0.8
Pasta, whole wheat, ½ cup cooked	1
Quinoa, ½ cup cooked	1.4
Rice, brown, ½ cup cooked	0.4
Wheat germ, 2 tablespoons	0.9
Vegetables (½ cup cooked unless otherwise indicated)	
Asparagus	0.8
Beet greens	1.4
Bok choy	0.9
Brussels sprouts	0.9
Collard greens	1.1
Peas	1.4
Pumpkin	1.7
Spinach	3.2
Sweet potatoes, mashed	1.2
Swiss chard	2.0
Tomato juice, 1 cup	1.0
Tomato sauce	1.2
Fruits	
Apricots, dried, ¼ cup	0.9
Prunes, ¼ cup	1.2
Prune juice, 6 ounces	2.3
Raisins, ¼ cup	0.9
Legumes (½ cup cooked)	
Black beans	1.8
Black-eyed peas	2.2
Garbanzo beans	2.4
Kidney beans	2.6
Lentils	3.3
Lima beans	2.2
Navy beans	2.2

continues

IRON CONTENT OF VEGAN FOODS *continued*

Recommended intakes are 18 milligrams for women and 8 milligrams for men.*	
	Iron (in milligrams)
Legumes (½ cup cooked) *continued*	
Pinto beans	1.8
Split peas	1.3
Vegetarian baked beans	1.5
Soyfoods	
Edamame, ½ cup	2.25
Soymilk, 1 cup	1.1–1.8*
Tempeh, ½ cup	1.3
Tofu, firm, ½ cup	2.0–3.5**
Textured vegetable protein, ¼ cup, dry	1.4
Veggie "meats," fortified, 1 ounce	0.8–2.1**
Nuts and Seeds	
Almonds, ¼ cup	1.3
Almond butter, 2 tablespoons	1.1
Cashews, ¼ cup	1.9
Peanuts, ¼ cup	1.7
Peanut butter, 2 tablespoons	0.6
Pecans, ¼ cup	0.7
Pine nuts, 2 tablespoons	0.95
Pumpkin seeds, 2 tablespoons	0.25
Sunflower seeds	0.9
Tahini	1.3
Other Foods	
Blackstrap molasses, 1 tablespoon	3.6
Dark chocolate, 1 ounce	3.4
Energy bar, 1 bar	1.4–4.5**

*Requirements may be considerably higher for vegans.
**Amount varies by brand.

Moreover, in addition to being unrealistic, this amount is probably unnecessary. While vegans need to consume more iron than people who eat meat, how much more depends on your overall diet. For example, iron in soyfoods is very well absorbed because it's in a form that isn't affected by phytate.[14] Vegans who consume vitamin C–rich foods with their meals and who avoid coffee, tea, and calcium supplements with meals are likely to need much less iron than the amount specified by the National Academies. Pairing iron-rich foods with vitamin C-rich foods isn't at all difficult and chances are you already do it. A stir-fried dish with tofu and broccoli, a bowl of oatmeal topped with strawberries or with a glass of orange juice, or bean soup with added leafy green vegetables are all examples of meals that make use of this strategy. See "Maximizing Iron and Zinc in Vegan Diets" on page 116.

If you are diagnosed with iron-deficiency anemia, it doesn't mean you should start eating meat. Iron deficiency, even in meat-eaters, is usually treated with supplemental iron, not more meat. Large doses of iron should be taken only under a doctor's care, however, since megadoses of any mineral can be harmful. There may also be an advantage to taking supplements of the amino acid L-lysine since, in one study of women whose iron stores were not improved with supplements, adding 1.5 to 2 grams per day of L-lysine to their diet increased their iron stores.[15]

ZINC

Zinc is needed for at least 100 different enzymatic reactions in the body. It's required for protein synthesis, cell growth, blood formation, immune function, and wound healing. While overt zinc deficiency is rarely seen in Western countries, it's possible that some people—especially children in low-income families—suffer from marginal deficiency. Poor growth in children is one sign of a marginal deficiency. But because zinc is used for so many functions, there might be other suboptimal health conditions related to low zinc intake that we don't really understand yet. It's also somewhat difficult to measure zinc status accurately.

As a result, we have some unanswered questions about zinc. And one of those questions is: how much zinc do vegans need?

Factors Affecting Zinc Requirements

The adult RDA for zinc is 11 milligrams for men and 8 milligrams for women. But because absorption from plant foods is quite a bit lower than from animal foods, the National Academies suggests that zinc needs could be as much as 50 percent greater for vegans. That means that vegan zinc needs would be 16½ milligrams for men and 12 milligrams for women. Vegan intakes often fall somewhat below these recommendations.[6,7,16]

While there is no evidence that vegans and other vegetarians suffer from zinc deficiency and there is evidence that they could adapt to lower intakes, it's still important to optimize zinc absorption. As with iron, phytate is one of the important factors affecting zinc bioavailability, so many of the food preparation techniques that boost iron absorption also work for zinc. (Note, however, that vitamin C does not appear to enhance zinc absorption despite its very beneficial effects for iron.)

See "Maximizing Iron and Zinc in Vegan Diets" on page 116 for guidelines on getting enough zinc. If you think that your diet may fall short on well-absorbed zinc, consider taking a multivitamin that contains zinc. Or if you are already taking calcium tablets, choose one with zinc.

ZINC CONTENT OF SELECTED FOODS

Recommended intakes are 8 milligrams for women and 11 milligrams for men.*	
	Zinc (in milligrams)
Breads, Cereals, and Grains	
Barley, pearled, ½ cup cooked	0.65
Bran flakes, 1 cup	2.0
Bread, white, 1 slice	0.3
Bread, whole wheat, 1 slice	0.6
Oatmeal, instant, 1 packet	1.0
Oatmeal cooked from rolled oats, ½ cup	1.2
Quinoa, ½ cup cooked	1.0
Rice, brown, ½ cup cooked	0.8
Wheat germ, 2 tablespoons	1.7
Vegetables (½ cup cooked, except where noted)	
Asparagus	0.5
Avocado, fresh, ½ of a medium-sized fruit	0.5
Broccoli	0.4

continues

ZINC CONTENT OF SELECTED FOODS   *continued*

*Recommended intakes are 8 milligrams for women and 11 milligrams for men.**	
	Zinc (in milligrams)
Vegetables (½ cup cooked, except where noted) *continued*	
Corn	0.5
Mushrooms	0.7
Peas	0.3
Spinach	0.7
Legumes (½ cup cooked)	
Adzuki beans	2.0
Black-eyed peas	1.1
Chickpeas	1.3
Kidney beans	0.9
Lentils	1.3
Lima beans	0.9
Navy beans	0.9
Pinto beans	0.8
Split peas	1.0
Vegetarian baked beans	2.9
Soyfoods	
Edamame, ½ cup cooked	0.8
Tempeh, ½ cup cooked	1.0
Tofu, firm, ½ cup	1.0–2.0
Veggie "meats," fortified, 1 ounce	1.4–1.8**
Nuts and Seeds (2 tablespoons)	
Almond butter	1.0
Cashews	0.9
Peanuts	0.9
Peanut butter	0.8
Pumpkin/squash seeds	0.8
Sunflower seeds	0.9
Tahini	1.4
Other Foods	
Chocolate, dark, 1 ounce	1.0
Energy bar, 1 bar	3.0–5.2**

*May be higher for vegans (see page 114).

**Amount varies by brand.

MAXIMIZING IRON AND ZINC IN VEGAN DIETS

- Use the tables on pages 111 and 114 to make sure you're choosing plenty of foods rich in iron and zinc. Good sources of iron are beans, leafy green vegetables, and dried fruit. Good sources of zinc are beans, nuts, peanuts, peanut butter, pumpkin seeds, sunflower seeds, bran flakes, wheat germ, and tempeh.
- Include a good source of vitamin C at every meal to increase iron absorption. Among the best sources are oranges, broccoli, strawberries, grapefruit, leafy green vegetables, bell peppers, Brussels sprouts, and cauliflower.
- Consume coffee and tea between meals rather than with meals.
- Take calcium supplements between meals rather than with meals.
- Toast nuts before adding them to recipes.
- If you enjoy sprouting beans and grains, this is another way to boost mineral absorption.
- Choose leavened breads and sourdough bread more often than flatbreads and crackers. Refined grains like white bread have much lower amounts of phytate, and while they may be fortified with iron, they have far less zinc than whole-grain products. Even though absorption is lower from whole grains, the total amount of zinc absorbed is usually greater from whole grains.

IODINE

Most people don't give a second's thought to iodine, a mineral that is needed for healthy thyroid function. But throughout the world, iodine deficiency is a serious public health problem. Deficiency in pregnancy is especially serious since it can impact brain development in the fetus.

Eating either too much or too little iodine can cause the thyroid gland to become enlarged, which is called a goiter. When iodine intake is too low, it causes hypothyroidism, resulting in slowed metabolism, elevated cholesterol, and weight gain. Too much iodine can cause either hypothyroidism or hyperthyroidism.

In the United States, most people get enough iodine by using iodized salt or eating fish or dairy products. Milk and other dairy foods aren't necessarily good sources of iodine, but iodized solutions are used to clean the cows' teats and dairy equipment, and the iodine ends up in the milk itself. Commercial plant milks, including those based on soy, almonds, rice, coconuts, pistachios, walnuts, hemp, and cashews, are very low in iodine.[17,18] Plant milks fortified with iodine have an iodine content similar to cow's milk but only a few products are iodine-fortified.[19]

The iodine content of most plant foods is variable, though, because it depends on the iodine content of the soil. Foods grown closer to the ocean tend to be higher in iodine and in some parts of the world, sea vegetables (seaweeds) provide iodine. (In fact, even ocean mist can provide iodine, although it's not a reliable or measurable source.) In some parts of Europe, where salt is not iodized at high enough levels (or at all) and the iodine content of plants is poor, iodine can be a concern for vegans. There is some evidence that vegans in Europe who do not supplement show signs of abnormal thyroid function[20,21] or inadequate intakes.[22-24] In the United States, Boston-area vegans had lower levels of iodine in their urine, an indication of low iodine intake, but their thyroid function was normal.[25]

Naturally occurring compounds known as goitrogens, which are found in soybeans, flaxseeds, and raw cruciferous vegetables (broccoli, Brussels sprouts, cauliflower, and cabbage), counteract the activity of iodine. A diet high in goitrogens can cause hypothyroidism if the diet is too low in iodine. But as long as your diet is adequate in iodine, there is no reason to avoid soyfoods or other sources of goitrogens. See Chapter 9 for more discussion on the safety of soyfoods.

Iodine and Sea Vegetables

While sea vegetables can be very rich in iodine, the content varies dramatically. Researchers measured iodine content of sea vegetables they collected from United States, Canada, Tasmania, and Namibia and found that amounts ranged from 16 micrograms to a remarkable 8,165 micrograms of iodine per gram of food.[26] To put those numbers into perspective, the RDA for iodine is 150 micrograms and the National

Academies has set 1,100 micrograms per day as the maximum amount per day that people can safely consume. This means that some sea vegetables may not provide enough iodine to meet needs and others may provide far too much. Like all minerals, iodine can be toxic at very high levels. Labels may not always accurately reflect the amount of iodine in sea vegetables since any number of factors can affect this including the water temperature, mineral content of the water, and how the sea vegetables are stored.

It's fine to enjoy sea vegetables in your vegan diet as people in coastal regions have been doing for centuries. But because of the variations in their iodine content, we recommend consuming them just two or three times a week and suggest not depending on them for meeting iodine needs.

Meeting Iodine Needs

The recommended iodine intake for adults is 150 micrograms per day. Vegans can get adequate iodine if they do any one of the following:

- If you use added salt on your foods, choose iodized salt. One-quarter teaspoon provides 76 micrograms of iodine, which provides enough to ensure that you're meeting needs since plant foods will provide at least some iodine. Different "natural" salt preparations, including sea salt, have variable amounts of iodine and aren't dependable unless they are iodized. The salt added to processed and fast foods is rarely iodized. Nor is the salt used to make soy sauce, tamari, or miso.

- If you prefer not to use salt, take a modest iodine supplement providing 75 to 150 micrograms of iodine three to four times per week. If you take a vegan multivitamin, check the label since it probably contains iodine. Using a supplement is our favorite way to get iodine since it is reliable (unlike sea vegetables) and harmless (unlike salt). Don't overdo it with supplements, though, since the range of safe iodine intake is relatively small, and it's important to avoid intakes above the upper limit for safety. We suggest not using kelp supplements to meet iodine needs because the amounts of iodine in these supplements do not always match what is on the label,[27] and in some studies, vegans using kelp supplements have been shown to have poor thyroid status (which may have been due to either inadequate or excess iodine intake).[21,22] Look instead, for supplements that list potassium iodide on the label.

RDAs AND UPPER LIMITS FOR IODINE INTAKE

Age (years)	RDA (micrograms)	Upper limit (micrograms)
1–3	90	200
4–8	90	300
9–13	120	600
14–18	150	900
Over 18	150	1,100
Pregnant		
18 or younger	220	900
Over 18	220	1,100
Lactating		
18 or younger	290	900
Over 18	290	1,100

VITAMIN A

The active form of vitamin A is retinol and it is found only in animal products. But plants have more than fifty compounds called carotenoids that the body can convert to vitamin A. The most common is beta-carotene. Because there are so many forms of vitamin A, the vitamin A content of foods is stated as retinol activity equivalents (RAE). Think of these as the amount of potential vitamin A activity in a food. The RDA for vitamin A is 900 RAE for men and 700 RAE for women.

In addition to their role as vitamin A precursors, the carotenoids have antioxidant properties and other potential benefits for reducing chronic disease. The preformed vitamin A in animal foods doesn't have those advantages.

In 2000, based on new evidence about the conversion of beta-carotene into active vitamin A, the Food and Nutrition Board doubled their estimate of how much beta-carotene it takes to produce adequate vitamin A. That means that the RAE content of plant foods is only half of what was previously thought. Where we once thought that vegan diets automatically provided enough vitamin A, it's now clear that getting enough requires at least some diligence.

A varied diet that includes plenty of brightly colored vegetables will ensure that you meet vitamin A needs. Just 1 cup of spinach or a ½ cup of carrot juice or a ¼ cup of sweet potatoes is enough to meet needs for the entire day. Both cooking and added fat increase the absorption of beta-carotene, so there is a benefit to eating some of these vegetables cooked with a little bit of oil, avocado, nuts, or a nut-based sauce.[28]

VITAMIN A CONTENT OF SELECTED FOODS

Recommended intakes are 700 RAE for women and 900 RAE for men.	
	Vitamin A (in retinol activity equivalents or RAE)
Vegetables (½ cup cooked unless otherwise indicated)	
Beet greens	276
Broccoli	60
Bok choy	180
Butternut squash	572
Carrots, 1 medium, raw	509
Carrots, ½ cup cooked	665
Carrot juice, 1 cup	2,256
Chicory greens, 1 cup raw	166
Collard greens	361
Dandelion greens	356
Hubbard squash	343
Kale	443
Mustard greens	369
Pumpkin, canned	953
Spinach	472
Sweet potatoes, mashed	1,291
Swiss chard	268
Tomato, 1 medium	76
Tomato juice, 1 cup	56
Fruits	
Apricots, 3 fresh (not dried)	101
Cantaloupe, 1 cup chunks	270
Mango, 1 medium	80
Papaya, 1 small	74

VITAMIN K

Although vitamin K was discovered in the early part of the twentieth century, its exact function in the human body wasn't understood until 1974, which is pretty recent in the world of nutrients.

Vitamin K is essential for blood clotting, and most people get enough to support that function. It's possible that vitamin K may contribute to bone health and reduce risk of fractures, but the research on this is conflicting.[29,30]

The best sources of vitamin K are leafy green vegetables. Soy, canola, and olive oils are also good sources. Since vitamin K is fat soluble, cooking greens in a small amount of oil or using a fat-rich dressing on raw leafy greens can help your body absorb more.

There isn't much information about the vitamin K intake of vegetarians or vegans, but what we know about vegan diets and about blood clotting in vegans suggests that people eating plant-based diets get plenty.[31] So why have we singled it out for discussion? The answer has to do with claims that have been made about vitamin K from those who question the adequacy of vegan diets.

The term "vitamin K" actually refers to two slightly different compounds with vitamin K activity. One, called phylloquinone or vitamin K_1, is found in both plant and animal foods. The other, menaquinone or vitamin K_2, is produced by bacteria and found in animal foods. The only plant food known to contain vitamin K_2 is natto, a type of fermented soy food that is popular in Japan but is rarely consumed elsewhere. While some have claimed that vitamin K_2 is a separate vitamin with its own role in the body, the evidence that there are any benefits to consuming this version of the vitamin are limited.

A study comparing blood-clotting rates (a measure of vitamin K activity) showed no difference between vegans and meat-eaters, which suggests that vegans are getting plenty of vitamin K without any sources of vitamin K_2.[31]

A few studies from the Netherlands have found that vitamin K_2 may reduce risk for heart disease,[32,33] but other research suggests that it could actually be K_1, the type of vitamin K found in plant foods, that is protective and that K_2 actually raises risk.[34] But even if vitamin K_2 were to have beneficial effects, it might make more sense to get it from a supplement rather than choosing vitamin K_2-rich animal foods, which are associated with greater risk for heart disease.

And it's probably not quite true that vegans have no source of vitamin K_2. It is produced by bacteria in our colon and appears to be absorbed into the blood.[35] Finally, the National Academies has not established any specific recommendations for vitamin K_2. We can say with assurance that vitamin K_2 is not a separate nutrient, and vegans do not need it in their diet.

A FEW MORE VITAMINS AND MINERALS OF INTEREST TO VEGANS

Riboflavin

Over the years, there has been some discussion about riboflavin (vitamin B_2) in a vegan diet since the main source of this nutrient in American diets is milk. But while riboflavin is found in only small amounts in many plant foods, a varied diet of grains, legumes, and vegetables provides plenty. Soyfoods are a particularly good source of riboflavin and so are fortified cereals. We don't have a great deal of information about vegan intakes, but the few studies that have been done show that vegans meet the RDA for riboflavin. Choosing soy (or other plant) milks that are fortified with this nutrient can provide extra insurance, but we don't think that vegans need to worry about riboflavin. We've listed the riboflavin content of plant foods on page 123.

Selenium

The amount of selenium in your diet depends on where you live—or where your food comes from—since the amount of selenium in plant foods is dependent on the amount in the soil where the foods are

RIBOFLAVIN CONTENT OF FOODS

Recommended intakes are 1.1 milligrams for women and 1.3 milligrams for men.	
	Riboflavin (in milligrams)
Breads, Cereals, and Grains	
Barley, whole, ½ cup	0.05
Bran flakes, ¾ cup	0.6
Corn flakes, 1 cup	0.74
Pasta, enriched, ½ cup	0.1
Pasta, whole wheat, ½ cup	0.03
Quinoa, ½ cup	0.1
White bread, 1 slice	0.7
Whole wheat bread, 1 slice	.05
Vegetables (½ cup cooked or 1 cup raw)	
Asparagus	0.1
Beet greens	0.2
Collard greens	0.1
Mushrooms	0.14
Peas	0.07
Spinach	0.21
Sweet potatoes	0.08
Fruit	
Banana, 1 medium	0.09
Legumes (½ cup cooked)	
Kidney beans	0.05
Split peas	0.06
Soyfoods	
Edamame, ½ cup	0.14
Soymilk, 1 cup	0.5
Veggie "meats," 1 ounce	0.17*
Miscellaneous	
Nutritional yeast, Vegetarian Support Formula, 1 tablespoon	4.8
Marmite yeast extract, ½ teaspoon	0.42

*Amount varies by brand.

grown. Evidence suggests that vegans in the United States and Canada get enough selenium. In parts of northern Europe, the selenium content of the soil is fairly low, however, and vegans may need to supplement.[36,37] The table on page 124 reflects selenium content of plant foods grown in the United States.

SELENIUM CONTENT OF FOODS

Recommended adult intake is 55 micrograms.

	Selenium (in micrograms)*
Breads, Cereals, and Grains	
Barley, pearled, ½ cup cooked	6.8
Bran flakes, 1 cup	4.1
Bread, whole wheat, 1 slice	7.2
Grape-Nuts, ½ cup	5.3
Oatmeal, ½ cup cooked	6.3
Pasta, enriched, ½ cup	20
Pasta, whole-wheat, ½ cup cooked	18.1
Rice, brown, ½ cup cooked	9.6
Legumes and Soyfoods (½ cup cooked)	
Chickpeas	3
Lima beans	4.2
Pinto beans	5.3
Soybeans	6.3
Tofu, firm	12.5
Nuts and Seeds	
Brazil nut, 1	95

*These numbers are from USDA and may not apply outside of the United States. People in other countries should check the selenium content of local supplies.

Choline

Choline is an essential part of every cell in your body since it's found in all cell membranes. It's also needed for production of the neurotransmitter acetylcholine, which plays a role in brain functions including memory and muscle control. Because choline is needed for the metabolism of fats, getting too little of this nutrient can cause accumulation of fat in the liver, which can interfere with liver function.

Until just twenty years ago, we didn't even have a government dietary recommendation for choline, and research on its health effects is still evolving. But getting enough choline may be important in prevention of cardiovascular disease and in protecting cognitive function with aging.

Even though Americans often don't meet choline recommendations, overt deficiency is rare. This is most likely because we make at least small amounts of choline ourselves. Even so, it's important to emphasize choline-rich foods in your diet, especially since choline needs seem to vary depending on genetic factors.

Recommended choline intakes are 500 milligrams per day for men and 425 milligrams for women. Although plant foods are considerably lower in choline in general compared to meat, dairy, and eggs, you can get plenty of choline with just a little bit of attention to food choices.

The best sources of choline in vegan diets are peanuts and peanut butter, beans, soyfoods, quinoa, asparagus, spinach, and vegetables in the cabbage family like broccoli and cauliflower. Choline content of other plant foods tends to be on the low side, but if you emphasize a few good sources of choline daily, the rest of the foods in your diet should contribute enough to help you meet recommended intakes. You can see the choline content of some popular vegan foods in the table below.

CHOLINE CONTENT OF FOODS

	Choline (in milligrams)
Recommended intake for an adult female	425
Recommended intake for an adult male	500
Legumes	
Roasted soybeans, ¼ cup	53
Kidney beans, ½ cup	45
Navy beans, ½ cup	41
Peanuts, ¼ cup	24
Peanut butter, 2 tablespoons	21
Soymilk, 1 cup	58
Vegetables	
Asparagus	23
Broccoli, ½ cup	31
Brussels sprouts, ½ cup	32
Cauliflower, ½ cup	24
Mushrooms, shiitake, ½ cup	58
Nuts and Seeds	
Almonds, ¼ cup	18
Pistachios, ¼ cup	24
Sunflower seeds, ¼ cup	19
Grains and Starchy Vegetables	
Potatoes, red skin, 1 large potato with skin	57
Quinoa, cooked, ½ cup	22
Wheat germ, 1 ounce	51

AND ALL THE REST

Every single nutrient is important to your health, but most are so readily supplied in vegan diets that we don't need to even think about them. If you're curious about where vegans get the rest of their nutrients, the chart on page 128 serves as a quick guide to nutrients that are particularly important to health and that we have not covered elsewhere in this book.

PUTTING IT ALL TOGETHER

It's good to know the different sources of individual nutrients and how to meet your needs for each one. But planning a healthy diet by tracking intake of individual nutrients can quickly become overwhelming and confusing. And it's not necessary for vegans or anyone else to do so. In Chapter 10, we'll provide simple guidelines for planning menus that bring together the information we've talked about so far. It's the Vegan for Life Food Guide—and it makes planning vegan diets a breeze.

VEGAN DIETS, MINERALS, AND HAIR LOSS

Every so often, we hear from women who believe that they have been losing hair since going vegetarian or vegan. While there are no studies of this issue in vegans, there is research on general nutrition factors and hair loss.

Reasons for hair loss vary among individuals, and they are not necessarily related to diet. About one-third of all younger (premenopausal) women experience some hair loss at one time or another (and the vast majority of these women are not vegan). And it is an unavoidable fact of life that hair thins as we age. Women going through menopause may notice a significant thinning of their hair. Stress can also result in some hair loss.

Hair loss can be associated with certain medical conditions, including thyroid problems, so if you are convinced that you are losing hair at an unusual rate, it's important to see a physician. Sometimes a dermatologist can diagnose the problem.

Rapid weight loss can cause an increase in hair loss, and the hair growth should return to normal after the weight loss ceases. Women who become vegan sometimes initially lose weight quickly and this might account for the hair loss.

At one time, there was a widespread belief that zinc deficiency was a common cause of hair loss, but zinc supplementation has not been shown to help. Some studies have linked low iron status to hair loss in women, and it is possible that iron levels that are at the lower end of normal may not support optimal hair growth.

The essential amino acid L-lysine plays a part in the absorption of iron and zinc, and vegans who don't eat many legumes could find themselves falling short on lysine. Iron supplementation alone doesn't always increase iron stores. But in one study, iron supplementation plus a supplement of 1.5 to 2 grams per day of L-lysine increased iron stores and decreased hair loss by half.[15] Other supplements, like excessive intakes of vitamin E and folic acid, can adversely affect hair growth.

Finally, women who feel they are losing hair may choose to shampoo less frequently in the belief that this will preserve their hair. This hasn't been shown to prevent hair loss. In fact, since everyone loses some hair on a daily basis, if you shampoo less often, you'll see more hair in the tub each time you shampoo, which may convince you that you are losing more hair.

VITAMINS

Nutrient	Best vegan sources	What it does
Vitamin C	Blackberries, broccoli, Brussels sprouts, cabbage, cantaloupe, guava, grapefruit, kiwifruit, mango, papaya, pineapple, raspberries, red peppers, strawberries, potatoes, cabbage	Acts as an antioxidant, protecting cells from damage by free radicals; required to make collagen, a component of connective tissue and needed for wound healing; plays a role in immune function; aids absorption of iron from plant foods
Vitamin E	Avocado, spinach, Swiss chard, mango, nuts and seeds, peanut butter, safflower oil, sunflower oil, some margarines	Protects fatty acids from oxidation; stabilizes cell membranes; involved in immunity and helps keep lining of blood vessels healthy
Thiamin (Vitamin B$_1$)	Whole and enriched grains, legumes, nuts, seeds, nutritional yeast	
Niacin	Beans, tempeh, tofu, nutritional yeast, yeast extract (Marmite), peanuts, peanut butter, fortified cereals, mushrooms, barley	The B-vitamins thiamin, niacin, pantothenic acid, pyridoxine, and biotin are all involved in metabolism of carbohydrate, fat, and protein and needed for energy production
Pantothenic acid	Beans, nuts, seeds, avocados, mushrooms, whole grains	
Pyridoxine	Avocado, potatoes, sweet potatoes, spinach, soybeans, bananas	
Biotin	Oatmeal, oat bran, barley, corn, mushrooms, spinach, sweet potatoes, beans, textured vegetable protein, almonds, peanut butter	
Folate	Avocado, broccoli, collard greens, spinach, turnip greens, oranges, beans, peanuts, yeast extract (Marmite) fortified cereals, enriched grains	Needed to make genetic material and help cells divide

MINERALS

Nutrient	Best vegan sources	What it does
Chromium	Whole grains, dark chocolate, oranges, broccoli	Enhances action of insulin and involved in metabolism of carbohydrate, fat, and protein
Copper	Whole grains, beans, nuts, potatoes, tofu, tempeh	Copper works with iron to help the body form red blood cells. It also helps keep the blood vessels, nerves, immune system, and bones healthy. Copper also aids in iron absorption.
Manganese	Whole grains, wheat germ, collard greens, spinach, sweet potato, pineapple, beans, tofu, tempeh, almond butter, tea	Acts as an antioxidant. Involved in metabolism of carbohydrates, amino acids, and cholesterol.

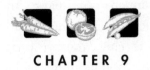

CHAPTER 9

Soyfoods in Vegan Diets

T ofu, soymilk, miso, and tempeh are traditional staples of Asian cuisine. But soybeans have also given rise to a new generation of products that include substitutes for ground beef, chicken nuggets, luncheon slices, hotdogs, cheese, and sour cream.

There is no doubt about it: both the traditional and the more modern soyfoods have made it easier than ever to be vegan. And aside from their practical benefits, soyfoods may offer some unique health advantages—but there have also been questions about their safety.

It's no small topic: approximately two thousand soy-related papers appear in medical and scientific journals every year. This chapter, which looks at both the potential benefits of soy as well as some of the more controversial issues, will help clarify the findings so you can make an informed decision about how these foods fit into your diet.

SOY NUTRITION

Soybeans are unique among legumes. They're higher in protein and fat and much lower in carbohydrate than other beans. While much of the fat is the polyunsaturated omega-6 type, soybeans are one of the few good plant sources of the essential omega-3 fatty acid ALA.

The carbohydrate in soybeans is composed largely of oligosaccharides, which are sugars that humans can't digest. They travel intact to the colon where they stimulate the growth of healthy bacteria.

The soybean's claim to fame, though, is its protein content. Soy protein is highly digestible, and its amino acid pattern closely matches human requirements. The quality of soy protein is comparable to protein from animal foods. According to the protein rating system that ranks proteins based on their amino acid pattern and digestibility, it is the most highly rated of all plant proteins.[1]

Soybeans are also a good source of iron, potassium, and folate. Although they contain phytate and oxalate, both inhibitors of mineral absorption, absorption of calcium from both tofu and fortified soymilk is as good as absorption from cow's milk.[2,3] Much of the iron in soy is present in a form called ferritin, which isn't affected by phytate and appears to be well absorbed.[4,5]

SOY ISOFLAVONES AND THE ESTROGEN QUESTION

Soybeans and traditional soyfoods like tofu, soymilk, and tempeh are uniquely rich sources of phytochemicals called isoflavones. Isoflavones are commonly classified as phytoestrogens or plant estrogens. They bind to the same receptors in cells—a necessary step for biological action—to which the hormone estrogen binds. This has led to a misconception about isoflavones—namely, that they are the same as estrogen. They're not. Instead isoflavones are among a group of complex compounds called SERMs, or selective estrogen receptor modulators.

It's the word "selective" that describes how different isoflavones are from estrogen. There are two types of estrogen receptors in cells called estrogen receptor *alpha* and estrogen receptor *beta*. Estrogen binds with equal affinity to both but isoflavones preferentially bind to estrogen receptor beta. As a result, they can act very differently from estrogen.[6] Depending on the type of receptors in a given tissue, SERMs can have estrogen-like effects or anti-estrogenic effects or no effects at all. There is evidence that compounds like isoflavones that preferentially bind to estrogen receptor beta could have anti-cancer properties.[7]

One issue regarding isoflavones is of particular interest to vegetarians and vegans. Isoflavones are metabolized differently among individuals and this difference could impact their health effects. For example, one type of isoflavone in soybeans is metabolized by intestinal bacteria to a compound called equol, which may be especially beneficial to health.[8,9] But only around 25 percent of Westerners have equol-producing bacteria in their intestines, compared to roughly 50 percent of Asians.[8] Some evidence indicates that vegetarians are more likely than meat-eaters to be equol producers.[10–12] This means that vegetarians and vegans may stand to gain more benefit from soyfoods than people eating a typical American diet.

SOY AND HEALTH

Heart Disease

Because soybeans are low in saturated fat, replacing meat and dairy with soyfoods can reduce blood-cholesterol levels by as much as 3 to 6 percent.[13] But there is much more to the story about soy and heart health because the protein in soy has a direct effect on blood-cholesterol levels, too.

It takes as much as 25 grams of soy protein per day (the amount in about three servings of traditional soyfoods) to have an effect, and the effect is modest, producing around a 4 percent reduction in LDL-cholesterol (the bad cholesterol).[13–15] In addition to this benefit from soy protein, the healthy fats in soy can make a significant contribution toward lowering heart disease risk.[15]

The impact of soy is even greater when it is teamed up with other heart-healthy components. The Portfolio Diet is an experimental approach that derives much of its protein from soy and includes plenty of fiber, nuts, and foods fortified with plant sterols (compounds with natural cholesterol-lowering properties). This approach lowers LDL-cholesterol by nearly 30 percent; it's as effective for reducing cholesterol as some drug therapies.[16] Also, soy protein may impact LDL-cholesterol in ways that make it less harmful and less likely to cause clogged arteries.[17]

Finally, the isoflavones in soy may also have a direct effect on the health of the arteries in ways that reduce heart disease risk.[18] Since many people who suffer heart attacks don't have elevated cholesterol, these additional potential benefits of soyfoods could mean that they offer protection even for people with low cholesterol levels.

Bone Health

Since estrogen therapy reduces bone loss and fracture risk in post-menopausal women, it's reasonable to ask whether isoflavones might have similar benefits. More than twenty-five clinical trials, mostly in postmenopausal women, have looked at this question.[19,20] Some have found improvements in bone-mineral density, but others haven't shown any benefit.

It may be that soy isoflavones simply aren't protective. Or it could be that a protective effect requires lifelong soy consumption. In the clinical studies, women typically consumed soy for two years at the most. But studies in Singapore and China found that women with the highest soyfood consumption—approximately two servings per day—were one-third less likely to fracture a bone.[21,22] It is reasonable to assume that these women consumed soyfoods throughout their lives.

Since most soyfoods are rich in protein and many are good sources of calcium, they are a good choice for bone health. But whether the isoflavones add additional protection remains to be determined.

Hot Flashes

Although hot flashes are relatively common among Western women as they go through menopause, women in Japan seldom report having them. One reason might be that they benefit from the estrogen-like effects of isoflavones. Nearly fifty studies have examined the effect of soyfoods and different types of isoflavone supplements on hot flash incidence and/or severity and, again, the results are inconsistent. The varied responses might be due in part to the fact that individuals metabolize isoflavones differently.

But a more likely explanation is that some isoflavone supplements are more effective than others when it comes to hot flashes. Soybeans contain several different types of isoflavones and the supplements consistently shown to have a benefit for hot flashes are those with an isoflavone profile similar to soybeans themselves.[23,24] Soyfoods are typically rich in an isoflavone called genistein and supplements where genistein accounts for at least half of total isoflavones are very effective.

The amount of isoflavones in about two servings per day of traditional soyfoods can reduce frequency and severity of hot flashes by about 50 to 60 percent. In women who have as many as seven to ten hot flashes per day, a 50 percent reduction can provide significant relief.

Breast Cancer

In 1990, the National Cancer Institute began looking at soyfoods and isoflavones as a possible way to reduce the risk of cancer. While their interest was in all cancers, they placed particular focus on breast cancer since most breast tumors are stimulated by estrogen. In addition, the historically low rates of breast cancer in Asia suggested that there was something about an Asian lifestyle that was protective.

Thirty years later, we have encouraging findings on soy, especially as it affects women who have had breast cancer. Although soy detractors question whether soy is protective or even safe for these women, this is based on certain types of studies in mice. But humans and mice have very different physiologic responses to isoflavones, which means the relevance of these findings to humans is uncertain.[25] Studies in humans show that neither whole soyfoods nor isoflavone supplements have harmful effects on indicators of breast cancer risk, such as breast cell proliferation and breast tissue density.[26]

The position of the American Cancer Society and American Institute for Cancer Research is that women with breast cancer can safely consume soyfoods.[27,28] Furthermore, the World Cancer Research Fund International suggests that soyfoods consumption might possibly improve survival in women who have had breast cancer.[29] Their stance is based in part on studies of soy intake in more than eleven thousand breast cancer survivors.

While eating soy may improve the prognosis for women who have breast cancer, it's less clear that soy helps prevent breast cancer from occurring in the first place. Adding soy to the diets of adult women isn't associated with a lower risk for breast cancer. In contrast, there is intriguing evidence that as little as one serving of soyfoods per day during childhood and/or the teen years reduces the risk for breast cancer later in life by as much as 50 percent.[30,31] Since girls in Asian countries grow up eating soyfoods, this may in part explain the lower breast cancer rates in these populations.

At present, we can say that in healthy women, soyfoods don't raise breast cancer risk, and, while it remains speculative, they may offer benefits for women who have had breast cancer. The most promising findings, though, are that girls who consume soy could have a lower lifetime risk of getting breast cancer.

Prostate Cancer

The rates of prostate cancer are low in countries where soyfoods are commonly consumed compared to Western populations. More importantly, men who consume higher amounts of soy are about 30 percent less likely to develop prostate cancer than those who consume little soy.[32] Also, some studies show that isoflavones accumulate in the prostate and possibly help to control the spread of prostate cancer.[33] Since prostate tumors are slow growing and are typically diagnosed late in life, anything that delays tumor onset or growth can profoundly impact prostate cancer mortality. But a lot more research is needed before any definitive conclusions about the role of soy in preventing and treating prostate cancer can be made.

There is some evidence that a diet high in dairy products could raise the risk for prostate cancer. So it may be that men who adopt a vegan diet and replace cow's milk with soymilk will have added protection against prostate cancer.

Cognitive Function

Estrogen may help maintain cognitive function in older age, and there has been speculation that soy isoflavones could have a similar benefit. However, results from a study of Japanese men living in Hawaii—the Honolulu-Asia Aging Study—which was published in 2000, showed that men who ate the most tofu had more signs of mental decline in their seventies through their nineties.[34] The study wasn't designed to look specifically at cognitive function, and it had plenty of other key weaknesses. In the decades since that study was published, other research has shown mixed results on soyfoods and cognition with some indicating that soy is protective.[35] For example, among older people in Taiwan, those who consumed soy at least once per day were less than half as likely to experience cognitive decline compared to subjects who didn't eat soy.[36] In a clinical trial of people between the ages of forty-five and seventy-five, subjects who were given soy protein experienced marked improvement in cognitive function in comparison to those who consumed whey protein from dairy foods.[37]

Although it's premature to suggest that soyfoods will improve cognitive function, the bulk of the evidence suggests that there is no reason for older people to avoid these foods.

Thyroid Function

Many foods, including soyfoods, millet, cruciferous vegetables, and some herbs, contain goitrogens. These compounds interfere with thyroid function (and in extreme cases can cause an enlarged thyroid, which is called a goiter). Generally, they cause problems only in parts of the world where iodine intake is low, since iodine is an essential nutrient needed for thyroid function. The effects of iodine deficiency can be worse if the diet is high in goitrogens. For Western vegans, this shouldn't be a problem as long as we consume enough iodine—an easy task if you use small amounts of iodized table salt every day or take an iodine supplement.

Concerns about the effects of isoflavones on thyroid function derive mostly from studies in test tubes and in rodents. In humans, the
evidence clearly shows that neither soyfoods nor isoflavones adversely
affect thyroid function in healthy people.[38,39] This research includes
studies that lasted as long as three years and that used high doses of
isoflavones.[40,41] The FDA, the European Food Safety Authority, and
the German Research Foundation have all rejected concerns about
isoflavones and thyroid function.[38,42,43]

About 10 percent of older people have subclinical hypothyroidism—
they have normal thyroid function, but higher than normal levels of
one of the thyroid hormones. This raises the risk of progressing to
overt hypothyroidism or low thyroid function. While older research
found that relatively modest amounts of isoflavones caused a minor
increase in the progression of this disease, when the same group of researchers did a follow-up study using a much larger dose of isoflavones
it had no effect on thyroid disease.[44,45]

Finally, there have been questions about the effect of soyfoods
on people who have hypothyroidism and take synthetic thyroid hormones. While soyfoods may reduce absorption of these synthetic hormones, this is true of high-fiber foods in general, as well as many herbs
and supplements. This is why synthetic thyroid hormones should be
taken on an empty stomach.

Reproductive Health and Male Feminization

Stories that make their way around the internet about the alleged feminizing effects of soyfoods are not supported by the research. A comprehensive analysis published in 2010 showed that neither soyfoods
nor isoflavones affect testosterone levels.[46] Studies published since
then support this finding.[47,48] Similarly, the evidence indicates that
neither soyfoods nor isoflavones, when consumed in amounts even
greatly exceeding typical Japanese intake, have any effect on estrogen
levels in men.[47–49]

In a small study of soy intake and sperm/semen characteristics, researchers found that sperm counts in men with higher soy intakes did

not differ from those who ate no soy. While men who ate more soy had lower sperm concentrations, this was partly due to a higher semen volume.[50] Even when isoflavone doses are ten times greater than what Japanese men typically consume, clinical studies show no effects of isoflavones on sperm or semen.[51-53] Soyfoods have been a part of Asian diets for centuries and there has never been any indication that they affect reproduction in these populations. The current research on this issue supports what history has long shown.

SOYFOODS AND SKIN HEALTH

As skin ages, it becomes thinner and less elastic, resulting in the inevitable crows' feet, laugh lines, and deep wrinkles. Some of these changes are driven by genetics and sun damage, but the reduced estrogen production that occurs with aging also plays a role.

Skin is packed with estrogen receptors and in particular, the type of estrogen receptors that isoflavones activate. As a consequence, the cosmetics industry has shown considerable interest in isoflavone-enriched face creams. Not only is there evidence that these topical creams help slow skin aging, but isoflavones may also work from the inside.[54] In postmenopausal women, isoflavone supplements have been linked to improved skin thickness and elasticity, and even a decline in small wrinkles.[55] Benefits have been seen with an amount of isoflavones that you could get from just a serving of traditional soyfoods like a half-cup of tofu or tempeh per day. It's not the fountain of youth, but if you enjoy soyfoods in your vegan diet, this is one more small perk of consuming them.

HOW MUCH AND WHAT KIND OF SOY TO EAT

Where do soyfoods fit into healthy diets? We can look to traditional Asian diets for guidance, staying mindful that a couple of common beliefs about Asian soyfood consumption—that soy is consumed mostly as fermented foods and used only as a condiment—are both wrong.

Fermented foods, such as miso, were the first soyfoods consumed in Asian countries, but it's not true that people in Asia consume mostly fermented soyfoods. Nonfermented foods like tofu have been a part of Asian diets for at least one thousand years and continue to play a significant role in these cultures. In China, soymilk and tofu make up the bulk of the soyfoods in diets. In Japan, about half the soy intake is from the fermented foods miso and natto and the other half comes from unfermented foods like tofu.[56]

A number of vegan foods, including veggie burgers and other meat analogues, are made from isolated soy protein or soy protein concentrate. They have been the target of some criticism because they are processed, but a large number of studies have used them and found there is nothing unsafe about them. In fact, most of the research on the quality of soy protein—which looks at the ability of soy protein to support protein balance in humans—used isolated soy proteins.

Surveys show that people in Japan and urban areas of China, such as Shanghai, typically consume around 1½ servings of soyfoods per day—providing about 10 grams of soy protein—although there is a wide range of intakes.[56] It's interesting to note that some of the health benefits associated with soy have been seen in people who consume the most soyfoods.

There is no requirement to include soy in your diet, but there is no reason to avoid it either. Since variety is an important factor in planning healthy diets, we recommend limiting soyfoods to three to four servings per day. Veggie burgers and other foods made from soy protein can be part of an overall healthy diet, but to get the full nutritional—and culinary—benefits of soy, be sure to explore some of the more traditional foods such as tofu and tempeh. The Soyfoods Primer on pages 38 to 42 can help familiarize you with these foods.

ISOFLAVONE, PROTEIN, AND
CALORIE CONTENT OF SOYFOODS

Soyfood	Isoflavones (in milligrams)	Protein (in grams)	Calories
Tofu, firm, ½ cup	31.5	10	88
Tofu, regular, ½ cup	29.3	10	94
Silken tofu, ½ cup	34.6	8.6	77
Natto, ½ cup	52	15.6	186
Soymilk, 1 cup	11.6	4.56	65
Miso, 1 tablespoon	6.4	1.75	30
Tempeh, ½ cup	36.1	15.3	160
Soy nuts, ¼ cup	55	17	194
Soybeans, ½ cup, cooked	47	14.3	149
Soybeans, green, ½ cup, cooked	17.7	15.7	180
Isolated soy protein, 1 ounce	28.7	22.6	95
Soy protein concentrate, 1 ounce	3.5–28.6 (varies depending on processing)	16.2	93
Soy flour, full fat, ¼ cup	37.4	7.2	92
Soy flour, defatted, ¼ cup	32.8	11.7	82.5

CHAPTER 10

The Vegan for Life Food Guide

ood guides have been a part of nutrition education in the United States for nearly one hundred years. They've come a long way, too. The first one, published in 1916, had five food groups: fruits and vegetables; meat, fish, and milk; cereals; simple sweets; and butter and wholesome fats. It was produced by the US Department of Agriculture (USDA), the same group that produces the MyPlate guide for Americans today.

While pressure from agriculture and the food industry shapes current food guides and keeps them friendly to animal foods, the trend has been toward a greater emphasis on plant foods. Vegetarians can use many of these guides with ease, but they are not especially useful for vegans. This is mainly because government food guides emphasize dairy foods for meeting calcium needs. Our food guide takes advantage of the fact that calcium is available in a wide variety of foods, which means that it's suitable for vegans and also represents a more accurate approach to meeting needs for this nutrient.

It's not the final word on planning a healthy vegan diet, though. No single food guide represents the only way to meet nutrient needs. And you don't need to follow these guidelines with meticulous attention every day. You won't keel over and die if one day you have only six servings of fruits and vegetables!

Our guide is meant to point you toward a diet that is based on a variety of whole grains, legumes, nuts, fruits, and vegetables. It doesn't include items like chocolate chip cookies, potato chips, and wine. But that doesn't mean you can't have them. They just don't fit into the food groups that should be at the center of your diet.

THE VEGAN FOOD GROUPS

To translate nutrition information into simple menu-planning guidelines, we've divided foods into the following groups:

Whole Grains and Starchy Vegetables

These foods are high in fiber, and provide protein, iron, zinc, and B vitamins. We've included starchy vegetables like potatoes and sweet potatoes because their calorie content and nutrient profiles are similar to those of grains. Although it's always a good idea to choose whole grains, products like fortified cereals can sometimes make important contributions to the diet, especially for children and some athletes. We recommend aiming for four servings of grains per day because these foods are excellent sources of fiber and iron. Whole grains can also be an important source of zinc in vegan diets.

Legumes and Soyfoods

These are the most protein-rich of all plant foods, and they are among the few good dietary sources of the essential amino acid lysine for vegans. We recommend at least three to four servings of these foods every day for adults. Generally, one serving provides around 7 to 8 grams of protein, but many of the soyfoods, such as tempeh, veggie meats, and some types of tofu, are quite a bit higher. These foods are also important sources of minerals like iron and sometimes zinc. If your diet is based on a variety of whole grains, vegetables, and nuts, then the three recommended servings from this group are plenty. If you like to spend some discretionary calories on desserts, added fats, or more servings of fruit (which are very low in protein), aiming for four servings of legumes per day will make it easier to meet protein and lysine needs.

If you are new to beans, keep an open mind about them. They are central to some of the world's best cuisine and can add great interest to your diet. Chapter 16 has tips for easy preparation and gas-free enjoyment of beans. We've also provided alternative ways to meet protein needs. See "If You Don't Like Legumes" on page 154.

While you don't have to eat soyfoods, they can be valuable in vegan diets. Not only are they nutritious, but they are convenient for replacing meat and dairy products in meals. They make it super-easy to plan vegetarian diets that are healthful, varied, and delicious.

Although the legume group includes soymilk and milk made from pea protein, it doesn't include almond, hemp, oat, or rice milk since they are almost always low in protein. You might be surprised to find peanuts and peanut butter in this group. While they may seem to be more closely related to tree nuts, they are actually part of the legume family. Like beans and soyfoods, they are an excellent source of protein.

Nuts and Seeds

Some vegans shy away from nuts and seeds because of their high fat content. But moderate nut consumption improves cholesterol levels and can even help with weight control (see Chapters 15 and 17 for more on this). These foods are concentrated in calories, though, so a serving is small—just two tablespoons of a nut or seed butter or whole seeds, or ¼ cup of nuts. We suggest consuming one to two servings of these foods every day. Choose nuts more often than seeds; they usually have a healthier fat profile and their health benefits are impressive. But if you are allergic to nuts, choose seeds or add another serving from the legumes and soyfoods group to your meals.

POWERFUL NUTRITION FROM TINY SEEDS

Flax, chia, and hempseeds are quickly becoming staples in the kitchens of health-conscious cooks. All three are excellent sources of the essential fatty acid alpha-linolenic acid (see page 99) and they provide plenty of fiber and iron, too. Store them in the refrigerator to keep them fresh. Here is a quick guide to using these seeds in your vegan diet.

CHIA SEEDS are very tiny seeds with a long history, dating back to the Aztec culture. (And yes, they are the same seeds that were used to create the popular leafy chia pets of the 1980s.) They absorb liquid easily, swelling up to create tapioca-like particles. Add chia seeds to overnight oatmeal or puddings to create a thick texture.

HEMPSEEDS, sometimes called hemp hearts, are from a type of cannabis plant, but they are too low in THC to provide any drug-like effects. With their mild flavor, hempseeds go with just about anything. Sprinkle them on salads, grains, or vegetables. They also blend well into smoothies. Or grind them in a food processor to make hempseed butter.

FLAXSEEDS come from beautiful blue wildflowers that grow in northern climates (and that are part of the same family of plants that provide linen for clothing). These brown or golden seeds have a hard protective hull and need to be ground into a powder before you can absorb their nutrients. You can grind them yourself in a clean coffee grinder or food processor, or purchase flaxseed powder. Combining ground flaxseeds with water creates a thick viscous liquid that makes a good binder in vegan loaves and pancakes. Always store ground flaxseeds in the freezer to prevent it from getting rancid.

Vegetables

Vegetables are among the best sources of vitamins C and A and contain thousands of plant chemicals that might improve health. All vegetables are good for you, but leafy greens like kale, collards, spinach, and turnip greens pack an especially powerful nutritional punch. They are rich in vitamins A, C, and K, potassium, iron, folate, sometimes calcium, and a host of plant chemicals that are linked to everything from reduced risk for heart disease to better eyesight with aging. Most people who grew up eating greens feel they can't live without them, and many newcomers to these foods agree. If, however, you need a more gradual introduction to them, try mixing small amounts of greens into soups and stews.

If you are pressed for time, frozen vegetables are a good alternative to fresh. They are almost always comparable in nutrient content and, in fact, sometimes have even higher levels of nutrients.

Fruits

Fruits are good sources of vitamins C and A as well as certain minerals, and they provide plenty of phytochemicals. While fruit juices can be a valuable source of nutrients, they should be used in moderation. Fresh, raw fruit is always a good choice, but frozen fruit is nutritious as well. Dried fruit can be particularly good sources of some nutrients and also fiber, although they are also high in calories. Be sure to brush your teeth after eating dried fruit.

Fats

Added fats aren't essential in healthy vegan menus, but small amounts of the right ones can fit in a well-balanced diet. We've placed them on the side to indicate that they are optional, but by no means off limits. Two or three servings per day (note: a serving is just a teaspoon) is a reasonable amount for most people. People with very high calorie needs may consume quite a bit more. You might want to read over the guidelines for choosing healthy fats in Chapter 7.

Plant Milks

While milks made from soybeans and peas are good sources of protein and are a part of the legumes food group, other milks don't have a logical place in a vegan food guide. If they are fortified, they can be excellent sources of calcium. But other than that, many are fairly low in nutritional value. They are also placed to the side of the plate since they don't fit into any of the food groups, but still play a role in many vegan diets.

Where's the "Calcium Group"?

All of the food groups in this guide include foods that provide calcium, so there is no need to create a separate "calcium," or "dairy alternatives" group. In the chart on page 149 we point you toward calcium-rich foods in each of the food groups.

DO YOU NEED TO EAT GRAINS?

Grains in some form or another sit at the center of most traditional world cuisines. But are they absolutely essential in a vegan diet? We've recommended four servings of these foods per day because they represent an easy way to ensure that you are getting adequate fiber and iron. When you choose whole grains, they are also a good source of zinc. But the truth is that legumes provide more iron than grains, and they are just as good a source of fiber and zinc.

There is no magic formula here. We would say that you should eat at least seven servings total per day of grains plus legumes and that at least three of those servings should be legumes. If you would rather cut back on grains and eat another serving or two of legumes, that's fine with us. The key is to make sure you're eating enough of these mineral-rich foods overall, and to ensure that you aren't skimping on legumes.

USING THE VEGAN FOR LIFE FOOD GUIDE

Aim for the minimum number of servings from each food group listed in the chart on page 149. Adults with higher calorie needs will need more. We provide recommendations for pregnant women and for children in Chapters 11 and 12.

Make the most of the food guide with these tips:

- Fill half your plate with fruits and vegetables.
- Choose good sources of vitamin C and vitamin A from the fruits and vegetables group.
- Eat plenty of protein-rich beans, soyfoods, and/or peanuts.
- Choose whole grains and starchy vegetables more often than refined grains.
- Opt for foods that provide omega-3 fats when you make choices from the nuts and seeds and the added fats groups.
- Focus on calcium-rich foods by aiming to eat at least 3 cups per day of some combination of fortified plant milks, fortified juices, calcium-set tofu, oranges, low-oxalate leafy green vegetables like kale, mustard greens, turnip greens, bok choy, and collard greens.
- Make water your main beverage.
- Make sure you meet needs for vitamin B_{12}, vitamin D, iodine, and omega-3 fats.

It's easy to use the food guide to pull together vegan menus that are healthy and delicious. The chart on page 149 offers guidelines for food choices and three menus on pages 151 to 154 show what meals might look like at three different calorie levels.

The Vegan for Life Food Guide

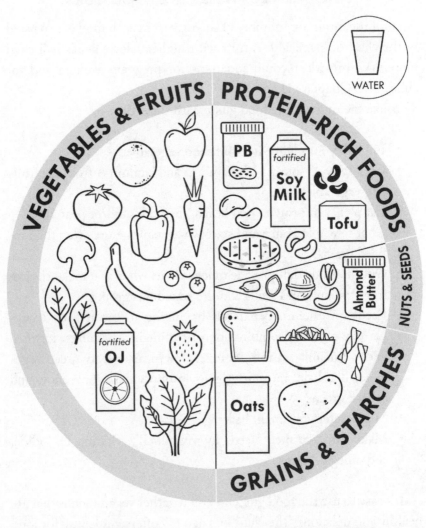

WATER

VEGETABLES & FRUITS

PROTEIN-RICH FOODS

PB

fortified Soy Milk

Tofu

NUTS & SEEDS

Almond Butter

fortified OJ

Oats

GRAINS & STARCHES

OTHER ESSENTIALS

B-12

vitamin B₁₂ • vitamin D • pinch of salt

OPTIONAL EXTRAS

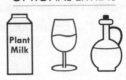

Plant Milk

Eat at least 3 cups of a combination of calcium-rich foods: fortified plant milks and juices, tofu, oranges, and leafy greens like kale, turnip greens, collards, and bok choy.

DIETARY ESSENTIALS

Foods	Aim for at least this number of servings	Examples of a serving	Choose these foods often
Vegetables and fruits	8	▸ 1 medium fruit ▸ ½ cup cut-up fruit ▸ ½ cup cooked vegetable ▸ 1 cup raw vegetables ▸ ½ cup fruit or vegetable juice	Choose vegetables more often than fruit. Choose whole fruit more often than juice. For vitamin C: oranges, grapefruit, strawberries, green leafy vegetables, bell peppers, cauliflower, broccoli For vitamin A: leafy green vegetables, carrots, winter squash For calcium: bok choy, broccoli, kale, collard greens, turnip greens, figs, navel oranges, fortified juice
Beans, soyfoods, peanuts	3	▸ ½ cup cooked beans, tofu, tempeh, TVP, soy yogurt ▸ ¼ cup soynuts or peanuts ▸ 2 tablespoons peanut butter; 1 cup soy or pea milk, 3 ounces veggie meats	For calcium: fortified soymilk or yogurt or pea milk, calcium-set tofu, white and black beans
Grains and starchy foods	4 It's okay to replace some servings of grains with legumes.	▸ ½ cup cooked grain, cereal, pasta, corn, potatoes, plantain, or sweet potato ▸ 1 slice bread or small tortilla ▸ 1 ounce ready-to-eat cereal	Choose whole grains and starchy vegetables in their skin most often.

continues

DIETARY ESSENTIALS *continued*

Foods	Aim for at least this number of servings	Examples of a serving	Choose these foods often
Nuts and seeds	1	▸ ¼ cup nuts ▸ 2 tablespoons seeds or nuts or seed butter	For calcium: almonds, almond butter, tahini For essential fatty acids: ground flaxseeds, hempseeds, chia seeds, walnuts
Water	Enough to satisfy thirst. Make it your main beverage of choice.		

Optional

Foods	Servings per day	Examples of a serving	Choose these foods most often
Oils and margarine	1–3 per day. More is okay if you have very high calorie needs.	▸ 1 teaspoon oil, margarine, mayonnaise	For essential fatty acids: canola, flaxseed, hempseed, or walnut oil
Plant milks made from tree nuts, flaxseeds, hempseeds, rice and oats		▸ 1 cup	For calcium: fortified brands

OTHER ESSENTIALS

VITAMIN B$_{12}$:

- Two servings per day of fortified foods providing 2 to 3.5 micrograms of vitamin B$_{12}$ per serving OR
- 25 to 100 micrograms per day from a chewable or sublingual supplement OR
- 1,000 micrograms twice per week from a chewable or sublingual supplement

IODINE:

- 75 to 150 micrograms three to four days per week (or ¼ teaspoon of iodized salt per day)

VITAMIN D:

- 600 International Units (15 micrograms) per day unless you are certain you are getting adequate sun exposure

OMEGA-3 FATS:

- ALA: Be sure to include a good source of ALA in your diet every day. The best choices are canola, flaxseed, hempseed, and walnut oil; walnuts, flaxseeds, chia seeds, or hempseeds.
- DHA: Consider a supplement providing 200 to 300 milligrams of DHA (or DHA plus EPA combined) from algae every two or three days.

SAMPLE MENUS BASED ON THE VEGAN FOR LIFE FOOD GUIDE

ABOUT 1,600 CALORIES

BREAKFAST

- ½ cup oatmeal
- ½ cup fortified soymilk
- 1 slice whole wheat toast
- 1 tablespoon jam

SNACK

- Apple slices with 2 tablespoons almond butter

LUNCH

- 1½ cups tomato-lentil soup
- Green salad with vinaigrette dressing with 1 teaspoon olive oil

SNACK

- ½ cup ready-to-eat cereal
- 2 tablespoons chopped walnuts
- 1 cup calcium-fortified nondairy milk

DINNER

- Veggie burger
- Small baked sweet potato
- 2 cups broccoli and cauliflower sautéed in 1 teaspoon olive oil

ABOUT 2,000 CALORIES

BREAKFAST

- Scrambled tofu: ½ cup tofu and ¼ cup mushrooms cooked in 1 teaspoon margarine
- 1 slice whole wheat toast
- 1 tablespoon peanut butter
- 1 cup strawberries

SNACK

- Oatmeal cookie

LUNCH

- 2 small whole wheat pita pockets with ½ cup hummus
- Chopped tomatoes and lettuce
- 1 cup pineapple chunks

SNACK

- ¼ cup mixed nuts
- ½ cup grapes

DINNER

- 5 ounces red wine
- 1 cup baked beans topped with 2 tablespoons shredded vegan cheese
- 1½ cups mixed quinoa and corn with 1 tablespoon ground flaxseeds
- 2 cups steamed collard greens sautéed in 1 teaspoon olive oil

ABOUT 2,500 CALORIES

BREAKFAST

- 1 cup granola or muesli topped with 1 teaspoon ground flaxseeds
- 1 cup fortified almond milk
- Banana

SNACK

- 1 cup instant lentil soup

LUNCH

- Tempeh BLT: 2 slices rye bread, 3 ounces marinated tempeh strips or tempeh bacon, lettuce and tomato, 2 teaspoons vegan mayonnaise
- 1 ounce baked tortilla chips
- 1 cup honeydew melon cubes

SNACK

- ½ cup vanilla soy yogurt
- ½ cup blueberries

DINNER

- Pasta Primavera: 1 cup pasta; 2 cups steamed broccoli, carrots and snow peas; ½ cup cannellini beans; 2 teaspoons olive oil; 1 tablespoon toasted pine nuts
- 3 fresh figs
- Green salad with vinaigrette using 1 teaspoon olive oil

SNACK

- 1 small brownie

IF YOU DON'T LIKE LEGUMES . . .

If you're beginning a transition to a vegan diet you may not have much experience with beans or soyfoods. Most Americans rarely eat them. Soyfoods and other legumes make it especially easy to meet protein needs on a vegan diet, but they aren't absolutely essential to balanced meal planning. The real issue when you drop these foods from your diet is that it becomes more of a challenge to meet the needs for the essential amino acid lysine. If you choose not to eat legumes, you'll need to add three servings of other lysine-rich foods to your diet. A serving is 1 cup of quinoa or ¼ cup of pistachios. This is in addition to the four servings of grains and one serving of nuts that are already recommended in the food guide.

Consider introducing beans to your meals gradually if they are new to your diet. Start out with one serving of legumes per day—maybe a hummus sandwich or bean burrito—plus one serving of a soyfood. Replace the third recommended serving with a lysine-rich food like ¼ cup of pistachios. Remember, too, that peanut butter is part of the legume group and can stand in for beans.

Because legumes are the most protein dense of all foods, diets require a bit more attention to planning when legume intake is limited. If you aren't consuming any legumes or soyfoods, make sure you are getting most of your calories from whole grains, vegetables, and nuts. Limit fruit and other low-protein foods like added fats, desserts, and alcohol.

ALLERGIES AND INTOLERANCES

Food allergies are an immune response to a protein that the body perceives as "foreign." The immune system reacts by producing antibodies, which can trigger skin rashes, nausea, or respiratory symptoms. Approximately 6 to 8 percent of children have food allergies and at least half outgrow them by adulthood. Food allergies affect only 2 to 4 percent of adults. As an adult, you may no longer be allergic to foods that caused problems for you as a child.

If you think you might be allergic to certain foods, it's a good idea to get tested by a qualified health professional and possibly get a second opinion from a professional who does a different type of testing. Be aware that the test that measures a blood antibody called IgG is not reliable because having IgG antibodies in the blood doesn't indicate a food allergy. Unfortunately, due to these tests, the number of people who believe they have allergies is much higher than the number who actually test positive for them with more reliable tests.

Although any protein can cause allergies, nine foods account for more than 90 percent of food allergies: milk, eggs, fish, shellfish, tree nuts, peanuts, soy, sesame, and wheat. Peanut and tree nut allergies are the ones that are most likely to persist beyond childhood. Allergies to soy are relatively uncommon in both children and adults, and they are also unlikely to cause severe symptoms like respiratory problems.

There is no treatment for food allergies; if you have them, the only solution is to avoid all foods that cause reactions. Vegans who have multiple allergies face some challenges, but once you understand what you can and can't eat, and begin to explore alternatives, you may find that planning healthy and satisfying meals is easier than you think.

For people with allergies to plant foods like nuts, peanuts, soy, sesame, and wheat there are plenty of foods to enjoy on the menu, such as quinoa, oats, rice, potatoes, millet, corn tortillas, certain types of Asian noodles, sunflower seeds, tahini, beans, vegetables, and fruits.

People with allergies should carefully read labels, of course, since soy, wheat, and nuts can turn up where you might not expect to find them. Food labels include a list of common allergens at the end of the ingredient list.

Although it's easy to be vegan without shopping outside of conventional supermarkets, people with allergies may want to explore natural foods stores and Asian, Indian, and Latin American groceries as a way of expanding their choices. The following is one example of a vegan menu for someone with allergies to soy, tree nuts, peanuts, sesame, and wheat.

BREAKFAST

- Oatmeal with toasted sunflower seeds, chopped dried figs, and calcium-fortified rice milk
- Fresh fruit

SNACK

- Coconut milk yogurt

LUNCH

- Tostadas: Corn tortillas, refried pinto beans, avocado, salsa, chopped raw vegetables, vegan cheese made without soy or nuts
- Fresh fruit

SNACK

- Rice crackers with sunflower seed butter

DINNER

- Rice noodles tossed with steamed vegetables and a sauce of white beans blended with sun-dried tomatoes and lemon juice
- Salad with vinaigrette dressing

Food Intolerances

Food intolerances are different from allergies. Allergic reactions involve the immune system and are usually an all-or-nothing proposition. Even tiny amounts of the offending food can cause a problem. Food intolerances can be dose-related, meaning that the offending food can sometimes be consumed in small quantities. Intolerances are the result of different factors, such as decreased production of a particular enzyme, and they often cause digestive problems. The most common by far is lactose intolerance—a decreased ability to digest the sugar in milk (obviously, vegans don't have to worry about this!). New vegans may experience discomfort in response to an increase in fiber intake or to foods like beans. We talk about how to deal with those issues in Chapter 16.

WHOLE VS. PROCESSED FOODS: FINDING A BALANCE

It's easier than ever to plan healthy and interesting vegan meals because of the ever-growing selection of veggie meats and cheeses and the array of convenience products like boxed and frozen dinners. Although many forms of processing strip away nutrients from foods, processed foods have a long and nutritionally important history in many world cuisines. Tofu and soymilk are two examples of processed foods that play a significant role in Asian cuisine.

While it is a good idea to build your diet around a variety of whole plant foods, moderate amounts of foods that don't carry the "whole foods" label can play a role, and sometimes an important one, in healthy vegan diets. For many, including veggie burgers, fortified plant milks, pasta sauce from a jar, instant soup, and other convenience foods makes vegan meal planning more realistic. It can improve the chances that you will meet nutrient needs and thrive on a vegan diet, and it can be especially important for children. Athletes and others with high calorie needs can also benefit from more processed foods.

Too often we have seen an unwavering commitment to eliminating all processed foods from meals morph into a restrictive eating pattern that is marginal in protein and fat and falls short of providing enough calories. Sadly, the result is that many people on this kind of regimen decide that a vegan diet is ruining their health or they find their meals unsatisfying and difficult, and they return to eating animal foods. On the other hand, we have rarely seen these kinds of problems in vegans who are more liberal in their food choices—enjoying veggie burgers, a drizzle of olive oil on salads, a sweet treat now and then, and whatever convenience products it takes to keep their vegan diet nutrient-rich and realistic. It's unfortunate to see people returning to animal foods when they might have been able to stay happily vegan by simply broadening their selection of plant foods.

The point isn't that you must eat processed foods to be healthy; it's that there is a reasonable way to balance healthy food choices with convenience if you wish to do so. A diet based on veggie meats and energy bars is not the best way to meet nutrient needs. But if a moderate use of processed foods makes it easy to stick with a vegan diet, then enjoying them will help you reap the health benefits of plant-based eating and support your commitment to a diet that reduces animal suffering.

STOCKING THE VEGAN PANTRY

Your vegan pantry will depend on your food preferences, of course, as well as your cooking style. Gourmet cooks may have shelves filled with specialty condiments and exotic ingredients from international grocery stores, while noncooks may opt for a little (or a lot) more convenience.

You can find the majority of these foods in any conventional grocery store. A few require a trip to a natural foods store, and depending on where you live, some may be available only by mail order.

Pantry Basics

Dried and canned beans: You'll find black, navy, garbanzo, kidney, pinto, and lima beans, plus lentils, black-eyed peas, and split peas in most grocery stores. Check specialty stores for some other interesting options, including red adzuki beans, maroon and white speckled Anasazi beans, and mung beans (great for sprouting).

Grains: Because grains have a long shelf life, you can keep lots of them on hand. Each has its own unique taste and texture, and they are a great way to add interest to meals. Here are a few choices:

- **Amaranth:** A tiny seed with a nutty flavor, it has a high protein content. It's often mixed with other grains.
- **Barley:** One of the oldest cultivated foods in the world, this has a chewy quality and mild taste. Pearled barley has the outer bran removed and cooks more quickly but is still high in fiber.
- **Bulgur:** A fast-food type of grain, this is whole wheat that has been precooked and then dried. It's common in Middle Eastern cooking, where it's used to make tabouli.
- **Couscous:** Common in the cooking of North Africa, this is made from steamed, dried wheat and it cooks very quickly.
- **Millet:** Americans think of this as birdseed, but it's widely used in African and Asian cuisines.
- **Quinoa:** This high-protein grain was a staple in the diet of the Incas, who called it the "mother grain." Quinoa is fast-cooking and high in protein, which has made it very popular among modern cooks. It has a natural soap-like coating to protect it from pests. This is sometimes but not always removed, so check the package to see if you need to rinse the quinoa before cooking.
- **Rice:** Choose brown rice most often and look for long-grain varieties since they are more slowly digested, producing a more gradual rise in blood glucose. But you may want to also keep

basmati and jasmine white rices on hand if you enjoy Indian and Thai foods.

- **Wheat berries:** A slow-cooking grain with a very chewy quality, it's usually mixed with other grains.
- **Italian pasta:** This type of pasta comes in a host of wonderful shapes, and many are available in whole wheat versions.
- **Asian pasta:** Modern choices include mung bean noodles, soba noodles (Japanese buckwheat noodles), ramen, and udon.
- **Bean pasta:** Made from chickpeas, black beans, lentils, or soybeans, these can be used just like regular Italian pasta, but they are higher in fiber and protein and are gluten-free. Look for them in the pasta section of the grocery store.
- Rolled or steel-cut oats and other hot cereals
- Breads and whole-grain crackers
- Whole wheat and corn tortillas

Nuts: This list includes almonds, cashews, hazelnuts, peanuts, walnuts, pecans, and pine nuts. Peanuts are an honorary member of this group since they are actually legumes. So are soynuts, which are soybeans that have been soaked and roasted until they are crunchy.

Seeds: Sesame, flax, chia, hemp, sunflower, and pumpkin seeds

Vegetable oils: Extra-virgin olive oil and canola oil are basics that will cover most of your food preparation needs. You might also keep flaxseed or hempseed oil on hand as a source of omega-3 fats, and toasted sesame oil and walnut oil for their interesting flavor profiles. See Chapter 7 for an extensive discussion of oils.

Canned tomato products: Prepared pasta sauce, tomato paste, whole and diced tomatoes, crushed tomatoes, and tomato sauce are all handy for making soups, stews, and other dishes.

Vegetable broth: If you don't have time to make homemade vegetable stock, vegetable broth or bouillon cubes or powder are available.

Textured vegetable protein (TVP™): A dry soy-protein product; re-hydrate with boiling water and add to spaghetti sauce for a ground beef substitute.

Soy curls: A dehydrated product made from whole soybeans by But-ler Foods. Once they have been rehydrated in hot water, they can be flavored and sautéed as a substitute for chicken or bacon.

Sea vegetables: These include dulse, arame, nori, hijiki, kombu, la-ver, and others. Most are available in dried form and are a quick addi-tion to soups. Nori is used to make the wraps for sushi.

Coconut milk: Look for coconut milk in the international foods sec-tion of the grocery store. It's an essential addition to many Thai and Indian dishes.

White and sweet potatoes

Onions and fresh garlic

Refrigerator Basics

This list includes items that must always be refrigerated as well as those that should be refrigerated after they have been opened.

Nut butters: Peanut and almond butters are staples. There are plenty of other choices, too, although they tend to be pricey. Nut butters are good for sandwiches or to spread on apple slices, but they also can be thinned with water and seasoned to make great sauces for grains and vegetables.

Sesame tahini: An essential ingredient in homemade hummus that is equally good for sauces and dressings.

Miso: Absolutely essential in Japanese cooking, it is also considered a staple by most vegans to add saltiness and depth to sauces and soups.

Fortified plant milks: Soymilk and pea milks are the most nutritious and protein-rich, but you might also enjoy almond, oat, hempseed, flax, and rice milk. Choose brands that are fortified with calcium.

Fresh or aseptically packaged tofu: Choose firm tofu for scrambles and stir-fries, soft or silken for sauces and soups.

Tempeh: An ancient food from Indonesia, this cake of fermented soybeans has an indescribably delicious flavor. It's a great protein source to toss into stir-fried dishes. You can read more about tempeh and other soy products in Chapter 2.

Vital wheat gluten: A flour made from wheat protein, it's used to create seitan, which has a chewy, meat-like texture. You can also buy prepared seitan.

Dried fruits: Figs, apricots, prunes, and raisins

Vegan mayonnaise: There are several brands on the market, but Vegenaise, made by Follow Your Heart, is well liked.

Vegan margarine: Most vegan cooks swear by the Earth Balance brand, which is widely available and does not contain hydrogenated oils.

Veggie meats: Look for these in the frozen and refrigerated section of grocery stores. Be sure to check labels since some contain dairy and eggs.

Vegan cheeses, cream cheese, sour cream, and yogurt: These are made from soy, almonds, cashews, hempseed, and even coconut.

You'll find cheeses that mimic American cheese and other sandwich slices as well as aged, cultured cheeses made from nuts.

Fruits and Vegetables

Lemons and limes

Condiments: Ketchup, mustard, relish, pickles, salsa, barbecue sauce, black and green olives—the same condiments that you'll find in the refrigerators of most omnivores, vegetarians, and vegans alike.

Freezer Basics

Frozen corn and peas: Nice to have on hand to toss into grain salads. They do not need to be cooked.

Premade pizza shells

Vegan ice cream

Veggie burgers and other veggie meats

Backup: The freezer is a good place to store extra packages of tempeh, seitan, and veggie meats, as well as nuts and seeds (which can turn rancid in the cupboard and even in the refrigerator after a long enough time).

Basic Condiments

Iodized salt: Many vegan cookbooks suggest using sea salt. But sea salt has the same effects on blood pressure and calcium loss as any other salt—and it's not a reliable source of iodine. So use salt sparingly, and when you do, choose plain iodized salt.

Vegan Worcestershire sauce: Traditionally, this sauce is made with fish (anchovies), but low-sodium Worcestershire sauce is often vegan. Or look for one that says "vegetarian" on the label.

Jams, jellies, and preserves

Tamari: A more authentic version of soy sauce

Nutritional yeast: Look for Red Star brand Vegetarian Support Formula because that's the type that provides vitamin B_{12}.

Vinegars: Apple cider, balsamic, and white wine vinegar will cover most of your needs, but there are many others available. Rice vinegar is great for adding an authentic Asian flavor to stir-fried dishes.

MORE LUXURIOUS CONDIMENTS

Cooking enthusiasts will want to have these on hand, but even if you don't consider yourself a "gourmet" chef, they can add fast, easy flavor to basic grain, bean, and tofu dishes.

- Chile paste
- Hoisin sauce
- Teriyaki sauce
- Chutney
- Curry paste
- Artichoke hearts
- Sun-dried tomatoes packed in oil
- Roasted red bell peppers
- Olive tapenade
- Capers
- Liquid smoke
- Mirin
- Dried shiitake mushrooms

Baking

In addition to baking essentials like enriched and whole-grain flours, baking soda, and baking powder, vegan cooks often stock the following:

For replacing eggs in baking: Ground flaxseeds or full-fat soy flour

Agar powders or flakes: Boil this seaweed in water or juice to produce a gelatin-like product. You'll find it in natural foods stores or Asian markets.

Other thickeners: Arrowroot powder and cornstarch

Chickpea flour: Natural foods and specialty stores are packed with all kinds of flours. Chickpea flour is a "basic" because when it is used to thicken vegetable broth, it makes a wonderful gravy to pour over mashed potatoes and vegan Thanksgiving stuffing. In Indian groceries, it's usually called *besan*.

Unsweetened cocoa powder

Sweeteners: There are plenty of great vegan sweeteners on the market, including organic sugar (which is usually processed without animal byproducts), rice syrup, barley malt syrup, maple syrup, blackstrap molasses (a good source of iron and calcium), and regular molasses (which has a milder flavor than the blackstrap variety but is not as nutritious).

Vanilla and lemon extracts

Bread crumbs

Wheat germ

Herbs and Spices

The sky's the limit when it comes to herbs and spices, especially if you love to cook and experiment with ethnic dishes. If you want just the basics, here's what to keep on hand:

- Allspice
- Basil
- Bay leaves
- Cayenne powder
- Chile powder
- Cinnamon
- Coriander
- Cumin
- Curry powder
- Garlic powder
- Ginger
- Nutmeg
- Onion powder
- Oregano
- Paprika
- Parsley
- Rosemary
- Savory
- Thyme
- Turmeric

Beverages

Coffee, tea, wine, beer, soft drinks, juices, and whatever else is popular in your home. Don't forget about water, which is the best choice as your main beverage.

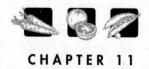

CHAPTER 11

A Healthy Start

*Vegan Diets in
Pregnancy and Breastfeeding*

Family members, friends, and even your health-care provider might express surprise and concern at the idea of a vegan pregnancy. After all, good nutrition and a healthy lifestyle are more important during pregnancy than at any other time of life. Fortunately, vegan diets that focus on appropriate food and supplement choices can easily meet nutrient needs. Even more than thirty years ago, a study of 775 women living in a vegan community in Tennessee found that pregnant women had adequate weight gain and gave birth to babies with normal weights, two important measures of a healthy pregnancy.[1] In fact, these women actually gained a little bit more than women in the general meat-eating population. And the longer they had been vegan, the better their weight gain. One other finding was surprising: pre-eclampsia, a potential complication of pregnancy that occurs in 5 to 10 percent of pregnant women, was nearly nonexistent among vegan pregnant women in this community.

In some studies of women following very restrictive diets, particularly macrobiotic diets, infants sometimes had lower birth weights. In these cases, it wasn't a vegan diet that was to blame. Rather, the diets at issue were too low in fat and calories. It's important to note that the findings about poor pregnancy outcomes are from older studies when vegans had less access to nutrition information and a variety of vegan foods. That's all changed dramatically in the past several decades, and today it's easier than ever to have a healthy vegan pregnancy. As long as you pay attention to meeting nutrient needs, especially for vitamin B_{12} and iron, a vegan diet can support a healthy pregnancy.[2,3]

WHEN YOU ARE PLANNING A PREGNANCY

The best time to start eating for the health of your baby is before you are pregnant. The American College of Obstetricians and Gynecologists recommends taking a prenatal multivitamin if you are contemplating a pregnancy. At the very least, it's wise for all women, vegan or not, to take a supplement of the B vitamin folic acid since adequate intake of this nutrient is vital in the early days of pregnancy. There is also evidence that folic acid can be helpful for women who are having trouble getting pregnant.[4] A diet rich in antioxidants may help as well. Women with conditions that are associated with infertility like PCOS and endometriosis as well as unexplained infertility tend to have increased markers of oxidative stress in their blood. Piling your plate with antioxidant-rich fruits and vegetables is always a good choice, and in this case, it may help you get pregnant.[5-7] You also might get your blood levels of vitamin D and iron checked to make sure you're getting enough of these nutrients. And if you aren't already taking vitamin B_{12}, this is the time to get on track.

Being significantly over- or underweight is associated with greater risk for pregnancy complications and having a preterm baby. If you are underweight, aim to put on a few pounds before becoming pregnant. Losing significant amounts of weight can be much more of a challenge, but even a few pounds could make a difference.[8,9]

Finally, think about cutting alcohol out of your diet, if there is any chance you might become pregnant, and if you are a coffee drinker, now is the time to cut back to one or two cups a day.

GETTING ENOUGH CALORIES

Although adequate weight gain is important for a healthy vegan pregnancy, eating for two doesn't mean eating twice as many calories. On average, pregnant women need an extra 340 calories per day during the second trimester and 450 extra calories during the third trimester. But needs for certain nutrients increase by as much as 50 percent (see table on page 177), so packing a lot of good nutrition into that little bit of extra food is important.

Pregnant women can follow the vegan food guide in Chapter 10 with just a few adjustments that we've shown in the Food Guide for Pregnant and Breastfeeding Women on page 178. An added serving of leafy green vegetables and two additional servings of protein-rich foods (beans, peanuts, and soyfoods) and grains will give you needed calories and help meet nutrient needs during the second trimester. During the last trimester, when your baby is growing fastest, add one more serving of either whole grains or legumes/soyfoods.

Calorie-counting during pregnancy isn't an exact science, but your health-care provider will help you stay on track by monitoring your weight gain. Average weight gain for a healthy pregnancy is between 25 and 35 pounds, but, depending on your weight at the start of pregnancy, your health-care provider may suggest a smaller or greater weight gain. Almost all of the weight gain will take place during the second and third trimesters. Poor weight gain during pregnancy is associated with low-birth-weight babies, who are at risk for health problems.

NUTRITION CONSIDERATIONS
IN VEGAN PREGNANCY

Vitamin B_{12}

When you read news stories about vegan babies with nutritional deficiencies, it's more than likely that vitamin B_{12} is at the center of the problem. Often the mothers of these infants had poor vitamin B_{12} status during pregnancy or inadequate intakes while they were breastfeeding.

Inadequate intake can result in birth defects or place newborns at high risk of serious B_{12} deficiency. Although we store some vitamin B_{12} in our livers, it appears that this stash of B_{12} doesn't make its way across the placenta. Your baby's vitamin B_{12} comes directly from your diet. For vegans, supplements and fortified foods are the only source of this nutrient.

To meet needs for vitamin B_{12}, take a daily supplement providing at least 25 micrograms and up to 250 micrograms of vitamin B_{12} in the form of cyanocobalamin. Check the label of your prenatal supplement to see if it already provides this. If it contains less than 25 micrograms, you'll need to include an additional source of vitamin B_{12}. Alternatively, you can get enough vitamin B_{12} by consuming two servings of B_{12}-fortified foods every day, with each serving providing at least 2.5 micrograms of B_{12}. (See chart on page 92 for examples of foods.) If you choose to do this, it's a good idea to also take an occasional supplement in addition.

Protein

Protein needs increase by almost 50 percent in pregnancy and, beginning with the second trimester, the RDA for pregnant women is 25 grams higher than for nonpregnant women. Vegan protein needs are slightly higher (see Chapter 4) but this translates to just 3 additional grams of protein per day, for a total of 28 grams.

Most nonpregnant omnivore women consume enough protein to meet the needs of pregnancy, but that may not be true of all vegan women. A nonpregnant vegan woman who starts her pregnancy at 130 pounds would require 80 grams of protein per day beginning in her second trimester (52 grams to meet nonpregnant needs plus 28 grams for pregnancy). This means you may need to give a little extra attention to protein by including at least five servings per day of legumes (beans, peanuts, peanut butter, soyfoods) in your daily menus. Including these foods, which are rich in the essential amino acid lysine, is especially important since lysine needs may increase as pregnancy progresses.[10]

Folic Acid/Folate

Also known as vitamin B_9, this vitamin is called "folate" when in food and "folic acid" in supplement form. Along with vitamin B_{12}, it is needed for development of the embryo's nervous system in the first weeks of pregnancy, and folic acid supplements appear to reduce the risk of having a baby with a nervous system defect. This early development of the nervous system takes place usually before a woman knows she is pregnant, which is why pre-pregnancy nutrition is so important. Many vegans are able to meet the increased needs for this nutrient by including plenty of leafy green vegetables, beans, and citrus fruits in meals. But to ensure adequate intake, a supplement is advised beginning in the months before you become pregnant and continuing throughout at least the first trimester.[11,12] Choose a prenatal supplement that provides 400 micrograms of folic acid.

Iron

Iron absorption—especially of the nonheme iron found in plant foods—increases significantly during pregnancy while the lack of menstruation reduces iron losses. Even so, iron requirements nearly double during pregnancy. It's especially important during the last trimester when the fetus is accumulating stored iron. Most of the increase in iron needs is to support the mother's blood volume, which can expand by as much as 50 percent during pregnancy. Theoretically, vegans could be at higher risk for iron deficiency in pregnancy due to smaller iron stores, but the truth is that all women are at risk. It's difficult to plan diets for either vegans or omnivores that meet iron needs of pregnancy. For that reason, a supplement providing 30 milligrams of iron is almost always recommended for pregnant women.[13] In addition to taking the supplement that your health-care provider recommends, it's important to continue eating iron-rich foods and maximizing absorption by including a good source of vitamin C at meals and snacks.

Zinc

It's difficult to assess zinc status in pregnant women, but there is evidence that many women, vegetarians and meat-eaters alike, have zinc intakes that are lower than recommendations, unless they are taking supplements. Zinc absorption may increase with pregnancy, but it's still important to aim to meet needs.[14] The benefits of zinc supplements in pregnancy aren't known, but they may be helpful for pregnant vegans since zinc absorption from plant foods is lower than from meat. Choose a prenatal supplement that provides around 15 milligrams of zinc to ensure adequate intake.

Vitamin D

Vitamin D requirements don't change with pregnancy but getting enough is important for both the mother's and baby's health. If you live in a warm climate and get regular sun exposure throughout your pregnancy, this may be enough to ensure good vitamin D status. But keep in mind that even people who live in sunny climates sometimes have levels of vitamin D that are too low. Fortified foods can provide some vitamin D but are unlikely to meet requirements. This is another nutrient that is most likely provided by your prenatal supplement, but check the label to be sure. The RDA is 600 International Units (or 15 micrograms).

Iodine

Iodine is needed for development of the growing fetus's brain and nervous system and deficiencies are linked to poor cognitive function and development. Throughout the world, iodine deficiency is the most common cause of preventable brain damage. Fortunately, it is easy for pregnant and breastfeeding vegans to get enough iodine through supplements or iodized salt. Check to make sure your prenatal supplement provides at least 150 micrograms of iodine. If it doesn't, you'll need to get iodine from an additional supplement or from small amounts of iodized table salt. Because sea vegetables may provide too little or too much iodine, we don't recommend relying on them for meeting needs. In rare cases, regular consumption of sea vegetables has resulted in iodine toxicity in pregnant women.[15,16]

Omega-3 Fats

Although synthesis of the long-chain omega-3 fatty acids DHA and EPA may be enhanced during pregnancy, vegetarians who don't consume direct sources of these fats have lower blood levels.[17] We don't know whether that's a problem, but there is some evidence that DHA intake during pregnancy is associated with lower risk of premature birth.[18] Experts recommend that pregnant women consume 300 milligrams of DHA and EPA combined per day.[19-21] We suggest choosing a supplement that is mostly or all DHA since this is the omega-3 fat that is significantly lower in the blood of vegans.

TIPS FOR A HEALTHY PREGNANCY

While it might seem as though there is a lot to think about in choosing healthy meals during pregnancy, we can summarize the information with just a few guidelines:

- Begin taking a prenatal supplement while you are planning a pregnancy. Look for one that provides iron, folic acid, zinc, vitamin D, and iodine.
- If your prenatal supplement does not provide at least 25 micrograms of vitamin B_{12}, take an additional supplement or use a combination of supplement and fortified foods.
- Talk to your health-care provider about your weight-gain goals. If you have trouble gaining weight, emphasize foods with a little more fat, such as tofu, nut butters, and avocados.
- Use the Food Guide for Pregnant and Breastfeeding Women on page 178 in making daily food choices. It's based on the food guide in Chapter 10 but with a little extra emphasis on legumes and grains.

- Protein needs go up by about 28 grams beginning with the second trimester. It's not difficult to meet those needs on a vegan diet, but it might require extra attention. Take a look at the list of protein-rich foods in Chapter 4. Aim for at least 15 to 20 grams of protein in each meal and choose a few protein-rich snacks as well.
- Eat plenty of iron-rich foods and include a good source of vitamin C at every meal to boost absorption. Most health-care professionals recommend iron supplements for all pregnant women. This can be especially helpful for vegans since iron needs are higher for those on plant-based diets.
- Avoid alcohol, tobacco, and recreational drugs while you are pregnant. Limit coffee and caffeinated tea to one or two cups per day. Also avoid foods like sprouts and unpasteurized juice and cider since they can be a potential source of bacterial contaminants.

NAUSEA IN PREGNANCY

Although it is usually called morning sickness, nausea associated with early pregnancy can occur at any time of day. In addition to being unpleasant, nausea can keep you from eating healthfully. Here are a few tips to help you deal with pregnancy-induced nausea:

- Eat frequent small meals since an empty stomach can make nausea worse. (Small meals can also help with heartburn, which can be a problem for some pregnant women.)
- Eat something immediately upon waking, when your stomach is likely to be empty. Keep carbohydrate-rich foods like crackers, raisins, or whatever appeals to you on the bedside table.
- Avoid liquids with meals if you find that this increases your nausea.
- Identify healthy foods that are less likely to make you feel sick. You'll need to follow your own instincts, but good choices to

continues

NAUSEA IN PREGNANCY   *continued*

consider include whole grain breads, dry cereals, cooked or dried fruits, and white or sweet potatoes. Try adding small pieces of vegetables and tofu to miso soup to make them saltier and easier on your stomach. Frozen fruit juice bars can help keep you from being dehydrated.

- Drink ginger tea or sip ginger ale or snack on gingersnaps.
- If your prenatal supplement upsets your stomach, try taking it before bed instead of during the day.
- Some women have found relief with use of Sea Bands, a type of acupressure cuff that you can buy online.[22]
- Vitamin B_6 supplements may also be effective but be sure to talk with your health-care provider before taking any additional supplements to what we've recommended in this chapter.[23]

VEGAN NUTRITION FOR NURSING MOMS

The rate of breastfeeding is higher among vegan mothers than in the general population. And that's nice for their babies since breast milk is the ideal food for infants. Ideally, babies should be fed human milk for at least the first year of their lives and preferably throughout the second year as well. But, even if you can't commit to breastfeeding for that long, doing so for a few months if possible will benefit your baby. Breastfed infants appear to have lower risk for infections and allergies, and breastfeeding may reduce their lifelong risk for some chronic illnesses—and possibly could reduce risk in the breastfeeding woman as well. A bonus for vegetarian women who breastfeed is that their milk might be lower in environmental contaminants.[24] Although we don't have recent data, a 1981 study of the breast milk of vegans found that levels of seventeen environmental chemicals were lower compared to the general population. In fact, the highest vegan value was lower than the lowest value in milk from the general population.[25]

Nutrient Needs in Breastfeeding

Nursing mothers need extra calories for the process of synthesizing milk and to provide the calories that babies need for growth. Energy needs, therefore, are higher during lactation than in pregnancy and many women will need as much as 500 calories more per day than they did when they weren't pregnant (or just a little bit more than needed during the third trimester of pregnancy). If you have post-pregnancy pounds to drop, a small reduction in calories can usually produce a gradual weight loss while still maintaining adequate milk volume. Don't decrease calories too much, though, as it can cause the milk supply to decrease as well. Drinking plenty of fluids is also important for producing adequate milk.

Needs for some nutrients go up slightly, so emphasizing nutrient-rich foods is as important as ever. You can see from the chart on page 177 that breastfeeding moms have higher needs for vitamin C, vitamin A, iodine, zinc, and some B vitamins compared to pregnant women. The requirement for folate is lower than during pregnancy but still higher than what a nonpregnant woman needs.

Note that iron needs drop after giving birth. As the blood supply goes back to normal pre-pregnancy levels and women are still not menstruating, at least in the early months of breastfeeding, iron needs are much lower than during pregnancy.

The two nutrients that require the most attention in diets of breast-feeding moms are ones that nutrition-savvy vegans are already focusing on—vitamin D and vitamin B_{12}. Deficiencies of vitamin B_{12} have been seen in babies whose mothers didn't follow recommended guidelines and can cause serious problems. One survey of the B_{12} content of breast milk found no difference in the levels among vegan, vegetarian, and nonvegetarian women, but overall, there was a risk of having levels that were too low in all groups.[26] Nursing women should continue to consume a daily vitamin B_{12} supplement.

The omega-3 fat DHA plays a role in both visual and mental development and it's common now for infant formulas to be fortified with this fatty acid. We recommend that you continue with a supplement providing 200 to 300 milligrams of DHA.

Many women continue with a prenatal supplement for the first few months of breastfeeding (but without the extra iron). It's also important to eat foods that provide plenty of folate and vitamin A. Choose plenty of orange and dark, leafy green vegetables to boost intake of these nutrients.

NUTRIENT RECOMMENDATIONS FOR NONPREGNANT, PREGNANT, AND BREASTFEEDING WOMEN

Nutrient	Nonpregnant	Pregnant	Breastfeeding
Protein (g)*	46	71	71
Thiamin (milligrams)	1.1	1.4	1.4
Riboflavin (milligrams)	1.1	1.4	1.6
Niacin (milligrams)	14	18	17
Vitamin B$_6$ (milligrams)	1.3	1.9	2.0
Folic acid (micrograms)	400	600	500
Vitamin B$_{12}$ (micrograms)	2.4	2.6	2.8
Vitamin C (milligrams)	75	85	120
Vitamin A (micrograms)	700	770	1,300
Vitamin D (International Units)	600	600	600
Vitamin E (milligrams)	15	15	19
Vitamin K (micrograms)	90	90	90
Calcium (milligrams)	1,000	1,000	1,000
Iodine (micrograms)	150	220	290
Iron (milligrams**)	18	27	9
Magnesium (milligrams)	310–320	350–360	310–320
Phosphorus (milligrams)	700	700	700
Selenium (micrograms)	55	60	70
Zinc (milligrams)***	8	11	12

*This is an average protein need since specific requirements are calculated based on your weight. Protein needs may be slightly higher for pregnant vegans. Use the guidelines in Chapter 4 to calculate your pre-pregnancy protein requirements and then add 28 extra grams of protein for pregnancy.
**The National Academies recommends 1.8 times this amount of iron for vegetarians and vegans but, as we explain in Chapter 8, we believe that recommendation is unnecessary.
***Zinc requirements for some vegans could be as much as 50 percent higher.

The following table offers guidelines for planning healthy vegan diets throughout pregnancy and breastfeeding. For more information, we recommend the book *Your Complete Vegan Pregnancy* by Dr. Reed Mangels, RD.

FOOD GUIDE FOR PREGNANT AND BREASTFEEDING WOMEN

Food group	Number of servings per day during pregnancy	Number of servings per day for breastfeeding
Grains and starchy vegetables	6	6
Legumes and soyfoods	5	6
Nuts	2	2
Vegetables	4 (include at least one leafy green vegetable)	4
Fruits	2	2
Fats	3	3
Calcium-rich foods	Eat at least 3 cups per day of some combination of foods that are good sources of well-absorbed calcium. These include fortified plant milks, fortified juices, calcium-set tofu, oranges, and low-oxalate leafy green vegetables like kale, mustard greens, turnip greens, bok choy, and collard greens.	

SUPPLEMENTS FOR PREGNANT VEGANS:

- Prenatal supplement that provides folic acid, vitamin D, zinc, iron, and iodine
- Vitamin B_{12} if your prenatal supplement doesn't provide at least 25 micrograms of cyanocobalamin
- A calcium supplement if you feel you are falling short of the 1,000 milligrams of calcium recommended during pregnancy
- 300 milligrams of DHA from algae

SUPPLEMENTS FOR BREASTFEEDING VEGANS:

- A daily vitamin B_{12} supplement providing at least 25 micrograms of cyanocobalamin
- 300 milligrams of DHA
- 150 micrograms of iodine

As always, let your health-care provider know about any supplements you are taking.

SAMPLE MENUS

You may very well feel like cooking up a storm during and after your pregnancy. But just in case you don't have the time or energy for much food prep, we've kept things simple with these sample menus. They are meant to illustrate the ease of planning healthy vegan menus without fuss. These menus utilize six mini-meals, which can be helpful with managing heartburn and nausea.

SAMPLE MENU FOR A PREGNANT WOMAN

BREAKFAST
- ▸ 1 cup fortified breakfast cereal
- ▸ 1 cup fortified soymilk
- ▸ Banana

SNACK
- ▸ Raw carrots with 2 tablespoons peanut butter

LUNCH
- ▸ Miso soup with ½ cup tofu and 1 cup cooked kale or collards
- ▸ Whole-grain crackers

SNACK
- ▸ Whole-grain bread with ½ cup hummus
- ▸ ½ cup fortified orange juice

DINNER
- ▸ 1 cup brown rice with 1 tablespoon ground flaxseeds
- ▸ ½ cup baked beans
- ▸ 1 cup steamed vegetables sautéed in 2 teaspoons canola oil

SNACK
- ▸ ½ whole grain English muffin with 2 tablespoons vegan cheese spread
- ▸ 1 cup fortified soymilk

continues

SAMPLE MENU FOR A BREASTFEEDING MOM

BREAKFAST

- ▸ ½ cup scrambled tofu cooked in 1 teaspoon canola oil
- ▸ 1 slice whole wheat toast with 1 teaspoon margarine
- ▸ 1 cup calcium-fortified orange juice

SNACK

- ▸ ½ cup grapes
- ▸ Whole-grain crackers with 2 tablespoons almond butter

LUNCH

- ▸ Veggie burger
- ▸ Whole wheat hamburger roll
- ▸ Slice tomato and lettuce
- ▸ Broccoli salad with ¼ cup chopped walnuts and ½ tablespoon vegan mayonnaise

SNACK

- ▸ Small bran muffin
- ▸ 1 cup fortified soymilk

DINNER

- ▸ 1 cup lentil soup
- ▸ 1 cup steamed collards
- ▸ Green salad with dressing
- ▸ Whole wheat bread

SNACK

- ▸ Smoothie: ½ cup fortified soymilk, ½ cup frozen fruit, ¼ banana

CHAPTER 12

Raising Vegan
Children and Teens

INFANTS

Even the most confident vegan adults might feel a little nervous about a vegan diet for their newborn baby. Infants typically triple their weight in the first year of life and need enough nutritious food to see them through this early growth spurt. Can a vegan diet satisfy their needs?

During the first months of a baby's life, this isn't even an issue. All infants start out as vegetarians. Or, to be more correct, they begin their lives as "lactarians." For the first six months or so, infants don't need anything other than breast milk or infant formula. Either is a complete food for young infants. Unless they are given B_{12} supplements (needed only if the breastfeeding mom's diet is inadequate), the diets of vegan babies are exactly the same as infants in omnivore families until they are around six months old.

The First Six Months

For the first six months of life, babies don't need—and shouldn't have—anything other than breast milk or infant formula.[1] They don't need any solid foods during this time, and certain vegetables can be dangerous to very young infants.

For a number of reasons, breast milk is the optimal food for babies, and most vegans choose it for their newest family members. Breast milk provides a nutrient balance that is close to ideal for growing infants. It also contains unique immune factors and reduces the risk for allergies. But sometimes breastfeeding isn't an option or isn't a family's preference. In that case, iron-fortified soy infant formula supports normal growth and development in babies and is approved by the American Academy of Pediatrics.[2,3] These formulas are not 100 percent vegan since they contain vitamin D derived from animals, but they are as close as we can get to a healthy vegan choice.

Infants should never be given homemade formulas and they should never be given regular soymilk or any other plant milk or cow's milk. In the rare cases where vegan infants have suffered from malnutrition, it's because they were being fed homemade formulas or did not receive adequate supplements of vitamin B_{12} and vitamin D. Because babies have very specific nutritional needs, it's essential to feed them only breast milk or commercial infant formulas, which are manufactured to meet those needs.

Around age six months, babies start to show that they are ready for solid foods. One sign of readiness is the ability to sit up and maintain balance. Another is the ability to use the tongue to move food to the back of the mouth for swallowing. Babies who are ready to explore solid foods will show interest in what other family members are eating, often trying to grab these foods to put in their own mouths. Your pediatrician will help you decide when your baby is ready for solid foods. Introducing these foods too soon, before four months of age, may raise risk for allergies and also for obesity later in life.[4,5] Most babies should start having some solid foods around the age of six months. Experimenting with these foods helps with your baby's development and social skills and supports the ability to learn to enjoy a variety of foods with different textures and flavors.

Infants also need the iron that these foods supply. Breast milk is generally low in iron and infants depend on their own body stores, which begin to decline by the age of four months. Depending on when your baby begins to eat these foods and how much is consumed, some infants may need supplemental iron drops beginning at four months. Your pediatrician will give you guidance on this.

First Solid Food Adventure

"Solid" is a bit of an overstatement for the first nonmilk foods a baby eats. Most infants begin with something that is more like a thick liquid but fed from a spoon, not a bottle.

First foods for an infant should be ones that are good sources of iron and zinc. The best choice is an infant cereal that is fortified with these nutrients and mixed with breast milk or infant formula. Once your baby is familiar with the experience of eating pureed cereal and is consuming about ⅓ to ½ cup per day, begin to offer a variety of other mashed or pureed foods. These might include mashed potatoes, well cooked, mashed beans, soft tofu, and mashed vegetables and fruit.

Since humans are born with a preference for sweet flavors, it's important to help children learn to enjoy vegetables, which have more bitter flavors, in infancy.[6] To help your baby become accustomed to new flavors, mash or puree vegetables and mix them with a familiar food like breast milk, formula, cereal, or with something bland like avocado or silken tofu. If your baby doesn't like a new food, give it another try a few days later. Be persistent because it can take many, many times for infants to accept a new food.[7]

You may want to keep a few jars of commercial baby food on hand for convenience sake, but most vegan parents make their own baby food. Not only does it save money, but it allows for greater variety in your baby's diet. Simply cook and then mash the food and freeze in an ice cube tray for individual portions. Thaw in the refrigerator before serving. Don't salt or sweeten the foods that you prepare for your infant.

Many parents begin offering finger foods right away, providing a baby with a varied diet of milk, pureed/mashed foods, and foods that they can feed themselves. To ensure experience with different textures and optimal development, make sure your baby is eating some finger foods by the age of eight or nine months. Choices for vegan babies include cooked pasta, strips of bread with the crust removed, pieces of ripe fruit without peel or skin like avocado, banana, peach, pear, kiwi, melon, or quartered grapes; soft cooked vegetables like broccoli, cauliflower, carrots, yam, or squash; and tofu fingers.

To minimize risk of choking, avoid giving infants very small foods such as nuts and whole grapes, raw vegetables, hard fruit, including raw apple; popcorn; and foods cut into coins, such as veggie sausages or carrots. Choose foods that the baby can mash against the roof of the mouth. Nut butters should be thinned with a little bit of milk or water and spread very thinly on pieces of bread (see box on page 185 for information about allergies and babies). It's also important to make sure infants are sitting up when they eat and that they have control over what they put into their mouth. Never leave an infant alone with food.

During this period, breast milk or soy infant formula continues to play a major role in your baby's diet and will be a part of the menu until at least the first birthday. Breast milk or infant formula is especially important for providing zinc, which can otherwise be low in a vegan infant's diet. Older babies who are eating some solid foods typically eat six or more small meals throughout the day and breast milk or formula will likely be a part of each of them, at least until late infancy. Regular soymilk should never be offered to babies before the first birthday because, like cow's milk, it is a poor fit for an infant's nutritional needs.

A Few Things to Keep in Mind for Vegan Babies

- Talk to your pediatrician about supplements. Vitamin D is usually recommended for breastfed infants in both vegan and omnivore families. Iron is recommended beginning at around four months. The duration of iron supplementation will eventually depend on other foods in your baby's diet. Breastfed vegan infants need vitamin B_{12} supplements only if the mother's diet isn't adequate. The table on page 186 shows suggested supplements for breastfed vegan infants.

PREVENTING ALLERGIES

The foods most likely to cause allergies in babies and infants are milk, eggs, fish, shellfish, tree nuts, sesame, peanuts, wheat, and soybeans. These foods are not all equally allergenic, though. Milk allergy is by far the most common source of allergies in children, whereas soyfoods are the least allergenic among these nine foods.[8-11] With the exceptions of allergies to peanuts and fish, children tend to outgrow allergies by their teen years so that babies who are allergic to wheat or soy will not necessarily grow into children or adults who have these allergies.

Delaying the introduction of solid foods until at least four months of age can help reduce the risk of allergies. However, once your baby is eating some solid foods, there is no reason to delay foods like wheat and peanut butter. In fact some evidence suggests that eating these foods in infancy reduces the risk for later allergy.[12] Talk to your pediatrician about how to introduce these foods if there is a history of food allergy in the baby's biological family.

The key to identifying allergies in infants is to introduce solid foods one at a time and wait for three to four days before introducing the next new food. Look for signs of allergic reactions such as skin rashes, wheezing and runny nose, or stomach issues such as frequent vomiting and diarrhea.

Young babies sometimes also suffer from colic, which is defined as excessive crying and fussiness in infants who are otherwise healthy and well-fed. There is evidence that in breastfed babies, colic can sometimes result from a reaction to foods in the mother's diet. Vegans have an advantage since one of the primary culprits seems to be cow's milk. But there are other foods in vegan diets that may cause colic in your baby particularly onions and vegetables in the cabbage family. If you find that removing these foods from your diet is helpful, it doesn't mean that your baby is allergic to them.

- Never give babies unpasteurized juice or cider, or any kind of honey, all of which can cause serious illness.
- Avoid juices for your baby's first year.[13]
- Don't give babies foods with added salt or sweeteners.
- Don't give a baby any milk other than breast milk or infant formula before the first birthday. Regular soy, rice, hemp, and

almond milks (or cow's milk) don't have the right balance of
nutrients for infants and shouldn't be offered until your baby is a
year old (these milks can, however, be used in small amounts in
food preparation).

- Don't offer foods that can cause choking like whole vegan hotdogs, popcorn, nuts, hard candies, and grapes. Don't offer infants nut and seed butters by the spoonful or spread too thickly
on bread or crackers.

DAILY SUPPLEMENTS FOR BREASTFED VEGAN BABIES

Nutrient	Birth to 6 months	6 to 12 months
Vitamin D	400 International Units (10 micrograms)	400 International Units (10 micrograms)
Vitamin B$_{12}$	0.4 micrograms only if the mother doesn't have a reliable B$_{12}$ intake	0.5 micrograms only if the mother doesn't have a reliable B$_{12}$ intake
Iron	1 milligram per kilogram (0.45 milligrams per pound) of body weight beginning at four months	1 milligram per kilogram (0.45 milligrams per pound) of body weight unless infant is consuming sufficient iron from solid foods
Fluoride		0.25 milligrams if water contains less than 0.3 parts per million fluoride

---

SAMPLE MEAL PLANS FOR VEGAN BABIES

6 TO 8 MONTHS

MORNING
- Breast milk or formula
- Fortified infant oat cereal mixed with breast milk, formula, or water
- Mashed strawberries

MID-MORNING
- Breast milk or formula
- Small pieces of banana

---

continues

SAMPLE MEAL PLANS FOR VEGAN BABIES *continued*

NOON
- ▸ Breast milk or formula
- ▸ Mashed tofu
- ▸ Mashed cooked carrots

MID-AFTERNOON
- ▸ Breast milk or formula
- ▸ Applesauce

DINNER
- ▸ Breast milk or formula
- ▸ Small pieces of cooked butternut squash
- ▸ Mashed cooked pinto beans

EVENING
- ▸ Breast milk or formula
- ▸ Fortified oat cereal mixed with breast milk, formula, or water

9 TO 12 MONTHS

MORNING
- ▸ Breast milk or formula
- ▸ Fortified infant wheat cereal mixed with breast milk, formula, or water
- ▸ Cooked pear in small pieces

MID-MORNING
- ▸ Breast milk or formula
- ▸ Mashed avocado

NOON
- ▸ Breast milk or formula
- ▸ Small pieces cooked green beans
- ▸ Small pieces soft veggie burger

continues

SAMPLE MEAL PLANS FOR VEGAN BABIES   *continued*

MID-AFTERNOON

- ▸ Breast milk or formula
- ▸ Mashed kiwifruit

DINNER

- ▸ Breast milk or formula
- ▸ Pieces of well-cooked pasta
- ▸ Pureed lentils
- ▸ Kale blended with applesauce

EVENING

- ▸ Breast milk or formula
- ▸ Pieces of soft bread

VACCINES AND VEGAN CHILDREN

Even children eating healthy plant-based diets can get sick. But with the discovery of vaccines, we now have protection against life-threatening diseases like polio, measles, and tetanus.

Vegan parents may question the use of vaccines that are tested on animals or use animal products. But a vegan ethic asks us to find alternatives to animal products whenever possible and practical, and there are currently no vegan alternatives to vaccines. Given the protection they offer children, and the fact that a population of healthy vegan kids benefits all animals, vaccines are a responsible choice for vegan families. And as the demand for alternatives to animal testing grows, we can expect that we'll eventually have vaccines that are produced without harm to animals.

THE FIRST BIRTHDAY AND BEYOND:
VEGAN TODDLERS

After the mad growth spurt and enthusiastic appetite of the first twelve months, things begin to slow down. Toddlers can have sluggish appetites, and children aren't known for their adventurous eating habits at this stage. Picky and sometimes quirky eating behavior can make it difficult to get toddlers and preschoolers to eat anything at all, let alone to try new foods.

Full-fat fortified soymilk or milk made from pea protein can be introduced to a baby on the first birthday. Avoid using other milks made from rice, almonds, hemp, coconut, or oats as the main beverage, since they are too low in protein (and calories) for young children. If your child is a slow grower or an especially picky eater, it might be wise to continue with either breastfeeding or soy infant formula for a while.

Adequate intake of iron and zinc is especially important for your toddler. Good choices for toddlers include peanut butter, sunflower seed butter, bean spreads, puddings and smoothies made with soymilk, spaghetti sauce with lentils, and hummus on whole-grain bread.

The food guide on page 191 and table of suggested supplements on page 205 will help you plan healthy meals for toddlers. Don't worry if your child doesn't eat exactly this way every single day. Two or three days of nothing but peanut butter and banana sandwiches never hurt anyone—not even a three-year-old. And getting children to eat healthful foods like vegetables isn't a vegan problem; it's a universal problem for parents of young children.

If you feel like your little one isn't eating enough, focus on higher-calorie foods that he or she enjoys, such as avocado, nut and seed butters, tofu, and full-fat fortified soymilk. Low-fat diets are not appropriate for young children. Don't overdo it with fiber, which can fill up small stomachs. Avoid foods like bran cereal, which are very high in fiber. While it's good to serve mostly whole grains, it's also okay to include some refined grains, such as regular pasta, in a toddler's diet. Toddlers and preschoolers will benefit from several small meals throughout the day; nutritious snacks are especially important for this

age group. A multivitamin supplement that provides vitamin D, iodine, iron, and zinc may set your mind at ease about whether your
child is meeting nutrient needs and can be a good choice during the
picky eater stage.

As you explore new foods with your child, it's important to keep
an open mind. You'll hear over and over again: Oh, no three-year-old
will eat asparagus! Well, guess what? Some three-year-olds do. He
may indeed be the rare three-year-old, but he may also be yours! So
don't second-guess what your child will or won't eat based on what
most kids prefer. After all, toddlers in Mexico eat pinto beans, and
two-year-old Chinese kids dine happily on tofu.

Research shows that it takes as many as ten exposures to a new food
before a young child will try it, so be persistent. If your child turns her
nose up at baked beans, serve them again, in a different type of meal,
after a week or so. And again. And again. It can help to serve new
foods in small amounts alongside foods that are already familiar, and
it's also important for children to observe you enjoying the food you're
introducing.

Children are more likely to try foods that are easy to eat and that
they can pick up with their fingers. If a toddler or preschooler is going
through a picky phase and refuses to eat a variety of foods, it's okay to
sneak foods into the diet any way you can. Your child may turn up his
nose at a glass of soymilk but might be perfectly content to consume
it in mashed potatoes, pancakes, a smoothie or chocolate pudding.
Getting vegetables into the diet of a young vegan can be more of a
challenge. Here are ideas that parents have found helpful:

- Finely chop leafy green vegetables and add to spaghetti sauce.
- Mix chopped raw kale, collards, or broccoli with rice and roll up
  in a tortilla.
- Add raw kale to fruit smoothies.
- Mix finely chopped carrots, sweet red peppers, and broccoli into
  vegan cream cheese, roll it up in a soft tortilla, and slice into
  colorful pinwheels.

- Use raw vegetables to make salads in the shape of animals, or use cookie cutters to make fun-shaped sandwiches.
- Temper the strong flavor of kale and collards by blending them with bland foods such as avocado, tofu, or tofu cream cheese.

Tips for Feeding Vegan Toddlers

- Young children have small stomachs that can fill up quickly. Offer toddlers five to six small meals per day.
- Provide your child with a wide variety of plant foods and avoid restrictive diets. Low-fat diets and raw foods diets aren't suitable at this stage of life.
- Engage little ones in food preparation to pique their interest in new foods. Young children can slice a banana with a plastic picnic fork, layer granola, berries, and soy yogurt for a breakfast parfait, tear up lettuce for a salad, and help harvest peas from the garden.
- Let toddlers assert their independence by allowing them to choose among healthy snacks. Asking "do you want a banana or

FOOD GUIDE FOR VEGAN TODDLERS, AGES ONE TO THREE

Food group	Servings per day	Approximate serving sizes
Milk	2	1 cup breast milk, soy infant formula, fortified full-fat soymilk, or pea protein milk
Legumes and nuts	3 or more	¼ cup cooked beans, tofu, tempeh, textured vegetable protein; 1 ounce meat analog; ¼ cup soy yogurt; 1–2 tablespoons nuts, seeds, or nut or seed butter
Fruits	3 or more	½ medium piece of fruit; ¼ cup cooked or canned fruit
Vegetables	2 or more	¼ cup cooked or ½ cup raw vegetables
Grains and bread	6 or more	½ piece of bread, ¼ cup cooked cereal, ½ cup dry cereal, ¼ cooked grains or pasta
Fats and oils	2–3	1 teaspoon oil or margarine. Include ¼ teaspoon flaxseed oil, 1 teaspoon canola oil, or ½ tablespoon ground flaxseeds mixed into grains or hot cereal.

some cantaloupe" is a way to tap into a child's need for control while ensuring a healthy choice.

- Offer new foods along with familiar ones and do so without fanfare. If a food is refused offer it again a few days later. Let your child see you enjoying the food—but again, without making a display about it—to encourage their interest.

VALUABLE FOODS FOR VEGAN CHILDREN

Although there is no requirement for any type of milk in a child's diet, fortified soymilk or fortified milk made from pea protein can make it easier for vegan children to satisfy their nutrient needs. Other fortified milks, such as almond, oat, rice, or hemp milk, can be used in moderation, but since they are usually low in protein, they can displace protein-rich foods if used as the child's main milk.

Nuts and seeds and the butters made from them can also be important in the diets of young children since they are energy and nutrient-rich. Red Star brand Vegetarian Support Formula nutritional yeast is a good source of B vitamins, including vitamin B_{12}. Add nutritional yeast to bean dishes, veggie burgers, scrambled tofu, or mashed potatoes.

Blackstrap molasses (but not regular molasses) is a great source of calcium and iron. It has a strong taste and is likely to be more acceptable to children when mixed into other foods like smoothies, baked beans, or baked treats. It can also be mixed into peanut or almond butter and spread on crackers or bread.

ON THEIR OWN: VEGAN SCHOOL-AGE CHILDREN

The school years bring a new set of challenges as children encounter school lunches, birthday parties at McDonald's, and overnights with friends. Some kids may be savvy to the ways of the meat-eating world; others may have had less exposure to the idea that their diets are "different."

Will your child's vegan habits follow him as he heads out the door? Parents are likely to be faced with a series of personal decisions about

SAMPLE MENU FOR A TODDLER

BREAKFAST
- ½ cup Cream of Wheat with ½ tablespoon ground flaxseeds
- 1 cup fortified soymilk
- ½ cup mandarin orange segments

SNACK
- ½ slice whole-grain bread
- 1 tablespoon almond butter

LUNCH
- ¼ cup hummus
- 1 small whole wheat pita pocket
- ½ peach

SNACK
- Raw vegetables
- 1 ounce soft tofu blended with ¼ cup avocado

DINNER
- ½ cup macaroni
- ¼ cup white beans
- ¼ cup steamed butternut squash
- ½ cup stewed apricots

SNACK
- 1 cup fortified soymilk
- 1 graham cracker

this. Some parents believe that a 100 percent vegan approach is most in line with their family's values and least likely to be confusing to a child. Others might allow some flexibility in certain social situations. Regardless, as children grow older, there will be times when parents no longer have control over what goes into their young ones' stomachs.

At home, however, parents can provide well-balanced vegan meals by following the food guide in Chapter 10 with some modifications to the number of servings as we've shown on page 205.

In public schools, cafeterias are unlikely to have regular vegan choices, and lunches brought from home are usually the best option. In some school districts, there is a push for healthier school lunches, which may include more vegan offerings. Joining with like-minded parents and faculty to work with school food service can be a way to make more of these foods available to all children.

BROWN BAG OR LAPTOP LUNCHES FOR VEGAN SCHOOLCHILDREN

IDEAS FOR SANDWICHES OR WRAPS

- Hummus with chopped apples
- Almond butter with shredded carrots
- Tofu salad with vegan mayonnaise and chopped celery
- Vegan cheese, avocado, and veggies
- Chopped chickpea salad with vegan mayonnaise
- Peanut butter and apple slices
- White beans pureed with cooked carrots and mixed with chopped apples and walnuts
- Avocado blended with shredded vegetables
- Cashew cheese with shredded carrots
- BLT: tempeh bacon with lettuce and sliced tomatoes
- Crumbled tofu, shredded raw cabbage, and peanut butter dressing
- Lentils with corn and sunflower seeds
- Vegan turkey and cheese
- Pinwheels: chopped vegetables and vegan cream cheese rolled in a whole wheat flour tortilla and sliced into rounds

IN THE THERMOS

- Canned or homemade vegetarian chili
- Vegetable soup
- Beans and franks: vegetarian baked beans with tofu hotdogs

continues

BROWN BAG OR LAPTOP LUNCHES FOR VEGAN SCHOOLCHILDREN
continued

ON THE SIDE

- Fresh fruit
- Raw vegetables with tahini or tofu dip
- Baked tortilla chips
- Pasta or rice salad
- Bagel chips
- Vegetarian sushi

SWEET TREATS

- Peanut butter or oatmeal cookies
- Soy yogurt
- Dried fruit or trail mix
- Graham crackers
- Granola bars
- Pitted dates rolled in shredded coconut or finely chopped nuts
- Nutty fruit bites: dried fruit, nuts, and peanut butter blended in a food processor and rolled into bite-sized balls

---

VEGAN TEENS

Growth during the teen years is faster than at any other time except for infancy. During growth spurts—when teens can grow several inches over a period of a few months—calorie and nutrient needs are much higher than usual. Growth spurts are accompanied by increased appetite, and it's important to make sure your teen is consuming plenty of nutrient-rich foods.

Needs increase dramatically for calories, protein, calcium, and—for girls—iron. Meeting these needs can be a challenge since teens eat many meals on the go or on their own, and nutrition isn't always a high priority. Many adolescents, vegan or not, fail to get enough calcium and iron. Diets often are too high in fat and sugar and low in fiber.

Teens raised in vegan households might have an edge over omnivore teens since they are likely to be familiar with a wide range of
healthy plant foods. Some of these foods may offer unique benefits.
For example, girls who consume soyfoods during puberty and adolescence have a lifelong lower risk for breast cancer.[14]

On the other hand, vegan teens may have to pay even more attention to calcium and iron than their omnivore peers. It's critical that
teenagers regularly consume high-calcium foods like fortified soymilk,
fortified juices, or calcium-set tofu. You should also include beans,
a good source of iron, in foods that teenagers tend to enjoy, such as
baked beans, salads with chickpeas, hummus, and burritos.

The biggest challenge faces teenagers in omnivore families who have
chosen to adopt a vegan diet on their own. In that case, it's important
for parents to offer support by learning about vegan diets and making
sure the kitchen is well stocked with lots of teen-friendly vegan foods.

A different set of challenges may face vegan parents of teenagers.
Adolescence involves a degree of personal independence from parents,
and for some teens this may translate to experimenting with animal
foods. This may be less of a concern in homes where children are in-
vested in a commitment to animal welfare and animal rights. It may
also be less likely as vegan options become more mainstream and popular among young people. For better or worse, teens can join their
meat-eating peers at many fast food restaurants and can find plenty
of snack options in convenience stores and vending machines that are
vegan. Making vegan meals as easy and appealing as possible while allowing teens an appropriate level of freedom can help families weather
some of the conflict around food and meals.

The food guide on page 205 will help teens make healthful food
choices. All vegan teens should have supplements of vitamin B_{12} and
vitamin D and may require supplemental iodine depending on their
use of iodized salt. Vegan teens can meet other nutrient needs from
a well-planned diet. The truth, though, is that nutrition is not a high
priority for many teens, regardless of the family's diet choices. It can
be a challenge for teenage girls to meet iron needs and for both boys
and girls to meet needs for calcium. A multivitamin supplement that

provides low doses of iron, zinc, calcium, iodine, and vitamin D, in addition to a vitamin B_{12} supplement, can be good insurance during these years of rapid growth and high nutrient needs.

Since teens will choose many of their own meals and snacks, it's a good idea to have plenty of healthful foods available that can be quickly prepared or carried in a backpack. Some ideas that are likely to have teenager-appeal:

Dried fruits
Trail mix
Popcorn
Frozen vegan pizza slices and pizza pockets
Hummus on pita bread
Calcium-fortified juice or soymilk in individual serving cartons
Bagels
English muffins with almond butter
Burritos
Veggie burgers
Instant soups
Instant hot cereals
Ready-to-eat cereals
Smoothies with frozen fruit, soft tofu, and fortified soymilk

The widely varying nutrient and calorie needs of the teen years make it difficult to come up with a sample menu for this age group. We've offered a couple of different sample menus for different calorie levels on pages 210 and 211.

HELPING CHILDREN TRANSITION TO A VEGAN DIET

Children who have grown up in a vegan family are likely to be familiar with and enjoy a variety of healthful plant foods. But what about kids in families that are making a transition from meaty meals to a vegan menu? If you have recently decided to go vegan or to experiment with veganism, it may take your children a little longer to make the switch.

Since your primary concern is their health and happiness, opt to make gradual changes that ensure they are well-fed and meeting their nutrient needs.

With very young children, you can simply start introducing new vegan foods the same way that you introduce any food to a two- or three-year-old. With older children who already have well-established eating habits, these changes won't go unnoticed. Talking to them about why your family is leaving animal foods behind may help. Most young children have a natural affinity for animals and don't want to see them hurt. You don't need to (and shouldn't) expose your child to graphic images of factory farms, but you can help them see pigs, cows, and chickens as loveable animals who deserve the same care as cats and dogs. For example, you might plan a family visit to animals at a farm sanctuary. Check this list to find one near you: https://www.vegan.com/sanctuaries/. Or introduce them to books that celebrate the bond between humans and farmed animals. The classic, beloved *Charlotte's Web* is an ideal choice.

Help children explore new plant foods through fun family activities that involve preparing and tasting different vegan versions of favorite menu items. You might taste-test a variety of plant milks served over favorite cereals or hold a mini chili cook-off comparing chili recipes made with beans and TVP. Or compare grilled cheese sandwiches using different vegan cheeses. Your child will develop cooking skills while also getting to exert some control over new meals.

Every meal doesn't have to be an adventure, though. You can also focus on foods they already enjoy like peanut butter and banana sandwiches, spaghetti with marinara sauce, and hummus wraps.

REAL VEGAN CHILDREN

We asked parents to share their experiences in raising vegan children. We were especially interested in hearing about what their kids like to eat, and whether they experience social challenges in being vegan. Parents told us that their kids are happy, active, and thriving. They are sometimes picky about food (just like nonvegan kids) but mostly enjoy a variety of foods, including some treats. And while there are sometimes challenges at school and birthday parties, both the parents and children believe that the joys of a compassionate vegan lifestyle are worth any extra effort. Here are a few of the responses we received:

CLARENCE TAN IS RAISING THREE VEGAN CHILDREN WITH HIS WIFE NG SHWU HUEY IN SINGAPORE:

"Our eldest, Jude (who is now 6) surprised even us when as a toddler he would polish off handfuls of leafy greens. Four-year-old Julia is different and prefers carbs, especially bread, but she and her brother both love broccoli. Baby Julianne is six months old and just discovering new tastes, like avocado and steamed carrots. She likes everything so far.

The two older kids went to a Montessori kindergarten that was very respectful of our dietary choices. When friends asked why he was vegan, Jude would say, 'Because I don't want to kill animals,' and that was that. Home-packed lunches for the older children might be various stir-fries, pastas, wraps, sandwiches, and congee. We make sure to include greens, beans, grains, fruits, and seeds in their daily diet.

Our children are very active (cycling, swimming, football, and skating) and hardly ever fall sick, which goes a long way to convincing relatives and friends that this really is a nutritious and healthful diet."

LESLEY AND RAY PARKER-ROLLINS HAVE BEEN RAISING SEVENTEEN-YEAR-OLD TYLER, SIXTEEN-YEAR-OLD WILL, AND ELEVEN-YEAR-OLD MAYA VEGAN SINCE BIRTH. LESLEY SAYS THAT THEY ARE LIVING EXAMPLES OF HAPPY, HEALTHY VEGAN CHILDREN:

"The freezer and cabinets are regularly stocked with vegan desserts and snacks so the kids can enjoy themselves at birthday parties, sleepovers, and school events. They also enjoy veganized versions of some of the kid-friendly staples like chicken nuggets, macaroni and cheese, pizza, and burgers. At home, some favorite dishes are tofu-vegetable stir-fries, spinach lasagna, vegan drummies, and tacos.

Tyler plays varsity football at his high school and is beginning his college search. Will likes playing video games and photography, and Maya enjoys the running club and drama club at her school.

I love that our children don't believe that animals are here for our use. Throughout their lives, their father and I have made sure they know that they can come to us with any questions, concerns, or ideas they may have regarding their experiences living in a not-yet-vegan world. I believe our children are grateful to us for teaching them to make compassionate choices for themselves, the animals, and the planet."

KELLY BERGEN IS A MOM OF TWO VEGAN CHILDREN, AGES THREE-AND-A-HALF AND SEVEN:

"They can be fussy eaters, despite being exposed to a great variety of foods from a young age, so we try to cram as much nutrition into their smoothies as possible each morning. They've been having smoothies (fruit and any combo of flaxseeds, hempseeds, pumpkin seeds, protein powder, peanut butter, cocoa powder, and nondairy milk or water) every morning for years. We eat a lot of whole grains and legumes, with Gardein for treat nights. We buy a lot of different fruits and vegetables, but which ones they'll eat depend on what phase they're in at the time. They're super healthy so far and the oldest is excelling in school and enrolled in soccer. Our kids do get their fair share of colds but recover quickly and have only needed to see the doctor a small handful of times.

Our kids know that we are vegan for ethical and environmental reasons and my oldest often writes about environmentalism and veganism in school. We teach them to lead by example and not criticize other people's choices in front of them. They're encouraged to discuss their feelings about other people's choices with us in private instead. We visit a farm sanctuary once a year to make sure they get to have positive interactions with animals and can put a face to the foods. Ruby Roth's books have been great resources for educating them at their level."

JOSIE AND MITCH STEIGER ARE RAISING THEIR TODDLER EVAN, WHO HAS BEEN VEGAN SINCE CONCEPTION. JOSIE SAYS THAT EVAN IS A SHINING EXAMPLE OF A HEALTHY VEGAN CHILD:

"Even now people have so many misconceptions about raising a child vegan. When people see my son, I know he combats those negative stereotypes. He's very interactive—constantly giggling and smiling—and people always comment on how big he is for his age. Evan has never been sick and loves to eat—everything from oatmeal mixed with fruit and nut butter to bananas to pizza to the occasional bite of cookie.

As my son grows older, I look forward to providing vegan treats for school and extracurricular activities to help open people's minds about how delicious vegan food is. But more than that, I want to empower my son with information so that he can explain why he's vegan. I think it's important to understand that it's okay to have to put in extra effort at times to do what's right."

MARY MARTIN IS CHIEF OPERATING OFFICER OF A THINK TANK FOR THE FINANCIAL SERVICES INDUSTRY AND A MOM TO A NINE-YEAR-OLD VEGAN DAUGHTER:

"My daughter was adopted on day 3 and has been vegan ever since. She is a green belt in Tae Kwon Do, an amazing swimmer, and a super curious, kind, funny, smart kid. She is in the 75th percentile for height and weight, rarely gets sick, and loves herself some no-flour black bean brownies. Cucumbers with toasted sesame oil and nama shoyu, topped with black and white sesame seeds is her favorite veggie. For the most part, parties, camps, school, and playdates are uneventful. If nothing else, moms and kids want to eat our food and want the recipes."

LILA IS A MOM OF TWO YOUNG VEGANS, AGES THREE AND FIVE:

"Our 5-year-old seems to understand why we don't eat animal products and is happy to shout it loudly including in the supermarket and at parties! It seems obvious to her why you would choose 'plant bacon' over 'pig bacon' and she hasn't asked to eat meat. 'Meat is animals' is all she seems to need. There are so many cultural references to things like 'sausages,' 'burgers,' 'nuggets,' etc. that I am really glad we have plant versions so they don't feel too different. Saying that, I think my 5-year-old does love being different in this way and takes pride in it."

LAWYER AND WRITER ANNA PIPPUS HAS TWO VEGAN CHILDREN, AGES THREE AND SIX:

"We keep it simple with the kids when it comes to communicating why we're vegan. Our main message is that we should treat others the way we want to be treated, and that includes animals. That makes sense to them. We sometimes add that animals on farms aren't very happy to be there. We also say things like, 'Just like my milk is for you, cows make milk for their babies.' The hard question from them, then, is, 'Well, why isn't everyone vegan?' We explain that people have been eating animals for a long time and that it can be hard to make changes, that some people are still learning about animal farming, and that it's our job to be positive ambassadors for animals and for veganism. We try to communicate as well that just because someone isn't vegan, doesn't mean they're not a good person, that we are all a work in progress."

MELISSA RESNICK IS A VETERINARIAN AND A MOM OF VEGAN TWINS:

"My kids are happy, healthy vegan third graders who excel at school, sports, and music. They're living proof you don't need animal products to thrive. There was no complicated explanation needed because no kid really wants to kill or harm an animal when there are so many other things to eat. Their lunches are sometimes a little different from their classmates but they still get plenty of treats. While we're vegan for the animals, good health is a pretty great side effect—I've never once had to ask my kids to eat their veggies and fruit!

I worry sometimes about them feeling different or left out but when I ask, they always tell me they're so happy they're vegan. It makes me so happy to see the joy they have for food that didn't come about from animal suffering. Their compassion extends from a bug found in our house that they'll catch and release, to our pets, and to the animals they don't eat.

For more stories of real vegan children, visit veganhealth.org/real -vegan-children/.

RAISING A NEW GENERATION OF BOYS, WITH A FOCUS ON COMPASSION

Mitch Steiger, father to a vegan toddler, views veganism as one way to challenge socially ingrained concepts of how men should behave. "As a father raising a son, I know that the pressure to be 'manly' or 'masculine' can be overwhelming and lead boys to make terrible decisions, from bullying people to hurting animals. While I can't save Evan from that pressure, I can help arm him with what he needs to withstand it: a good base of knowledge from which to build a solid moral compass and the self-confidence to defend those who need his help.

I also want to teach him that strength, independence, and deserving respect have nothing to do with gender, and physical strength is either useless or harmful without mental, emotional, and spiritual strength. Hopefully, I can successfully encourage him to develop all of these so that he can and will consistently stand up for what's right, despite what a lonely endeavor that can sometimes be, especially when it comes time to defend animals with his words or his actions."

CHILDREN AND WEIGHT

The incidence of overweight and obesity among children is at an all-time high, and vegan kids are not immune to this. Weight is a complex issue and with children especially, it's important to approach it in ways that encourage healthy habits as well as healthy self-esteem. Children should not be put on weight reduction diets and should never be criticized about their body size. To encourage habits that will reduce risk of obesity, consider these tips:

- Make it easy for kids to eat lots of fruits and vegetables by keeping washed, trimmed raw vegetables and hummus or bean dips in the refrigerator and a bowl of fruit on the counter.
- Limit sweet drinks, including juices. A splash of fruit juice in a glass of sparkling water is a fun, low-sugar option.
- Cancel the family's membership to the "clean plate" club. Children know when they are full and shouldn't be forced to eat more. Allowing them to say when they have had enough reinforces the idea that they should eat only when hungry.
- Put sweets and snacks in their place. Don't refer to them as "bad," but don't elevate them in the minds of your children by using them to reward behavior. Serve healthy foods most of the time and offer occasional treats.
- Encourage kids to be active either through organized sports, or creative play, or family activities like an after-dinner walk or weekend hikes.
- Limit screen time. The American Academy of Pediatrics recommends no more than one hour per day of high-quality programs for children between the ages of two and five years. For children six and older, place limits on screen time and also on the types of media viewed. The AAP's Healthy Children website offers a family media planning guide: https://www.healthychildren.org /English/media/Pages/default.aspx.
- Be a role model for healthful eating and exercise habits.

- Be a role model for a healthy body image. Avoid making negative comments about your own body or making either positive or negative comments about the bodies of others.

MEAL PLANNING GUIDELINES FOR PRESCHOOLERS, SCHOOL-AGE CHILDREN, AND TEENS

Food group	Servings	
	Four to eight years old	Preteens and teens
Grains	6–8	8–10
Protein-rich foods: Legumes and soyfoods	3	5
Nuts and seeds	1 or more	1 or more
Vegetables	4	4
Fruits	2–5	2–5
Fats	2	3
Calcium-rich foods	At least 3 cups per day of some combination of foods that are good sources of well-absorbed calcium. These include fortified plant milks, fortified juices, calcium-set tofu, oranges, and low-oxalate leafy green vegetables like kale, mustard greens, turnip greens, bok choy, and collard greens.	At least 4 cups per day of some combination of foods that are good sources of well-absorbed calcium. These include fortified plant milks, fortified juices, calcium-set tofu, oranges, and low-oxalate leafy green vegetables like kale, mustard greens, turnip greens, bok choy, and collard greens.

In addition to foods from the food guide, the following supplements can help your child meet nutrient needs.

SUPPLEMENTS FOR PRESCHOOLERS, SCHOOL-AGE CHILDREN, AND TEENS

Age	B_{12} in daily dose (micrograms)	B_{12} in two doses per week (micrograms)*	Iodine (micrograms)	Vitamin D (International Units)**	DHA (milligrams)
1–3 years	10–40	375	90	600	200
4–8 years	13–50	500	90	600	200
9–13 years	20–75	750	120	600–1,000	200
14–20 years	25–100	1,000	150	600–1,000	200

*If vitamin B_{12} supplement is taken twice a week rather than daily, use these amounts for each of the two doses.
**Current recommended vitamin D intake is 600 International Units for children over the age of one year. We've provided a range of intakes up to 1,000 International Units since some experts believe higher intakes are beneficial.

A NOTE ABOUT DHA

There are no studies measuring levels of the long-chain omega-3 fats EPA or DHA in vegetarian or vegan children. However, we do know that many healthy children have been raised on vegan diets without supplements of either the long-chain omega-3 fats or the essential fatty acid alpha-linolenic acid (ALA). It's possible that children who are vegan from birth are more efficient at manufacturing DHA and EPA. But until we know more, we recommend a DHA supplement of about 200 milligrams per day for children.

SAMPLE MENU FOR PRESCHOOLER/ KINDERGARTEN-AGE

BREAKFAST
- ½ cup oatmeal with 2 tablespoons chopped walnuts or 1 tablespoon ground flaxseeds
- ½ cup calcium-fortified orange juice
- 1 slice whole wheat toast with 1 tablespoon almond butter

SNACK
- ½ cup fortified soymilk
- 1 small carrot muffin

LUNCH
- Missing Egg Salad Sandwich: Small whole wheat pita pocket, ½ cup mashed tofu, ½ tablespoon vegan mayonnaise, shredded zucchini
- 1 orange

SNACK
- Fruit smoothie: ½ frozen banana, ½ cup strawberries, 1 cup fortified soymilk

DINNER
- Rice pilaf: ½ cup brown rice, ¼ cup lentils, 2 tablespoons raisins
- ½ cup steamed kale with 1 tablespoon sliced almonds
- ¼ cup vegan ice cream

SNACK
- ½ cup fortified soymilk
- 2 fig bars

SAMPLE MENU FOR AN EIGHT-YEAR OLD

BREAKFAST
- ▸ 1 ounce ready-to-eat cereal with ½ tablespoon ground flaxseeds
- ▸ ½ cup fortified soymilk
- ▸ ½ cup sliced strawberries

SNACK
- ▸ ½ peanut butter and banana sandwich
- ▸ ½ cup fortified soymilk

LUNCH
- ▸ Taco: 1 corn tortilla, ¼ cup refried black beans cooked in 1 teaspoon olive oil, ½ cup chopped lettuce and tomato, 1 ounce shredded vegan cheese
- ▸ ½ cup calcium-fortified orange juice

SNACK
- ▸ Red pepper strips
- ▸ 3 tablespoons guacamole

DINNER
- ▸ 1 cup macaroni
- ▸ ½ cup tomato sauce with ¼ cup lentils
- ▸ ½ cup cooked carrots

SNACK
- ▸ ½ cup fortified soymilk
- ▸ 1 graham cracker

SAMPLE MENU FOR A TWELVE-YEAR-OLD

BREAKFAST
- ▸ 2 whole-wheat pancakes cooked in 2 teaspoons margarine
- ▸ 1 cup blueberries
- ▸ 2 tablespoons chopped walnuts
- ▸ 1 cup fortified soymilk

SNACK
- ▸ 5 figs
- ▸ ½ cup soy yogurt

LUNCH
- ▸ No-Tuna Sandwich: 2 slices whole wheat bread, ½ cup mashed chickpeas with chopped celery and 1 tablespoon vegan mayonnaise, sliced tomatoes
- ▸ Banana

SNACK
- ▸ 1 whole wheat roll
- ▸ Veggie burger
- ▸ Sliced tomato and pickles
- ▸ 1 cup fortified soymilk

DINNER
- ▸ 1 cup brown rice
- ▸ 1 cup steamed broccoli
- ▸ ½ cup steamed carrots
- ▸ ¼ cup peanut sauce

SAMPLE MENU FOR A TEENAGER
(ABOUT 2,200 CALORIES)

BREAKFAST

- ▸ 2 cups raisin bran
- ▸ 1 tablespoon ground flaxseeds
- ▸ 1 cup fortified soymilk
- ▸ 1 banana
- ▸ 1 slice whole-grain toast
- ▸ 2 tablespoons peanut butter

SNACK

- ▸ ¼ cup hummus
- ▸ Whole-grain crackers
- ▸ Raw carrots

LUNCH

- ▸ Falafels: 3 falafel, 1 medium whole-grain pita, shredded lettuce and chopped tomatoes, 2 tablespoons lemon-tahini sauce
- ▸ Orange
- ▸ 2 oatmeal cookies

SNACK

- ▸ Smoothie: ½ cup fortified soymilk, 1 cup frozen mixed berries

DINNER

- ▸ Black bean burger
- ▸ Whole-grain hamburger roll
- ▸ Ketchup and pickles
- ▸ Green salad with vinaigrette dressing
- ▸ 1 cup steamed broccoli

SAMPLE 3,000-CALORIE MENU FOR TEENAGE GROWTH SPURT

BREAKFAST ON-THE-GO

▸ Protein-rich smoothie: 1 cup silken tofu, ½ cup calcium-fortified orange juice, 1 frozen banana, 1 tablespoon ground flaxseeds
▸ English muffin with 2 tablespoons peanut butter

SNACK

▸ ¼ cup trail mix

LUNCH

▸ Vegan sub sandwich: 6-inch whole wheat sub roll, 4 vegan deli slices, 2 slices vegan cheese, lettuce, tomato, pickles, 1 tablespoon vegan mayonnaise
▸ 1 cup fortified almond milk
▸ Apple

SNACK

▸ 2 oatmeal cookies
▸ 1 cup fortified soymilk

DINNER

▸ Burritos: 3 medium whole wheat tortillas, 1 cup refried beans, ½ cup mashed avocado, chopped tomato and lettuce, salsa
▸ 1 cup brown rice
▸ 2 cups steamed kale with dressing of 2 tablespoons tahini seasoned with lemon juice

SNACK

▸ 2 cups bran flakes
▸ 1 cup fortified almond milk

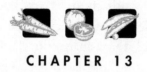

CHAPTER 13

Vegan Diets for People over Fifty

The process of aging begins early in life and some changes are taking place even when we are still in our twenties. Many age-related changes start to become most obvious in our fifties, though. The way you age and the speed at which you age is partly influenced by genetics, but lifestyle and environment play a much bigger role. Even if a healthy diet won't stop the clock, it can slow certain aging processes. For example, antioxidants, which are abundant in many plant foods, can counter some of the damage to cells that affect the aging process in skin, muscles, and your eyes. Diet and exercise may safeguard telomeres, which are protective caps at the end of DNA strands. Shortened telomeres are associated with aging and some evidence suggests that exercise, stress management, and plant-based diets, like a traditional Mediterranean pattern, are linked to greater telomere length.[1]

GOOD NUTRITION FOR HEALTHY AGING

The biggest issue for everyone, vegan or not, is that calorie needs for older adults decrease while nutrient needs stay generally the same or—in the cases of calcium, vitamin D, vitamin B_6, and possibly protein—go up. Needs increase for some of these nutrients in order to compensate for changes in digestion and absorption. Others are the result of slower protein synthesis and faster bone turnover that promote loss of both muscle and bone mass as you age.

The chart on page 222 shows changes in the RDAs for people over fifty. Some older omnivores and lacto-ovo vegetarians fall short on nutrient intake and we suspect that this is true for some vegans as well. Ensuring that nutrient needs are met can help protect bones, muscles, and cognitive function in aging.

KEEPING MUSCLE AND BONES STRONG

A common effect of aging is sarcopenia, which is the progressive loss of muscle mass and muscle strength. It's due to a number of factors, including lifestyle habits, disease, inflammation, hormonal changes, and age-related changes in muscle metabolism. Over time, sarcopenia can lead to frailty, problems with mobility, poor bone health, falls and fractures, decreased activity, and a loss of independence. The best strategies for preventing sarcopenia are exercise along with adequate protein and calorie intake.

There is some controversy, though, about how much protein older people need in order to maintain good muscle strength. Lower calorie intake results in slightly higher protein needs, and there is also evidence that protein is utilized less efficiently with aging. Many experts in protein nutrition and aging have called for an increase in the protein RDA for older people to at least 1 gram per kilogram of weight and perhaps as much as 1.2 grams.[2-4] Keeping in mind that vegans may have somewhat higher protein needs, this translates to about 0.5 to 0.6 grams per pound of healthy body weight. At the higher end of these recommendations, a woman weighing 130 pounds might need 78 grams of protein per day and a man weighing 160 pounds would need 96 grams.

This represents an increase of 25 to 50 percent more than the current RDA but it may be a reasonable goal. In one study, people with high protein intakes lost far less muscle after the age of seventy compared to those whose protein intakes were close to the current RDA.[5] Protein also protects bones and higher intake is linked to lower risk of hip fracture in postmenopausal women.[6]

Some experts also recommend emphasizing foods that are high in the amino acid leucine, which appears to help stimulate muscle synthesis. The best sources of leucine in vegan diets are the same foods we emphasize for protein in general: legumes. Research has shown that in vegetarians, getting protein from textured vegetable (soy) protein is just as effective as getting it from beef for muscle synthesis in older men.[7]

Although there is currently no consensus on protein needs of older people, it's clear that protein is important for maintaining muscles and that sarcopenia can be a very debilitating condition. A reasonable way to increase your protein intake without piling on extra calories is to replace some servings of grains in your diet with beans, soyfoods, and peanuts. Use the food guide in Chapter 10 but aim for just three servings of grains per day and five servings of legumes. The menu on page 222 shows one option for planning meals around these guidelines.

While there is still debate about the protein needs of older people, there are clear recommendations for increases in vitamin D and calcium. This is largely because synthesis of vitamin D from sun exposure declines and calcium absorption becomes less efficient with aging. By the time you're in your seventies, you may make only one-quarter the amount of vitamin D that your body produced back in your twenties.[8] The RDA for vitamin D is 800 International Units (20 micrograms) beginning at age seventy-one. Because it becomes so difficult to synthesize vitamin D from sun exposure as you get older, you'll need to get vitamin D from supplements and/or fortified foods. Fortified cereals and fortified plant milks can provide some vitamin D, but usually it isn't enough to meet the RDA. Talk to your health-care provider about how much vitamin D to take since some people need more than the RDA to maintain healthy blood levels.

Calcium needs increase from 1,000 to 1,200 milligrams per day after the age of fifty. This mineral is important not just for bone health but is also linked to better control of blood pressure and lower risk for colon cancer. Getting calcium from foods like leafy green vegetables, calcium-set tofu, and fortified milks is ideal. If you find yourself falling short of recommendations, consider a low-dose supplement just to make up the difference. Large doses of calcium that bring your intake above the RDA don't appear to have any benefits.

VITAMIN B$_{12}$: THE VEGAN ADVANTAGE

There is evidence that some signs of aging—such as loss of hearing, forgetfulness, confusion, and depression—could be related at least in part to inadequate vitamin B$_{12}$ since this vitamin affects the nervous system. A low intake of vitamin B$_{12}$ can also raise the risk for stroke, a problem in older people.

Both overt deficiency and marginal vitamin B$_{12}$ deficiency are common among older people eating different types of diets.[9] It may seem surprising that meat-eaters would develop a deficiency, but absorption of vitamin B$_{12}$ from meat, dairy, and eggs declines among a large percentage of older people due to digestive changes. Changes causing decreased absorption may affect as many as 30 percent of people over the age of fifty and 37 percent of those over the age of eighty.[10] However, most of these changes don't affect absorption of vitamin B$_{12}$ in supplements and fortified foods. Therefore, the National Academies advises all people over the age of fifty to get at least half of their B$_{12}$ from these sources. Many people, though, aren't aware of this recommendation. This is where vegans might have the edge, as we discussed in Chapter 6. Vegans who are educated about good nutrition are *already* taking B$_{12}$ supplements. Some research has shown that older adults need as much as 500 micrograms per day. If you have impaired kidney function, talk with your doctor about B$_{12}$ supplements.

PROTECTING COGNITIVE FUNCTION

We don't have any information about cognitive function in older vegans, but among Seventh-Day Adventists (See page 73 for more about health practices of the Seventh-Day Adventist Church), people who eat meat were more than twice as likely to develop dementia.[11]

Alzheimer's disease is the most common type of dementia. It's characterized by deposits of plaque and abnormal tangles of proteins in the brain. There is a genetic component to Alzheimer's but there is also evidence that certain factors like inflammation and oxidative stress, both of which are related to diet, can raise risk. We talk about oxidative stress on page 218.

Another type of dementia is the result of atherosclerosis (buildup of fats and cholesterol) in arteries leading to the brain, reducing the flow of oxygen to brain cells. Because a vegan diet is associated with both lower cholesterol and lower blood pressure, it offers a way to reduce risk for this type of dementia. See Chapter 15 for more information about how to protect the health of your arteries.

Meeting nutrient needs is essential for protecting cognitive function. Deficiencies in vitamin B_{12}, B_6, and folate can result in higher levels of homocysteine, which might raise the risk for cognitive decline.[12-15] Older people have higher requirements for vitamin B_6 and it appears that men need more than women—despite the fact that needs are identical for younger men and women. This means that, while older women only have a slight increase in needs, the recommendations for older men are 30 percent higher than younger men. Many plant foods have moderate amounts of vitamin B_6 and intakes among vegans are generally good.[16,17] The foods that are the best sources of vitamin B_6 are avocados, bananas, spinach, potatoes, sweet potatoes, fortified breakfast cereals, and soymilk. Beans all contain moderate amounts of vitamin B_6.

Finally, it's possible that supplements of the omega-3 fats DHA and EPA could help protect cognitive function, but overall, the evidence for this is slim.[18]

Nondietary factors play a significant role in keeping the brain young. Exercise seems to be especially important, as is challenging your brain as much as possible by reading, doing crossword puzzles, or learning new skills.

Tips for Protecting Cognitive Function:

- Yes, we sound like a broken record when it comes to this, but we can't say it too often: Make sure you have a reliable source of vitamin B_{12} in your diet.
- Choose foods that are good sources of vitamin B_6 (avocados, bananas, spinach, potatoes, sweet potatoes, fortified breakfast cereals, soymilk, and beans).
- Eat an antioxidant-rich diet by consuming lots of fruits and vegetables, including leafy greens and berries (frozen and fresh).
- Exercise your body with daily walking, weight training, or an exercise class.
- Exercise your mind: do crossword puzzles, play Words with Friends, master a new language, learn to play the piano, or write your memoirs for the grandkids. Even for people as young as fifty, these kinds of activities may help protect cognitive function.

ANTIOXIDANTS AND AGING

Foods that are rich in antioxidants may help protect your bones, muscles, brain, and even eyes by countering the effects of free radicals. Free radicals are normal products of metabolism and energy production. They have a short lifespan of about one-millionth of a second, but in that time, they can set off a chain reaction of cellular damage. This leads to oxidative stress, a condition linked to both muscle loss and osteoporosis.[19-21]

Plants have thousands of antioxidants, which are compounds that can put a stop to the damage from free radicals. Animal foods have antioxidants, too, but their content pales in comparison to plants. In one evaluation of more than 3,100 different foods, the average antioxidant content of plant foods was about sixty-four times higher than the average content of meat, dairy, and eggs.[22] Fruits and vegetables are antioxidant powerhouses, but these compounds also occur in beans, nuts, seeds, soyfoods, and whole grains, and even in olive oil, coffee, and tea. So it's not surprising that some research has found better antioxidant status or lower levels of markers of oxidative damage in people who eat more plant-based diets including vegans and vegetarians.[23,24]

Good antioxidant status may offer real advantages for older vegans. For example, a study in the United Kingdom showed that vegans had a much lower risk of developing cataracts, a common symptom of aging, compared to people who ate meat.[25]

Eating more antioxidant-rich foods may also offer protection against Alzheimer's disease. Researchers at Rush University Medical Center in Chicago and Harvard School of Public Health in Boston developed the MIND diet based on studies of dietary patterns that can lower risk for and delay progression of Alzheimer's disease. While the MIND diet is not vegan, it limits animal foods and places an emphasis on antioxidant-rich plant foods, especially leafy green vegetables, berries, nuts, whole grains, beans, and olive oil.[26,27]

Since some of these antioxidants need fat for their absorption, avoid letting your diet get too low in fat. Choosing a diet that meets nutrient needs and that is rich in antioxidants is a powerful way to protect health through the years.

IRON FOR OLDER VEGANS

Iron needs don't increase with aging. In fact, for women, they drop by roughly half since women no longer lose iron through monthly periods. Iron deficiency is still fairly common among people over the age of 65, though, and it's very common in people over the age of 85.[28] As at all other stages of the life cycle, vegans need to give extra attention to iron, ensuring not only generous intakes but also aiming to consume a good source of vitamin C at as many meals and snacks as possible to ensure iron is well-absorbed.

MEAL-PLANNING CHALLENGES

The challenges in planning healthy meals for older people aren't all related to changes in nutrient needs. Taste sensitivity declines with aging due to either a decline in the sense of smell or an actual reduction in the number of taste buds. It is a real phenomenon and can lead to over-salting of food or poor appetite. It's hard to eat if food doesn't taste good, but it's not difficult to add a burst of flavor to foods with a few simple tricks:

- Boost the umami in dishes by stirring nutritional yeast into bean dishes, blending sun-dried tomatoes into dips, and roasting vegetables with balsamic vinegar. See page 31 for more information about umami.
- Double up on the herbs and spices in your favorite recipes if they no longer taste as good as they used to.
- Add chopped or dried fruit to savory grain dishes for a contrasting sweet flavor.
- Add a few drops of liquid smoke to beans or to marinades for vegetables, tofu, or tempeh.
- If you like spicy foods, perk up meals with salsa or cayenne pepper, or add curry powder to beans.

Changes in living situations can have a significant effect on food choices, too. Older people who find themselves living alone may find that their interest in cooking and eating suffers. If your local senior center offers meals, call to see if there is a vegan option. (If enough people ask, they might just add one.) Check to see if your community has a local vegetarian group or a group devoted to animal rights or animal welfare issues. Many of these organizations hold potluck meals and offer cooking classes. Seventh-Day Adventist churches often hold free cooking classes and meals. The meetup.com website is an easy way to find all kinds of groups devoted to shared interests.

If you can't find a vegan group to join, you can still enjoy eating your own vegan food with others. Join a book group and bring a platter of vegan cookies or take a vegan dish to the next church potluck or coffee hour.

If getting out of the house is a problem, especially during cold weather, most grocery stores have deliveries. Meals on Wheels may have vegetarian foods, but vegan offerings are still fairly rare. Again, it can't hurt to ask, and it will plant the idea that people are looking for these options.

NUTRITION TIPS FOR OLDER VEGANS

- Keep an eye on calories. As calorie needs decrease with aging, it's important either to cut back on calorie intake or—a better idea for all-around health—to increase physical activity.
- Limit empty-calorie sweets and snack foods. This is good advice for everyone, but if you are cutting back on calories to manage your weight, it's important to get the most you can from the foods you are eating. Choose plenty of whole plant foods and fortified foods to meet nutrient needs.
- Eat plenty of vitamin B_6-rich foods like potatoes, sweet potatoes, bananas, figs, beans, veggie meats made from soy, avocados, spinach, fortified breakfast cereals, and soymilk.
- Take a vitamin D supplement. It's unlikely that older people—vegan or omnivore—can meet needs otherwise.
- Choose plenty of calcium-rich foods. If your diet regularly falls short of calcium, take a modest supplement.
- It goes without saying that no matter how old you are, a vitamin B_{12} supplement is essential.
- Give your diet a protein boost by consuming plenty of legumes, nut butters, and soy products. Choose quinoa instead of rice or barley because it is one of the most protein-rich grains.
- Don't forget to drink plenty of water. Many older people don't get enough liquids.

CHANGES IN NUTRIENT NEEDS WITH AGING

	Age 31–50		Age 51–70		Age 70-plus	
	M	F	M	F	M	F
Calcium AI milligrams	1,000	1,000	1,200	1,200	1,200	1,200
Vitamin D AI International Units	600	600	600	600	800	800
Iron RDA milligrams	8	18	8	8	8	8
Iron RDA milligrams, vegetarians	14	33	14	14	14	14
Vitamin B_6 RDA milligrams	1.3	1.3	1.7	1.5	1.7	1.5
Vitamin B_{12} RDA micrograms	2.4	2.4	2.4	2.4	2.4	2.4

THIS SAMPLE MENU FOR OLDER PEOPLE MAXIMIZES NUTRIENT INTAKE WITH AFFORDABLE, EASY-TO-PREPARE MEALS

BREAKFAST

- ▸ 1 ounce bran flakes with ½ cup chopped walnuts
- ▸ 1 cup fortified soymilk
- ▸ 1 banana, sliced

SNACK

- ▸ ½ whole wheat English muffin
- ▸ 2 tablespoons peanut butter
- ▸ ½ cup grapes

LUNCH

- ▸ 1 cup homemade or reduced-sodium canned black bean soup
- ▸ Tossed green salad with vinaigrette dressing

SNACK

- ▸ Smoothie with ½ cup tofu and ½ cup frozen strawberries

DINNER

- ▸ Bean burrito: 1 corn tortilla with ½ cup refried beans, topped with chopped tomatoes, avocado, and salsa
- ▸ 1 cup braised kale
- ▸ ½ cup vegan ice cream

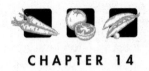

CHAPTER 14

Sports Nutrition for Vegans

There is no question that plant-based diets are suitable for athletes, including those involved in competitive sports. Some of the most talented athletes in the world in a variety of sports including football, weightlifting, tennis, and car racing have enjoyed successful careers eating diets built around plant foods.

Most of us aren't in their league, of course. If you're hitting the gym two or three times a week to work out, you probably don't need to change much about your vegan diet. However, exercise physiologists recommend higher protein intakes for building muscle mass. It's likely this affects even noncompetitive fitness buffs who want to get stronger. Iron is another nutrient that needs some attention in the diets of vegan athletes, and we'll also talk about the performance enhancers creatine, carnitine, and carnosine.

MEETING ENERGY NEEDS

Exercise efficiency, gender, non-exercise habits, body size, and genetics all affect calorie requirements. And because needs vary with every individual and depend on how much exercise you do, there is no set formula for determining your energy requirements; it's a matter of experimentation. Energy needs for athletes can range anywhere from 2,000 to 6,000 calories per day.

Endurance athletes like long-distance runners have higher calorie needs than strength athletes but for any athlete, inadequate calorie intake can result in muscle loss, increased risk of injury, and poor recovery from exercise. Female athletes who don't get enough calories can stop menstruating, which is linked to poor bone health.

In general, vegans tend to consume fewer calories than people who eat meat and teen athletes and others with high calorie needs may find it a challenge to eat enough. If you need help in meeting calorie needs, simple additions and adjustments to your diet can help boost calories:

- Include more refined grains in meals. While whole grains are normally the best choice for optimal health, athletes who eat a large quantity of food can afford to eat more processed foods than nonathletes. Because of their lower fiber content, processed foods are less filling. Pasta is a good option since, as long as it is cooked al dente, its carbohydrate is more slowly released into the bloodstream compared with other processed grains. Or choose pasta made from lentils, black beans, or edamame for an especially protein-rich choice.
- Use moderate amounts of oils on salads and for sautéing vegetables.
- Snack on nuts or trail mix or vegan yogurt with granola.
- Add avocado or nut butters to sandwiches to boost fat and calorie intake.
- Add tofu or tempeh to salads or mix it into grain dishes to increase calorie, fat, and protein content of meals.
- Add silken tofu to fruit smoothies.
- Carry energy bars with you for snacks-on-the-go.

PROTEIN

There is considerable agreement among experts in sports nutrition that both endurance and strength athletes require more protein than the RDA.[1,2] Recommendations for daily protein needs of athletes generally range from 1.2 to 2.0 grams of protein per kilogram of body weight. Some experts recommend that at minimum, athletes should strive to consume twice the RDA.[3] Keeping in mind that vegans have a slightly higher protein requirement, a vegan athlete should aim for about 1.8 grams of protein per kilogram of body weight (or 0.8 grams of protein per pound of body weight).

The exact protein requirement varies depending on a number of factors, though. Those who are just starting a training program and actively building muscle need more protein than athletes who are trained and maintaining muscle mass. Since getting enough calories spares protein for muscle synthesis, an athlete who is restricting calories to lose body fat will also need more protein. Those engaged in endurance sports are likely to need somewhat less protein than athletes attempting to build considerable muscle—although because of their high calorie intake, most endurance athletes are likely to end up with fairly high protein intakes.

The timing of protein intake has been a topic of much debate among sports nutritionists. Older recommendations were to consume a protein-rich meal within a couple of hours after exercise to maximize muscle protein synthesis. But newer evidence shows that muscle protein synthesis increases for at least twenty-four hours following strength training and there are similar increases following endurance exercise.[1] This means that consuming a big dose of protein right after exercise is probably not important. However, there does seem to be an advantage to dividing protein intake across several meals throughout the day.[3] A reasonable approach for vegans would be to consume four meals per day with each meal providing 0.2 grams of protein per pound of body weight. This translates to 26 grams of protein per meal for an athlete weighing 130 pounds and 34 grams per meal for one who weighs 170 pounds. It's fine to divide this protein into smaller doses across more meals if you prefer.

Although protein powders aren't essential for meeting needs and supporting muscle strength, many athletes find them to be an easy way to boost protein intake. Among nonvegans, whey protein is popular because it's high in leucine, an essential amino acid that stimulates protein synthesis.[4] But the evidence suggests that the source of the protein plays only a minor role in muscle synthesis. Soy protein has been found to be as effective as whey and other animal protein sources for muscle mass and strength.[3,5,6] We don't currently have information on the effects of other types of protein powders but successful body builders use powders based on pea, rice, and other plant proteins. Vegan athletes also have the option of adding a small leucine supplement to their diet. Keep in mind, though, that a mix of amino acids is needed for adequate muscle synthesis so taking a dose of leucine in place of food isn't the ideal approach.

While these recommendations are aimed at those who train rigorously, building and maintaining muscle mass is good advice for everyone. It's especially important with aging to guard against bone loss and to maintain balance and strength over the decades. Older muscles appear to be less sensitive to protein, which means that it takes more to stimulate muscle protein synthesis. The protein recommendations we make here for athletes are also most likely appropriate for anyone over the age of sixty who wants to build and maintain healthy muscles.

CARBOHYDRATE AND FAT

Carbohydrates serve as a primary fuel for both muscle and brain during intense workouts and people who try to cut back on carbs often compromise their performance. Just as for protein and calories, exact requirements for carbohydrates depend on training and calorie needs. Most athletes need between 5 and 12 grams of carbohydrate per kilogram of body weight per day or about 2.2 to 5.5 grams per pound of weight. Those engaged in endurance activities should aim for the upper end of that range. Vegans are in good standing in this regard, since plant-based diets are typically high in carbohydrates.

Very high-fat, low-carbohydrate diets seem to impair high-intensity athletic performance.[1] (We talk about some of the issues regarding keto diets in Chapter 15.) There is also no advantage to consuming a diet that is very low in fat. In their joint position statement on sports nutrition, the Academy of Nutrition and Dietetics and the American College of Sports Medicine recommend getting at least 20 percent of calories from fat.

IRON

Iron losses can occur with all types of intense exercise, particularly in endurance exercises like long-distance running. It's especially relevant to female athletes since their needs may be as much as 70 percent higher than the RDA.[7] This raises questions for female vegan athletes in particular since, as we discussed in Chapter 8, vegans and other vegetarians have higher iron requirements than meat-eaters. Unless you have been diagnosed with iron deficiency, however, routine iron supplements aren't recommended. All vegan athletes should give some attention to including plenty of iron-rich foods in their diets and to the strategies for maximizing iron absorption that we outlined on page 109. Including a good source of vitamin C at meals and snacks is the best way to ensure good iron absorption from your diet. Periodic screening to make sure your iron status is good is helpful for all athletes, but especially vegan women.

PERFORMANCE ENHANCERS

A number of supplements, which include amino acids and other protein-type compounds, are marketed to athletes to enhance their performance.

Creatine

Creatine is the only nutritional supplement that has been consistently shown to improve strength and muscle mass in strength athletes in a large number of clinical trials. However, showing benefits during a specific athletic event (other than weightlifting) has been more elusive. And even within weightlifting, there appear to be creatine "responders" and "nonresponders."

Creatine reduces fatigue during repeated, short bursts of intense exercise—the type that occurs with weightlifting, sprinting, soccer, rugby, and hockey. Less fatigue during sprinting and weightlifting can mean increased training and greater results. Creatine is associated with gains in muscle and with improved carbohydrate storage in the body for fueling endurance sports.[8,9]

Humans synthesize creatine in their liver and kidneys, and meat-eaters consume around 1 to 2 grams of creatine per day (although about 30 percent of it is destroyed in cooking). There is no creatine in vegetarian diets, though, and not surprisingly, vegetarians have lower levels of creatine in their blood, urine, red blood cells, and muscle tissue. One study found that vegetarians benefit more from creatine supplementation than meat-eaters.[10] It appears that athletes with higher levels of creatine derive less benefit from supplements.[11] Fortunately, for those who wish to try creatine supplements, they are vegan.

Creatine supplements are usually taken in two phases for loading and maintenance. Taking creatine with a carbohydrate-rich food like juice can help muscles absorb the creatine.

Loading: Take approximately 20 grams per day divided into four equal doses over the course of the day, for a total of six days.

Maintenance: The usual dose of 2 grams per day is meant for meat-eaters, which means that the dose for vegans may be closer to 2.7 to 3.4 grams per day.[12] Some researchers suggest taking creatine only every other month to maximize its effects.

The most common adverse effects of creatine supplementation are weight gain (which is due primarily to fluid gain).[13] Some athletes also experience gastrointestinal discomfort.[1] Although its use is widely debated, it is generally considered safe for adults.[14] That said, there have been anecdotal reports of dehydration, muscle strains or tears, and kidney damage, so it's important to let your health-care professional know if you are taking creatine.

Carnitine

Carnitine (also known as L-carnitine and acetyl-L-carnitine) is an amino acid found in meat and dairy products. It's needed for fat metabolism and is promoted for weight loss and improved performance. However, there is little evidence that it helps with either.

While there is very little carnitine in plant foods, it can be synthesized by the liver and kidneys. Vegans, vegetarians, and people who consume lower-fat, high-carbohydrate diets have lower blood levels of carnitine. There is no indication that this is unhealthy, and we don't know if it has any bearing on athletic performance. In one study, vegans who took supplements of 120 milligrams of carnitine per day for two months excreted more carnitine in their urine, but the levels in their plasma didn't increase significantly. This suggests that most of the carnitine was being lost in the urine.[15]

There is no evidence that vegans need to take carnitine, but since nonvegetarians typically eat 100 to 300 milligrams of carnitine per day, it is probably safe for vegans to take supplements providing that amount. Solgar brand carnitine is made by yeast fermentation of beet sugar and is one option available to vegans. If you take carnitine, watch for side effects, including nausea and diarrhea.

Carnosine and Beta-Alanine

Carnosine (also known as beta-alanyl-L-histidine) is a molecule made up of two amino acids, beta-alanine and histidine. Animals, including humans, produce it in various tissues, especially the muscles and the brain. Plant foods don't contain any, and one study has shown that vegetarians have 50 percent less carnosine than meat-eaters in their muscle tissue.[16] Exercise itself can boost carnosine levels, though, and one study found that high-intensity interval training increased muscle carnosine levels in vegetarian men who were not consuming beta-alanine.[17]

Although the amino acid beta-alanine isn't required in the diet (the body makes its own), beta-alanine supplements have been shown to increase muscle carnosine levels. Even though carnosine supplements are available, to our knowledge, only beta-alanine, not carnosine itself, has been tested on athletic performance in human subjects.

About half a dozen studies have shown that approximately 6 grams of beta-alanine in doses spread over a day, for a period of four or more weeks, results in improved ability to perform, particularly during bouts of cycling.[18,19] Not all studies have shown a significant benefit, though.[20]

The athletic performance of some individuals might benefit from beta-alanine supplementation, and vegetarians could possibly benefit more than nonvegetarians, although no studies have compared the two groups. Now Foods makes a vegan beta-alanine supplement.

Beta-alanine appears to be safe in amounts of 6 grams per day for up to ten weeks, although some people have reported mild numbness or tingling.

THE FEMALE ATHLETE: HEALTH ISSUES

The female athlete triad is characterized by low body weight, insufficient calories, and loss of menstruation, referred to as amenorrhea. It's especially common in sports that emphasize lean body size like gymnastics and figure skating, and activities with high calorie expenditure like running. In fact, more than half of young women who are long-distance runners may experience amenorrhea. Amenorrhea correlates strongly with poor bone health. Even though weight-bearing exercise protects bones, it doesn't compensate for the reduced bone formation that is seen in women who stop menstruating.

Vegan athletes may be at greater risk for low body weight and amenorrhea because vegans often consume fewer calories. The high-fiber content of plant foods can cause an athlete to experience a sense of fullness before consuming enough energy.

The best treatment for amenorrhea is to decrease exercise, increase calories, and, if necessary, increase body weight. Increasing calories by

200 to 300 per day and not exercising for one day per week is a reasonable approach to restoring a normal menstrual cycle.[21] Even with this approach, it can take many months and even as long as a year for women to begin menstruating again. It is also crucial for all female athletes to meet recommendations for calcium and vitamin D. Vegans may need to use supplements of both nutrients to meet needs.

FUELING COMPETITION

Staying hydrated and ensuring sufficient fuel are keys to success in athletic competition.

Many athletes involved in endurance events build their glycogen stores through carbohydrate loading by tapering off activity during the twenty-three hours before an event and packing their meals with carbohydrate-rich foods. Vegan meals are clearly ideal for this. Eating carbohydrates in the hours just before an event can increase glycogen stores even further, especially in the liver, and can also provide an additional source of fuel during competition from glucose that is still in the digestive tract.[1]

A pre-event meal should be low in fat and fiber, moderate in protein and rich in carbohydrates to allow the stomach to empty more quickly. Depending on your body size, aim to drink between 1½ and 3 cups of fluids in the two to four hours before an event. The goal is to achieve urine that is pale yellow in color while having enough time to empty your bladder before competing.

During endurance exercise of more than an hour, consuming 30 to 90 grams of carbohydrates from drinks or gels is associated with better performance. Most athletes need to drink about 0.4 to 0.8 liters of fluid per hour during competition. If your event is just an hour or less, you won't need to consume calories, but some research shows that simply exposing your mouth to small amounts of carbohydrate can stimulate the brain and enhance performance. For longer competition, consuming about 30 to 60 grams per hour (or 90 grams per hour for very long events) of carbohydrates from drinks, gels, and energy bars helps fuel performance.

After an event, the goal is to restore glycogen, ensure that you're well-hydrated, and fuel protein synthesis in your muscles. Choose a post-event meal that provides about ½ gram of carbohydrates per pound of your body weight plus 20 to 25 grams of protein. Over the next hours drink 1¼ to 1½ quarts of fluid for every pound of body weight lost. Continue to consume high carbohydrate foods over the next four to six hours.

MEAL PLANNING GUIDELINES FOR ATHLETES

Food group	2,500 calories	3,000 calories	4,000 calories
Legumes (beans, soyfoods, peanut butter, protein powders)	6 servings	7 servings	8 servings
Fruits and vegetables	10	12	15
Grains	8	10	14
Nuts/seeds	2	2	4
Oils	2	3	4

SAMPLE MENUS

2,500 CALORIES: FIVE MEALS

MEAL 1

▸ ½ cup baked tofu
▸ Whole-wheat toast with 1 teaspoon vegan margarine
▸ Banana

MEAL 2

▸ 1 cup navy beans cooked in ½ cup tomato sauce
▸ 1 cup brown rice

MEAL 3

▸ 1 veggie burger
▸ 1½ cups quinoa
▸ 1 cup cooked collards

MEAL 4

▸ Salad: 2 cups mixed greens, ½ cup kidney beans, ½ cup mixed nuts, 2 mandarin oranges, vinaigrette dressing with 2 teaspoons oil

MEAL 5

▸ 1 cup sweet potatoes with 1 teaspoon vegan margarine
▸ ½ cup baked tofu
▸ 1 cup steamed broccoli

3,000 CALORIES: FIVE MEALS

MEAL 1

▸ Smoothie: 1 scoop protein powder, ½ cup frozen strawberries, 1 banana, 1 cup soy or pea milk

MEAL 2

▸ Veggie burger
▸ Quinoa salad: 1½ cups quinoa, ½ cup almonds, 2 mandarin oranges, vinaigrette with 1 teaspoon oil

MEAL 3

▸ 2 cups rice
▸ 1 cup red beans
▸ 1 cup roasted green beans
▸ ½ cup squash

MEAL 4

▸ 1 slice toast
▸ 2 tablespoons peanut butter

MEAL 5

▸ Salad: 2 cups mixed greens, ½ cup chickpeas, 1 cup tomatoes, 2 cups chopped raw vegetables, ¼ cup walnuts, vinaigrette with 2 teaspoons oil
▸ Baked potato

4,000 CALORIES: SIX MEALS

MEAL 1

‣ Scrambled tofu and spinach: 1 cup tofu, 1 cup spinach, 1 teaspoon oil
‣ 1 cup roasted potatoes
‣ 1 whole-wheat toast with 1 teaspoon vegan margarine

MEAL 2

‣ 3 cups pasta
‣ 1 cup white beans cooked in 1 cup tomato sauce

MEAL 3

‣ Sesame cabbage salad: 2 cups shredded green and red cabbage, ¼ cup sliced almonds, ½ cup chopped apple, lemon tahini dressing with 2 tablespoons tahini
‣ 1 cup sweet potatoes
‣ 2 oatmeal cookies

MEAL 4

‣ Smoothie: 1 scoop protein powder, 2 tablespoons almond butter, ½ cup mixed frozen berries, 1 banana

MEAL 5

‣ Veggie sausage
‣ 3 slices avocado
‣ 1 whole-wheat roll
‣ Kale salad: 1 cup raw kale, 2 tablespoons pumpkin seeds, ½ cup sliced grapes, vinaigrette with 2 teaspoons oil

MEAL 6

‣ 1½ cups quinoa mixed with ¼ cup mixed nuts
‣ 1 cup lentils
‣ 1 cup cooked carrots

CHAPTER 15

Plant Food Advantages

Reducing Chronic Disease with a Vegan Diet

D iets built around plant foods can offer profound benefits for health. Time-honored patterns, like the traditional Mediterranean diet, are linked to a lower risk for cardiovascular disease, cancer, diabetes, and cognitive decline with aging. Plant-based diets, including vegan diets, have been used more recently as therapeutic approaches for managing heart disease and diabetes. While diet is just one part of a health-promoting lifestyle, there is no doubt about the fact that plant foods have some unique attributes:

- Plant foods contain fiber, which is associated with a lower risk for cancer, heart disease, diabetes, and obesity. High-fiber diets are associated with improved digestion and a lower risk for digestive cancers, lower blood cholesterol, better regulation of blood-sugar levels, and may help reduce calorie intake since fiber promotes a feeling of fullness. Animal foods contain no fiber, and people who follow a usual American diet based on meat and dairy generally don't get as much fiber as experts recommend.

Vegans typically consume as much as two times what the average American consumes.

- Plant foods are low in saturated fat. Most of the saturated fat in American diets comes from meat and dairy foods. High intakes of some types of saturated fat are associated with higher blood cholesterol levels and a greater risk for heart disease. In contrast, the unsaturated fats in plant foods support health. Replacing saturated fat in your diet with polyunsaturated or monounsaturated fat or fiber-rich carbohydrates helps reduce blood-cholesterol levels.
- Plant foods contain no cholesterol. Although dietary cholesterol has a much smaller effect on blood cholesterol levels than saturated fat, it may still contribute to disease risk.
- Plant foods provide phytochemicals. These are compounds found only in plants, and there are hundreds of thousands of them in vegan foods. Some are antioxidants while others have anti-inflammatory or anti-microbial activity. Phytochemicals in certain foods like leafy green vegetables can filter out harmful UV rays. Some phytochemicals appear to have direct effects on processes that detoxify carcinogens. Getting plenty of these health-promoting compounds is simple; it's just a matter of eating whole plant foods, especially plenty of fruits and vegetables.
- Plant foods are excellent sources of nutrients, such as folate, potassium, and vitamins C and E, which may be related to lower risks for chronic disease.

Given that people who emphasize fruits, vegetables, whole grains, legumes, nuts, and seeds in their diet tend to enjoy better health, it stands to reason that vegans—who eat diets that include only these foods—might have the best health of all. But determining disease rates is complex and this is especially true for vegans, who still make up a relatively small percentage of the population.

RESEARCH ON VEGETARIANS AND VEGANS

Much of the available information about the health effects of vegan diets comes from just two large epidemiologic studies. These studies are expensive, so there aren't very many of them.

- The Oxford branch of the European Prospective Investigation into Cancer and Nutrition (EPIC-Oxford) has about 65,000 participants and is unique because it recruited a high number of vegetarians and vegans in order to compare the health of these groups to omnivores.
- The Adventist Health Study-2 (AHS-2) is a study of members of the Seventh-Day Adventist church. It started in 2002 and has about 96,000 subjects from all fifty states and Canada. Because the Adventist church promotes healthful practices and encourages a vegetarian diet, this study population also includes a high number of vegetarians and vegans. Because Adventists also have low rates of smoking and drinking, they are a good population in which to compare vegetarians with meat-eaters. This is the only large group of vegetarians or vegans from the United States whose disease rates have been studied.

You'll see that we refer often to EPIC-Oxford and AHS-2 in the following pages because these two studies are responsible for a great deal of what we know about vegan health.

We also have studies going back to the 1980s that have provided information about certain aspects of vegan health like blood cholesterol levels. Finally, a number of studies have looked at the impact of using a vegan diet in treating diseases like heart disease and diabetes.

In this chapter, we look at the research on health of vegans, the use of vegan diets for treating chronic disease, and the broader body of research on diet and health in order to create guidelines for planning an optimal vegan diet.

VEGAN DIETS AND BODY WEIGHT

Scientists assess body weight by looking at the body mass index (BMI), which is a measure of weight based on height. It's not a perfect assessment, however, because it doesn't account for muscle mass (which weighs more than fat). For that reason, it's not a useful measure for older people, who often have low muscle mass, or for athletes with a high proportion of muscle. It also can't predict health on an individual basis. Keeping these caveats in mind, though, BMI is a helpful tool for comparing populations.

A BMI of 20 to 25 is labeled "normal," sometimes also described as a "healthy" BMI. Above 25 is overweight and over 30 is considered obese. In both the AHS-2 and EPIC-Oxford studies, vegans have a lower body mass index than meat-eaters, vegetarians, and semi-vegetarians. The most likely factor affecting weight in these populations seems to be fiber intake, which may affect weight in a number of ways. The tables below display the findings from these two studies.

BODY MASS INDEXES OF SEVENTH-DAY ADVENTISTS (FROM THE AHS-2 STUDY)[1]

Vegans	Lacto-ovo vegetarians	Pesco-vegetarians (they eat fish but no other meat)	Semi-vegetarians	Meat-eaters
24.1	26.1	26.0	27.3	28.3

BODY MASS INDEXES OF BRITISH VEGETARIANS (FROM THE EPIC-OXFORD STUDY)[2]

	Vegans	Lacto-ovo vegetarians	Pesco-vegetarians	Meat-eaters
Men	22.5	23.4	23.4	24.4
Women	22	22.7	22.7	23.5

It's not possible to draw conclusions about a person's health based on their BMI alone. But on a population basis, we know that very high BMIs are associated with higher risk for heart disease, hypertension, diabetes, and cancer. The lower average BMI of vegans is part of the reason for their reduced risk for certain chronic diseases. We'll see, though, that it is not the whole explanation.

CARDIOVASCULAR DISEASE

Cardiovascular disease (CVD) refers to conditions that involve narrowed or blocked blood vessels, raising the risk for heart attack and stroke. A diet built around plant foods has potential benefits for reducing risk of CVD. In particular, vegans have lower rates of hypertension and lower blood cholesterol levels, two factors that are strongly protective against having a heart attack or stroke.

Hypertension

Interest in the ability of vegetarian diets to lower blood pressure dates back to the early part of the twentieth century. In 1926, California physician Arthur Donaldson reported that the blood pressure of vegetarian college students increased within two weeks of adding meat to their diets.[3] Nearly one hundred years later, research on the blood-pressure benefits of plant-based diets continues to accumulate. Findings from both the AHS-2 and EPIC-Oxford show that vegans have lower blood pressure than people who eat meat and other vegetarians.[4,5] In the EPIC-Oxford Study, meat-eaters were 2½ times as likely as vegans to have hypertension.[6]

You might assume that the average lower body weight of vegans explains their lower blood pressure, but most experts believe that it is a combination of multiple factors. Lower sodium intake also accounts for only part of the difference in blood pressure among the different dietary groups. Diets high in fruits and vegetables are associated with lower blood pressure, and that may be part of the explanation for the protective effects of plant-based diets. It's also possible that plant proteins help protect against hypertension.

The power of dietary changes for reducing blood pressure has been well-studied using the DASH diet, a plant-based (but not vegan) pattern that emphasizes foods rich in potassium, magnesium, calcium, fiber, and plant proteins with a low intake of saturated fat and refined carbohydrates. This diet is extremely effective in quickly reducing blood pressure in people with hypertension even when it allows a sodium intake that is above current recommendations.[7,8] It's even more effective when sodium is restricted to 1,500 milligrams per day. A low-sodium DASH diet is equivalent to drug therapy for lowering blood pressure in people with moderate hypertension.[9] While the original DASH diet was moderately low in fat, further research found that including more unsaturated fats and proteins, especially from plants, produced even better results.[10]

Findings from the DASH study as well as research on other lifestyle factors that affect blood pressure can give us insight on planning a vegan diet that is maximally effective in preventing or reversing hypertension.

GUIDELINES FOR REDUCING BLOOD PRESSURE

- Eat generous amounts of fruits and vegetables. The DASH study recommends seven to twelve servings per day and the generally higher intake of these foods among vegans is very likely one reason for their lower risk of hypertension.
- Choose foods that provide potassium, magnesium, and calcium. Use the chart on page 81 to guide your choices.
  - Foods that are particularly rich in potassium include potatoes, sweet potatoes, spinach, zucchini, tomatoes, bananas, dates, figs, apricots, oranges, orange juice, cooked beans, and almonds. Aim for 4,700 milligrams per day—this is quite a bit higher than the current RDA for potassium but is the level that was used in the DASH study.
  - Magnesium is found in bananas, dates, figs, orange juice, prunes, corn, okra, potatoes, spinach, sweet potatoes, almond butter, peanut butter, almonds, cooked beans, and whole grains like barley, oatmeal, and quinoa. The DASH researchers recommend 500 milligrams per day, which is a little bit higher than the RDA.
  - The best sources of calcium are fortified plant milks, leafy green vegetables, calcium-set tofu, almond butter, fortified juices, navel oranges, and figs. DASH recommendations are for 1,250 milligrams per day.

- Get at least 30 grams of fiber per day. Vegan diets are naturally rich in fiber and it's easy to meet this goal when you choose mostly whole grains and eat plenty of legumes, nuts, seeds, fruits, and vegetables.
- Limit sodium to no more than 2,300 milligrams per day. Some people, especially African Americans and older people, may need to reduce it further to 1,500 milligrams per day to lower their blood pressure.
- Limit alcohol to no more than one drink per day.
- Engage in at least 30 minutes of exercise every day.
- If you carry extra fat around your middle, even a small weight loss of 10 pounds or so can help lower blood pressure. However, it's more important to focus on eating a diet rich in fruits and vegetables and low in sodium. In the DASH study, the subjects reduced their blood pressure without losing weight. And we also know that weight is only part of the explanation for the lower blood pressures often seen in vegans.

TIPS FOR REDUCING SODIUM INTAKE

- When purchasing canned beans, vegetables, and tomato sauce, look for reduced sodium versions.
- Rinse canned beans and vegetables to remove some of the sodium.
- Limit processed veggie meats and cheeses.
- Limit foods packed in brine like pickles, pickled vegetables, olives, and sauerkraut.
- Limit salty condiments like mustard, ketchup, barbecue sauce, soy sauce, tamari (even reduced-sodium varieties), and miso.
- Cook grains and beans from scratch more often and cook them without added salt.
- Use spices instead of salt. In cooking and at the table, flavor foods with herbs, spices, lemon and lime juice, vinegar, or salt-free seasoning mixes.

Vegan Diets and Risk Factors for Heart Disease

There has been much discussion in the media and among research experts challenging the long-held belief that saturated fat raises the risk for heart disease.[11,12] In part, it's because replacing saturated fat in the diet with refined carbohydrates doesn't lower heart disease risk; it increases it. This has led to the suggestion that the real problem is refined carbohydrates, not saturated fat.

Actually, the problem is probably both refined carbohydrates and saturated fat. We know from a large body of research that replacing saturated fat with healthy fats—polyunsaturated and monounsaturated—reduces blood-cholesterol levels and is associated with a lower risk for heart disease.[13] Similar but smaller benefits occur when saturated fat is replaced with carbohydrates from whole, unrefined plant foods. It's not a matter of giving up carbs or fats; it's a matter of choosing the right ones.

The issue is somewhat complicated by the fact that foods contain different types of saturated fats and only certain ones affect blood cholesterol levels.[14] While the research in this area is still evolving, it doesn't affect vegan food choices very much because vegans tend to have low saturated fat intakes overall.

It's possible to eat too much saturated fat as a vegan if your diet is high in coconut oil. We talked about this oil in Chapter 7. In short, it's fine to use it in small amounts but we recommend keeping intake low. We also recommend limiting foods, such as some vegan margarines, that have added palm oil or palm kernel oil, other plant sources of saturated fat.

Not surprisingly, vegans have lower blood cholesterol levels than both meat-eaters and other vegetarians. More importantly, they have lower LDL-cholesterol. This is the "bad" cholesterol that is responsible for increased deposits of plaque in the arteries, which causes them to narrow and even become blocked.

Studies published since 1980 have consistently shown lower cholesterol levels in vegans compared to meat-eaters and lacto-ovo vegetarians.[15] In the EPIC-Oxford Study, vegans not only had lower

THE FAMILY OF FATS

Foods contain three types of fatty acids—saturated, monounsaturated, and polyunsaturated—which have different effects on health.

Saturated fat raises blood cholesterol levels and has been linked to risk for heart disease and maybe other chronic conditions as well. With the exception of palm kernel oil and coconuts, plant foods have far less saturated fat than meat, whole dairy foods, and eggs.

Monounsaturated fats can help lower cholesterol levels and may be beneficial in reducing risk for a number of chronic diseases. Plant foods that are rich in monounsaturated fats include avocados, olives, most nuts (except walnuts), peanuts, olive oil, canola oil, high oleic sunflower and safflower oils, and almond oil.

Polyunsaturated fats are especially effective in lowering blood cholesterol levels and are associated with a reduced risk for heart disease. Seeds, walnuts, soyfoods, and many vegetable oils are rich in these fats. The essential omega-6 and omega-3 fats that we talked about in Chapter 7 are both polyunsaturated fats.

Sterols are fat-like compounds that are found in the membranes of cells. **Cholesterol** is a sterol found almost exclusively in animal foods. While every cell in the body needs cholesterol as part of its structure, we make plenty of it and have no dietary requirement. **Phytosterols** are plant sterols that may help lower blood cholesterol levels and protect against heart disease. Plant foods provide phytosterols, which the human body can't make. The best sources are vegetable, nut and olive oils; nuts and seeds; wheat germ; avocados; and beans.

cholesterol levels than all other groups, but they also had the lowest levels of a compound called apolipoprotein B. This is the main protein found in LDL-cholesterol.[16]

Vegans also have consistently lower levels of triglycerides, which act as temporary storage for unused calories.[15] Diets high in alcohol, refined carbohydrates and sugars, and fat can lead to elevated triglycerides, which raises risk for heart disease.

There is evidence, too, that vegans have reduced levels of chronic inflammation.[17] Unlike acute inflammation, which is a short-term response to injury and is part of the healing process, chronic inflammation occurs over a long period of time throughout the body. It can be measured by immune system markers, and it raises risk for heart disease, diabetes, cancer, and Alzheimer's disease. Lifestyle factors, including diet, are closely associated with the risk of inflammation.

Finally, vegan diets are rich in antioxidants. Although studies using antioxidant supplements haven't shown a protective effect against heart disease, there is reason to believe that an antioxidant-rich diet might have benefits, including a reduction in inflammation. With their lower inflammation and hypertension, and reduced levels of cholesterol and triglycerides, we can expect vegans to have considerable protection against heart disease. But the actual research is somewhat confusing. The only analysis to include subjects from both the United States and Europe was published in 1999. It found that vegans had a 26 percent lower risk of death from heart disease than meat-eaters. Surprisingly, though, risk was even lower for lacto-ovo vegetarians and pescatarians (who eat fish, but no other meat).[18]

More surprises have come from the AHS-2 study. While it found that vegan men had a remarkable 42 percent lower risk of dying from a heart attack than men who ate meat, both vegan and vegetarian women had the same risk as nonvegetarian women. And this was most likely not because vegan women were eating any differently from vegan men.[1,19] It may be that other factors are especially important for risk in women. For example, stress and depression can raise risk for heart disease and women are more likely than men to suffer from depression.

The only study that has looked at heart disease incidence in vegetarians—that is, how many vegetarians actually have heart disease as opposed to how many die from it—is the EPIC-Oxford study. It found that vegetarians (a group that included vegans) had a 30 percent reduced rate.[20]

But overall, the findings about heart disease in vegans are limited, and they are not quite what we would expect. One thought is that this might be related to low vitamin B_{12} levels although the theory that inadequate B_{12} raises heart disease risk has fallen out of favor over the years.[21,22] It's also possible that some vegans don't consume enough healthy fats for optimal heart health.

While the research hasn't shown consistently less heart disease among vegans, there is still considerable interest in using vegan and near-vegan diets as part of a lifestyle approach to treating people who already have heart disease. Based upon what we know about the overall health of vegans and especially markers for heart disease, it makes sense that a vegan diet that is planned to be as healthy as possible would be a good approach to treating heart disease.

Vegan Diets for Treating Heart Disease

Dr. Nathan Pritikin was an early advocate of a vegan diet that limited all fats as a way to prevent and treat chronic disease. His approach was effective in reducing cholesterol, blood sugar, and blood pressure levels.

A few years later and using a similar although not-quite-vegan diet, Dr. Dean Ornish launched a study called the Lifestyle Heart Trial.[23] The subjects were people with moderate to severe coronary heart disease. Some followed the usual diet that was recommended for heart disease while others adopted a comprehensive lifestyle plan, which included a very low fat vegetarian diet (consisting almost entirely of whole plant foods with the addition of egg whites and nonfat dairy), aerobic exercise, stress management, support groups, and smoking cessation.

The subjects who followed a standard cholesterol-lowering plan got worse over the course of the study (atherosclerosis increased by nearly 28 percent after five years), but the health of subjects in the lifestyle group improved. Atherosclerosis in this group decreased by nearly 8 percent after five years.

Because the Lifestyle Heart Trial included comprehensive lifestyle changes, we can't really say how much of an impact diet alone had. For example, the lifestyle group included only one woman, and she quit smoking (which is a powerful way to reduce heart disease risk) when she entered the program. So the study provides no findings on whether this diet works to reduce atherosclerosis in women. The types of relaxation techniques used in the program might also have been responsible for some of the improvements due to lowering blood pressure. Those following the lifestyle program also lost more weight than the subjects in the control group.

A program from the Cleveland Clinic also successfully used a very low fat vegan diet to reverse atherosclerosis. But, because it hasn't yet been tested with a controlled study and we don't have findings about weight loss and other changes among the participants, it's too early to draw conclusions about the diet.[24]

While one of the common characteristics of these diets is that they were all low in total fat, it's not clear that this is as important as a reduced *saturated fat* intake. Higher-fat plant-based diets like traditional Mediterranean patterns are very effective in reducing heart disease risk.[25] Healthy dietary fats reduce blood cholesterol levels and also may enhance the effects of HDL-cholesterol, the "good" cholesterol. HDLs act to reduce cardiovascular disease risk through a number of mechanisms that researchers are trying to more fully elucidate. The amount of HDL in your blood may be less important than the quality of your HDL, which refers to how well it functions.[26] A standard blood test won't tell you this and, therefore, you can't know what your HDL level might mean for your disease risk. Higher-fat foods like almonds, walnuts, and olive oil are all associated with improved HDL function.[26–29]

It's likely that the benefits associated with low-fat vegan diets are due to some combination of weight loss, reduced intake of saturated fat, and protective compounds like antioxidants in plants. One comparison of three diets varying in fat content found that it didn't matter whether subjects ate low-fat or low-carb. The factor that predicted reduced plaque in the arteries was reduced blood pressure, which was a result of weight loss.[38] It may be that simply eating a vegan diet that includes a variety of healthful plant foods, aimed in particular at reducing blood pressure and blood cholesterol levels, is the key to reversing heart disease.

BLOOD VESSELS AND ADDED FATS

The endothelium is a thin layer of cells that lines blood vessels. When it is damaged, the result can be inflammation and increased risk for heart disease. Factors that damage the endothelial lining include hypertension, high LDL-cholesterol levels, smoking, lack of exercise, and stress. The endothelial lining is very susceptible to oxidative damage, which means that antioxidants in plant foods may be important for keeping this crucial part of the blood vessels healthy.

Proponents of very low fat diets for preventing or managing heart disease suggest that dietary fat, especially added oils, may damage the endothelial lining of the arteries. But studies that raised questions about the effect of fats and oils on the endothelium generally used unhealthy meals that were extremely high in fat—as high as 83 percent of calories in one study—along with unhealthy refined carbohydrates.[30–32] On the other hand, there is evidence that certain fat-rich foods like sesame oil, olive oil, and walnut oil, have a protective effect on the endothelium.[28,33–35] This may be one reason why the traditional Mediterranean diet, which is built around plant foods and high in healthful fats, is linked to healthier endothelial function.[36,37]

The current evidence suggests that the optimal diet for heart health can include higher-fat foods. Tree nuts in particular, like almonds, walnuts, and pecans, provide the type of fats that reduce blood cholesterol levels. They are also especially high in arginine, an amino acid that is a precursor to nitric oxide, a naturally occurring compound that helps protect the endothelial lining. Many studies have linked regular nut consumption to lower risk for heart disease.[39]

Extra-virgin olive oil is a unique source of oleocanthal, the phytochemical that gives this oil its characteristic peppery bite. One theory is that the key benefit of good-quality olive oil is that it makes vegetables taste so good that people eat more of them. But oleocanthal adds more than flavor; it's an antioxidant that may reduce heart disease risk by lowering inflammation in the body.[40]

Other higher-fat foods like traditional Asian soyfoods may have some benefits for heart disease as we saw in Chapter 9. Based on the current evidence, higher-fat plant foods can play a role in a heart-healthy diet.

HOW CARBOHYDRATES AFFECT DISEASE RISK

Carbohydrates are an important source of energy for the body since they are the preferred fuel for the brain and central nervous system. Foods contain two types of carbohydrate: *simple sugars* and *complex carbohydrates.*

Simple sugars contain one or two molecules of sugar. Fructose is a single-molecule sugar that is abundant in fruit. Sucrose, which is common table sugar, is made from two single-molecule sugars, glucose and fructose. Dairy foods naturally provide lactose, another simple sugar.

Complex carbohydrates are long chains of sugars. Most of the carbohydrate in potatoes, beans, and grains is *starch*, a complex carbohydrate made of long chains of the simple sugar glucose. Plant foods also contain *non-starch polysaccharides*, which are long chains of glucose that can't be digested by humans and that are a type of dietary fiber. Refined carbohydrate-rich foods generally have most of their fiber stripped away, leaving just starch.

Oligosaccharides are short chains of sugars—longer than simple sugars, but shorter than starch. Some are not digested by humans and can cause intestinal problems in some people. We discuss these in more detail in Chapter 16.

All digestible carbohydrates, whether they come from natural sugars in fruit, table sugar, or bread, pasta, beans, and potatoes, are digested in the intestines to produce the single-molecule sugar glucose. This life-sustaining sugar passes into the blood where it provides energy to cells. As blood glucose levels rise after a meal, the pancreas releases the hormone insulin into the blood.

Insulin helps cells absorb glucose (and also fat) from the blood, allowing the cells to use these nutrients for energy.

Some carbohydrates are converted to glucose more gradually than others. The glycemic index (GI) is a measure of how quickly carbohydrates are broken down and absorbed into the blood. A food with a high GI causes a rapid increase in blood glucose leading to a surge in insulin, which is associated with increased risk for heart disease, diabetes, and possibly cancer.[41]

Foods with a low GI can help with weight control since they help promote the use of body fat for energy, and they also tend to be more satisfying.[42] This is one reason for the popularity of low-carb, high-protein diets. But vegans are typically closer to their ideal body weight than omnivores, despite their higher carbohydrate intakes. And some people experience weight loss and improved glucose control on carbohydrate-rich diets.

In fact, diets don't necessarily need to be low in carbohydrates to have a low GI. The key is not to avoid carbohydrate-rich foods, it's to choose carbohydrates that are digested more slowly. Choosing whole grains instead of refined grains, whole fruits instead of juices, cooked cereals like oatmeal instead of ready-to-eat cereals, and gently cooked or raw vegetables instead of canned vegetables, are some simple ways to do this.

DIABETES

Diabetes is a broad term that encompasses two different diseases. Type 1 diabetes is an autoimmune disorder in which the pancreas doesn't produce enough (or any) insulin. Without insulin, blood glucose can't get into cells, and the cells starve. People with this disease require lifelong insulin therapy. But the more prevalent type of diabetes is type 2, in which enough insulin is produced, but the cells become resistant to it. Type 2 diabetes accounts for as much as 95 percent of all cases of diabetes in the United States. It used to be called *adult onset* diabetes because it rarely occurred in younger people. That's something that has changed over the past decades, however, and we now see type 2 diabetes in a significant number of young adults and even children.

People of African American, Hispanic/Latino American, American Indian, or Alaska Native descent are at a particularly high risk for type 2 diabetes. Although there is a strong genetic component to type 2 diabetes, lifestyle and diet play an important role in the risk of developing this disease. Risk is strongly linked to abdominal fat and also visceral fat, which is fat that accumulates around the organs. Other factors like depression and a sedentary lifestyle raise the risk for type 2 diabetes. And diabetes raises risk for heart disease, so a heart-healthy diet is an important component of diabetes treatment.

Some people with type 2 diabetes take medication, but the condition can often be managed very well through diet and exercise. Sometimes, losing a few pounds is enough to improve glucose control.

In the AHS-2 vegans had about a 60 percent lower risk for developing type 2 diabetes compared to people who eat meat. Their risk was also lower than people eating other types of vegetarian diets.[43,44] The lower BMIs of vegans in this study explain some of the protection but even when we take BMI out of the picture, vegans still have a lower risk for diabetes. This tells us that there are aspects of vegan eating patterns that have direct benefits in lowering risk for diabetes.

For example, researchers associated with the Physicians Committee for Responsible Medicine (PCRM) looked at the effects of a low-fat vegan diet in people who were overweight but didn't have diabetes. These subjects experienced improvements in cell function of the pancreas (which produces insulin) and a decrease in body fat including fat around their organs.[45]

The same dietary approach was used in a group of subjects who did have diabetes. Those who consumed a low-fat vegan diet had better blood glucose control than those who consumed a conventional diabetes diet. They ate fewer calories and more fiber and they lost more weight. The differences in blood glucose control were due mostly to weight loss, but this study provides an important finding about diet: it helps disprove the idea that all people with diabetes should avoid carbohydrates. These subjects did well on a diet that was very high in carbohydrates from whole plant foods.[46,47] Both of these studies used diets that were very low in fat. But just as we saw for heart disease, it is likely that the amount of fat isn't the important factor.

In Korea, researchers put people with diabetes on either a vegan diet or a conventional diabetes diet that were both about 20 percent fat (which is moderately low). The subjects eating the vegan diet had a higher intake of fiber, though. The vegan group lost more weight and had better blood glucose control.[48] And a study in the Czech Republic used a high-fat, near-vegan diet (it allowed just one cup of low-fat yogurt per day) in people with diabetes. This diet also improved blood glucose control, and it reduced body fat and led to a reduction in diabetes medication use.[49]

What these studies tell us is that different types of vegan diets can be effective in controlling type 2 diabetes, especially if they promote weight loss. It's likely that vegan diets are a good choice for managing diabetes because they are high in fiber, low in saturated fat, and replace animal protein with plant proteins.

PUTTING IT ALL TOGETHER: FOOD CHOICES FOR MANAGING CHRONIC DISEASE

It doesn't matter whether you need to reduce heart disease risk or control diabetes, the guidelines on how to eat are generally the same.

- Reduce your saturated fat intake. Vegans are automatically off to a good start in this regard, since most plant foods are naturally low in saturated fat.
- Include one to two servings of nuts in your daily menu since they help reduce LDL-cholesterol and have other heart-healthy factors.
- Eat whole, fiber-rich plant foods rather than refined carbohydrates. The type of fiber in dried beans helps lower blood cholesterol and is beneficial for control of blood glucose.
- If you enjoy them, include soyfoods in your diet since soy protein can help lower LDL-cholesterol and soy isoflavones may improve the health of your arteries. See pages 131–132 for more on this.

- Eat plenty of fruits and vegetables, including abundant choices that provide potassium, magnesium, and calcium to help keep blood pressure in a healthy range. Make sure you are meeting the requirements for omega-3 fats as discussed in Chapter 7.
- Make sure you are meeting vitamin B_{12} needs.
- Talk to your doctor about alcohol. Moderate intake may improve the function of HDL-cholesterol. But for women, even low levels of alcohol consumption can put them at a higher risk for breast cancer.

DEPRESSION AND DIET

Everybody gets the blues now and then. That's different from chronic depression, which is a debilitating disease. Depression, along with stress and anxiety, takes a toll on your health since it raises risk for heart disease and diabetes. For most people, dealing with depression requires a comprehensive approach involving lifestyle changes, counseling, and sometimes medication. There is increasing evidence that diet can help, too.

Depression and stress can raise levels of inflammation in the body, which in turn raises risk for other chronic diseases. But this is a two-way street because it appears that inflammation may also be at the root of some types of depression. This tells us that a diet that reduces inflammation might help in managing depression.[50]

A low intake of vitamin B_{12} might also raise risk for depression through its effects on homocysteine levels, although there is a lot of debate about this (see page 89). Vitamin B_6 is important for mental health, too, since it is needed for the neurotransmitter serotonin.

Plant-based diets in general seem to have some benefits for people who suffer from depression. A traditional Mediterranean diet is linked to better mood and there is some evidence that both vegetarians and vegans experience better mood and less depression.[51-56]

On the other hand, one study found higher depression scores in vegetarian men, though this study wasn't designed to measure causation.[57] The researchers suggested that inadequate vitamin D was a plausible explanation. While, on average, vegans have vitamin D levels in the healthy range, they tend to be lower than omnivores. And we suspect that some vegans may struggle with depression for reasons that have nothing to do with their diet but are related more to a heightened sense of empathy and compassion.

Diet is not a cure-all for depression and it's not meant to replace other effective treatments including counseling, cognitive therapy, and medications. But lifestyle changes and tweaks to your vegan diet can be helpful parts of an approach to improve mental health.

- Follow our guidelines for healthful eating to reduce chronic disease on page 251. The same diet that lowers your risk for heart disease and diabetes can reduce inflammation and improve symptoms of depression. This means eating plenty of fruits and vegetables, focusing on slowly digested carbohydrates from unrefined foods, and choosing foods that provide healthful plant fats.
- If you use added fats in your meals, choose extra-virgin olive oil most often. Perhaps because of its anti-inflammatory properties, it has been linked to lower risk of depression.[58,59]
- Take supplements of vitamin B_{12} and vitamin D. Inadequate intakes of both could lead to depression.
- Make sure you get enough vitamin B_6. See page 217 for foods that are rich in this nutrient.
- If you have been diagnosed with depression, talk to your doctor about taking vegan EPA supplements as they have shown promise in treating depression.
- Get adequate sleep. Too little sleep may increase inflammation.
- Engage in daily exercise. Physical activity can be a powerful antidote to stress and depression. It's even better if you are able to exercise outdoors.
- Consider a daily meditation or prayer practice. The mindfulness-based stress reduction program developed at the University of Massachusetts has been well studied for its benefits to both mental and physical health. Their website provides resources and can help you find local classes: https://umassmed.edu/cfm.

- Connect with animals. A rescued pet can do wonders for relieving stress, anxiety, and depression. If you cannot currently adopt an animal, consider joining a foster program or volunteering to help socialize animals at a shelter. Or let friends know that you're available to help with pet sitting.
- Foster positive, fun, and supportive relationships. Social interaction is an important factor in overall health, including mental health.

VEGAN DIETS AND CANCER

The relationship of diet to cancer is somewhat difficult to study. It's a complex disease and there aren't many markers for cancer risk. While we can measure the effects of diet on blood-cholesterol levels and make predictions about how they will affect heart disease risk, we don't have many straightforward blood parameters related to cancer risk.

Despite this, we have gained some good knowledge over the past years about dietary choices to reduce risk for cancer. According to the American Institute for Cancer Research, choices to reduce cancer risk include a diet rich in whole plant foods and low in red meat, processed foods, sugary drinks, and alcohol.

There are some potential benefits of a diet built around fiber-rich plant foods as seen in studies of the intestinal health of people eating different kinds of diets. The environment of the colon in vegetarians—including the levels of different bacteria and enzymes—differs from meat-eaters in ways that appear to be protective against colon cancer.[60] This is due in part to a higher intake of fiber, which is linked to a lower risk for cancer.

In contrast to the possible protective effects of plant foods, certain animal foods may raise cancer risk. Red and processed meats are linked to a higher risk for colon, stomach, and possibly bladder cancer. There is also evidence to suggest that high calcium consumption raises the risk for prostate cancer, although conversely, it's associated with lower risk for colon cancer.

What we know about diet and cancer risk suggests that vegans should have some protection. But studies of diet and cancer sometimes take many years to produce results and we are just starting to see data on cancer rates of vegans. In the EPIC-Oxford study, vegans had a 19 percent lower risk for overall cancer, although the finding was just barely statistically significant.[61] In the Adventist Health Study, vegans had a 16 percent lower risk for overall cancer compared to meat-eaters which, like EPIC-Oxford, was barely statistically significant. Vegan women had lower risk for female-specific cancers and vegan men were less likely to have prostate cancer.[62,63]

While the findings on cancer rates in vegans are a little less exciting than what we would like, keep in mind that cancer is a disease that develops over a long period of time. There is evidence that how people eat in childhood is linked to their later risk for developing cancer. This makes it hard to uncover the links between diet and cancer risk without studying lifelong eating habits. And we can also assume that many of the vegans in these studies grew up eating nonvegan diets. Until we know more, it's safe to assume that a diet built around whole plant foods is a good choice for lowering cancer risk.

SPECIAL MEDICAL CONDITIONS

Two medical conditions—type 1 diabetes and kidney disease—are beyond the scope of this book. But we want to address them briefly, if only to assure you that people with these conditions can be vegan.

TYPE 1 DIABETES

While there is no research on vegan diets for people with type 1 diabetes, there is no reason why someone with this disease can't be vegan. As with any dietary approach to diabetes, it's wise to eat mostly fiber-rich, whole plant foods and avoid refined grains, added sugars, and sugary drinks. As with any dietary change in type 1

---

continues

diabetes, you'll want to work closely with your health professional to monitor blood-sugar levels and insulin needs.

KIDNEY DISEASE

Plant-based diets have been shown to be beneficial in reducing the markers of kidney disease, and people with moderate kidney disease may benefit from a vegan diet.[64] This may be due to their lower protein levels, but it could also be from their effect on blood cholesterol levels and blood pressure, and their antioxidant content. The lower absorption of phosphorus from whole plant foods may also be an advantage.[65] While vegetarian meats should be restricted for people with chronic kidney disease because of their high contents of sodium and protein, they can play a role in the diet of people on dialysis because they provide high-quality protein. See Veganhealth .org/kidney-disease for a list of vegetarian meats and their saturated fat, potassium, phosphorus, and sodium.

A vegan diet is more difficult for people on dialysis because of the need to restrict potassium and phosphorus, while at the same time ensuring adequate protein intake. Planning such a diet is beyond the scope of this book, but we recommend *The Vegetarian Diet for Kidney Disease* by Joan Brookhyser Hogan, a registered dietitian and board-certified specialist in renal nutrition.

PALEOLITHIC VS. VEGAN DIETS

Do you need to eat like your ancestors for optimal health? That's the theory behind the popular Paleolithic diet approach to food choices. Paleo advocates suggest that many of our modern-day chronic illnesses are the result of straying from the protein-rich, hunter-gatherer diet that sustained humans for hundreds of thousands of years.

The Paleolithic ("Old Stone Age") era began more than 2.5 million years ago with the emergence of the first tool-using hominids. It lasted until the advent of agriculture some twelve thousand years ago, which introduced grains and legumes (and in some cases, dairy foods) into diets. The transition from a hunter-gatherer society to one where people grew food and domesticated animals meant a significant change in dietary habits. Today's Paleo advocates shun those changes, choosing to eat only the foods that were presumably available to our ancestors: meat, fish, eggs, nuts, fruits, and vegetables. The theory is that this hunter/gatherer pattern is what we are genetically designed to eat.

But duplicating the true diet of early humans isn't quite so straight-forward as Paleo promoters would have us believe. For one thing, we simply don't have access to the same foods. Nearly every food consumed today, including fruits, vegetables, and meats, are drastically different from the foods that were available one hundred thousand years ago. Meat from factory farmed animals doesn't at all resemble meat from the wild animals that early humans hunted. And while modern Paleo dieters often seek out meat from grass-fed animals, this is not a viable option for feeding our global population and it's also not affordable for most people.

Anthropologists who research early diets suggest that grains may in fact have been part of Paleolithic diets. Dr. Anna Revedin, an archaeologist at the Italian Institute of Prehistory, found evidence of starchy grains from the roots of ferns and cattails on stones used as primitive grinding tools during the Paleolithic era. Her research group believes that these early, pre-agriculture humans consumed flour that underwent multistep processing involving peeling, drying, grinding and cooking.[66] Anthropologist Amanda Henry of the Max Planck Institute for Evolutionary Anthropology, in Leipzig, Germany, looked at remnants of food in plaque on ancient teeth and found evidence that early Neanderthals consumed grass seeds, legumes, and roots, and that some of these foods had been cooked.[67]

In fact, anthropologists believe that it's unlikely that there was one single Paleo diet. Instead, just like today, diets most likely varied over time and in different regions of the world. It's likely that most of these early diets were extremely high in fiber and low in saturated fat since the animals that early humans consumed were leaner than those raised on modern farms. They contained little added sugar (small amounts from honey only), were relatively low in sodium, and were rich in vitamin C, calcium, and potassium.[68] It's not surprising, then, that some studies have found that Paleolithic-inspired diets can improve blood pressure and glucose tolerance.[69] Compared to a modern Western diet that makes use of white flour, French fries, factory-farmed meat, and sugary sodas, the Paleolithic diet had distinct advantages. But those same benefits are hallmarks of well-planned vegan diets that emphasize fiber-rich plant foods.

In a 2002 article in *Scientific American*, anthropologist William Leonard of Northwestern University wrote: "We now know that humans have evolved not to subsist on a single, Paleolithic diet but to be flexible eaters, an insight that has important implications for the current debate over what people today should eat in order to be healthy. [. . .] What is remarkable about human beings is the extraordinary variety of what we eat. We have been able to thrive in almost every ecosystem on the Earth, consuming diets ranging from almost all animal foods among populations of the Arctic to primarily tubers and cereal grains among populations in the high Andes."[70]

This remarkable variety of eating patterns is good news for those of us navigating food choices in our increasingly complex world. Early humans had to be concerned only with getting enough food to survive through child-rearing years. Today, when we make dietary choices, we're thinking about the impacts not just on nutrient needs, but also on global warming, dwindling natural resources, world hunger, and animal welfare. A vegan diet is the most logical response.

It's easy enough to plan vegan meals that mimic what is best about Paleolithic patterns by getting fat from nuts, seeds, olives, and avocados, and by eating plenty of fiber- and nutrient-rich fruits and vegetables. Our modern food supply and kitchens mean we can also take greater advantage of certain foods, like legumes, that were less available to early humans and that we now know have demonstrated health benefits. We're fortunate to have all these choices because, in today's world, a diet built around plant foods is the best option for meeting nutrient needs, optimizing health, protecting the planet, and showing compassion for animals.

VEGAN KETO DIETS

While carbohydrate-rich vegan diets can be effective for weight loss and for managing symptoms of chronic diseases like diabetes, many people prefer a lower-carb approach. A number of studies show that cutting carbs can be effective for people with diabetes in particular. None of those studies have been in vegans, though, and we don't know that a low-carb intake has any advantages over the kind of carbohydrate-rich diet we talk about in this chapter. But just like meat-eaters, vegans have different dietary preferences, and we often hear from those who want to limit carbs or even explore a ketogenic diet.

Ketogenic diets are the very extreme of low carbohydrate intakes and they are nothing new in the world of weight loss. In the 1960s, the low-carbohydrate *Drinking Man's Diet* promised weight loss while allowing all the steak and martinis you wanted. Not surprisingly, it was among the most popular diets of the decade!

More recently, keto enthusiasts have adopted this eating pattern not just for weight loss but also for managing type 2 diabetes and other chronic illnesses.

Ketogenic diets restrict carbohydrates to extremely low levels, as little as 30 grams per day in some cases (compared to typical recommendations of about 225 to 300 grams). By depriving cells of the glucose that carbohydrates provide, ketogenic diets force the body to break down its own fat for energy. Some of the fats are converted in the liver to ketones. Because the brain can't directly use fatty acids for energy, the body provides ketones to fuel the brain.

In the short term, ketogenic diets work well for weight loss, although the reasons why aren't well understood. It may simply be because ketones help suppress appetite, or it could be that the diet speeds up fat breakdown. Metabolic changes that occur on ketogenic diets also take energy, which may help drive weight loss.[71]

Traditionally ketogenic diets have been built around meat, high-fat dairy products, eggs, and oils. So it might surprise you to know that there is a vegan version of this diet. It emphasizes healthy oils, coconut products, nuts, seeds, nut and seed butters, nonstarchy vegetables, tofu, tempeh, seitan, lupini beans, black soybeans, cashew cheese, vegan cream cheese, nutritional yeast, avocados, and (in moderation) berries. As challenging as this diet is, it has an enthusiastic following. The *Vegan Keto Made Simple* Facebook group has some 50,000 members.

How well ketogenic diets work for weight loss over the long term hasn't been studied. We also don't know much about their long-term impacts on health. There is evidence that they improve blood cholesterol and triglyceride levels in some people and can help in the management of type 2 diabetes.[72] However, we need more research to answer questions about the effects of these diets on intestinal bacteria and on bone and kidney health.

And, because a ketogenic diet is an extremely restrictive approach that eliminates whole categories of healthy plant foods, it's not likely to be a long-term solution for most people. That makes it more of a fad diet with a focus on weight loss than a lifestyle approach with a focus on health and enjoyment.

While we have reservations about ketogenic diets, we also recognize that some vegans who have not been satisfied with their health or weight on typical plant-based diets might be interested in trying a keto diet. And given the popularity of ketogenic diets in general, we're happy that a vegan option exists. If you are determined to try this way of eating, we recommend joining the *Vegan Keto Made Simple* group for support and guidance on food choices. The free *Keyto* phone app provides menus and shopping lists for a vegan ketogenic diet.

However, most vegans who are looking to eat a low-carb diet are likely to find that a more modest reduction in carbs is most realistic. A reasonable goal is to keep carbohydrate intake at around 30 to 40 percent of calories.

Here are some guidelines for tweaking your vegan diet to cut back (a little) on carbohydrates and boost protein intake.

- Emphasize beans over grains. Ultra-low carb diets discourage them, but that's a mistake since these foods have so many wonderful health benefits. Black soybeans and lupini beans are both especially low in carbohydrate compared to other options.

- Experiment with pasta made from beans. Those made from edamame (soybeans) are especially high in protein and low in carbohydrates.
- Choose higher-protein grains like quinoa.
- Since lower carbohydrate intake usually translates to higher fat, get good-quality fats from nuts and seeds.
- Include soyfoods and seitan (wheat protein) in meals.
- Emphasize vegetables over fruits.

Here is one example of a lower-carbohydrate diet for vegans. It provides around 1,800 calories and is 40 percent carbohydrate, 35 percent fat, and 25 percent protein.

BREAKFAST

- ½ cup pinto beans
- 4 slices tempeh bacon
- 1 cup spinach
- 1 small corn tortilla

SNACK

- Smoothie made with 1 cup frozen whole strawberries, 6 ounces silken tofu, 2 tablespoons orange juice, ¼ teaspoon vanilla extract

LUNCH

- 1 slice whole wheat bread
- ½ cup soy curls marinated in liquid smoke and tamari and sautéed in 1 teaspoon oil
- 1 cup collards topped with tahini dressing (made with 2 tablespoons tahini)

SNACK

- Rice cake with 1 ounce nut-based cheese
- Apple

DINNER

- ▸ 6 ounces seitan
- ▸ 2 cups chopped kale and mushrooms sautéed in 1 teaspoon oil
- ▸ 2 tablespoons chopped walnuts

CHAPTER 16

Plant Foods and Digestive Health

Your intestines are home to some 100 trillion microbes, most of which are bacteria. The vast majority live in the large intestine where they are referred to as *gut flora* or the *microbiota*. These bacteria depend on us for their survival and in return provide a host of benefits for our health.

A healthy and diverse colony of bacteria may lower risk for obesity, type 2 diabetes, colon cancer, and heart disease.[1]

A decade of research suggests that diet may be key to promoting growth of beneficial bacteria. Certain foods can shuttle microbes directly to the intestines while others provide the fuel that encourages good bacteria to thrive.

Probiotics are foods or supplements that contain active microbes that are delivered directly into your intestines. There's some evidence that consuming probiotics might lower the risk for inflammatory bowel disease, skin disorders, and even the common cold.[2] Vegan probiotics include nondairy yogurt containing active live cultures, sauerkraut, and fermented foods like tempeh, miso, and certain nut cheeses.

But more interesting than probiotics may be certain types of fermentable fiber, sometimes referred to as *prebiotics*, that stimulate the growth of healthy bacteria in the colon.

Because humans can't digest dietary fiber, it travels through the intestines and arrives in the colon intact. Some types of fiber provide bulk to the stool, speeding its passage out of the colon and helping prevent constipation. Other types of fiber are prebiotics, or food for bacteria—in fact, intestinal bacteria survive primarily through the fermentation of these types of fiber.

As bacteria ferment fiber, they produce various gases and short-chain fatty acids. While the gases pass out of the body, the short-chain fatty acids provide an important source of nutrition for the cells lining the colon. Short-chain fatty acids are also involved in regulating appetite and improving glucose metabolism. They are associated with reduced inflammation and some have anticancer activity.

There is intriguing research suggesting that there might be important differences in the microbiota activity of people eating plant-based diets compared to those who regularly eat meat. For example, a small study at the University of Pennsylvania found no difference between the microbiota of vegans and meat-eaters but did find evidence of higher levels of metabolites produced by gut microbes among the vegans.[3] Another example is that vegans might not generate TMAO, a compound that has been linked to risk for heart disease and that depends on intestinal bacteria for its production.[4] And vegetarians (including vegans) might have enhanced production of equol, a health-promoting compound that is created when intestinal bacteria metabolize isoflavones in soyfoods (see Chapter 9).

The products of fermentation also create a more acidic environment in the colon, which can inhibit the growth of pathogens. One study comparing microbial populations in vegans, vegetarians, and meat-eaters found that a vegan diet was associated with lower pH in the colon, which prevented the growth of harmful *E. coli*.[5]

While the impact of fiber-rich, plant-based diets on gut microbial activity and ultimately on health is still a somewhat new area of research, it's likely that the typically high fiber content of vegan diets offers benefits from the healthy products of gut bacteria.

But for newcomers to plant-based diets, the initial increase in fiber consumption and its related microbial activity sometimes causes discomfort.

FIBER, BEANS, AND GAS

Switching out meat, milk, and eggs for plant foods is almost guaranteed to increase your fiber intake. That's good news since a high-fiber diet is linked to a lower risk for many chronic diseases and can help with weight control. But a sudden increase in fiber intake can sometimes cause bloating, cramping, and gas. It's important to make sure you're drinking plenty of fluids to help relieve those symptoms. It may also help to include some refined grains in your diet along with well-cooked vegetables at the beginning of your transition to a vegan diet. Gradually increasing your consumption of fiber-rich plant foods can give your body time to adjust.

Some of the discomfort that new vegans experience is due to an increase in gas production in the colon as bacteria break down fermentable fibers. Dried beans are particularly rich in a type of fiber that promotes growth of healthy gas-producing bacteria, earning them the nickname "the musical fruit."

If you notice increased gas production when you start eating more beans, it means that your gut bacteria are engaged in activity that is good for you. But healthy or not, gas can be uncomfortable, not to mention embarrassing.

Not everyone who adds beans to their diet encounters these issues. One study found that just 50 percent of people who added beans to their daily diet suffered from uncomfortable gas.[6] But if you're new to beans and they give you problems, there are ways to alleviate the discomfort:

- Add beans to your diet gradually. Over time, changes in the bacteria in your colon may make bean digestion easier. In one study, most of the people who experienced increased gas after adding a half-cup of beans to their daily diet experienced a lessening of symptoms over several weeks.[6]

- Emphasize smaller beans like lentils and split peas, which tend to produce less gas.
- Rinse beans several times during soaking. Soaking beans not only helps them cook faster, it also leaches out some of the carbohydrates that cause gas. Here is the technique that is shown to work:
    - Place beans and soaking water in a large pot and bring the water to a boil. Boil for two minutes.
    - Drain the beans and add fresh water. Soak in the refrigerator for at least six hours.
    - Drain and add fresh water for cooking. This process can reduce the gas-causing fiber in beans by more than 75 percent.
- Add a pinch of baking soda to the cooking water when you cook beans. It helps soften their skins but be aware that it can also make the beans mushy if you add too much.
- Cook beans thoroughly since soft, well-cooked beans are easier to digest. Canned beans may be easier to digest because they are usually well cooked.
- If all else fails, consume a digestive enzyme supplement before eating beans. Products such as Bean-zyme contain an enzyme that breaks down the sugars in beans.

GLUTEN INTOLERANCE

Gluten is a family of proteins found in grains like wheat, rye, spelt, and barley. Gluten is responsible for the elasticity in bread dough and gives bread its ability to rise. It also adds texture to baked goods.

About one in one hundred people worldwide have celiac disease, which is an autoimmune reaction to gluten that damages the small intestine. In children, symptoms of celiac disease include abdominal bloating, chronic diarrhea or constipation, weight loss, fatigue, irritability, and delayed growth. Adults with celiac disease may have unexplained iron-deficiency anemia, fatigue, joint pain, osteoporosis, depression, tingling in hands and feet, and itchy skin. Symptoms can be mild, which means that many people with celiac disease remain undiagnosed. Treatment for celiac disease is complete avoidance of gluten.

Wheat allergy is a separate condition that involves an immune system response to one or more of the proteins in wheat. If you have an allergy to any of these proteins, you might experience breathing difficulties, nausea, hives, a bloated stomach, and an inability to focus after eating foods that contain wheat. Interestingly, gluten is less likely than other proteins in wheat to cause allergic reactions, so some people with a wheat allergy can eat nonwheat foods that contain gluten, like barley and rye.

While both celiac disease and wheat allergy can be diagnosed through established tests, a third condition, called gluten intolerance, is much harder to diagnose and remains controversial. Also referred to as nonceliac gluten sensitivity (NCGS), this is a reaction to gluten in people who have neither celiac disease nor wheat allergy. Reported symptoms include intestinal discomfort, fatigue, muscle and joint pain, skin problems, depression, and "foggy mind."

Within the medical community, there is considerable debate about NCGS. Some researchers believe that a small group of people may have an immune reaction to gluten or to something else in wheat. But others are convinced that these patients are in fact reacting to a group of poorly absorbed carbohydrates called FODMAPs. It's complicated because although wheat, rye, and barley contain both FODMAPs *and* gluten, these compounds aren't related—FODMAPs are carbohydrates while gluten is a protein.

Studies comparing the effects of gluten and FODMAPs in subjects who described themselves as gluten intolerant found that gluten was less likely to produce GI symptoms than the FODMAPs in wheat.[7,8]

To complicate things more, there are other components of wheat, rye, and barley that could be the real culprits. For example, some researchers believe that a group of proteins called amylase trypsin inhibitors might cause symptoms often attributed to gluten.[9]

Suffice it to say that we still have a lot to learn about what actually causes the conditions attributed to gluten intolerance.

Avoiding wheat and other gluten-containing grains adds a bit of complexity to your menu planning, but these foods are not essential for a healthy vegan diet. Our food guide in Chapter 10 calls for just four servings (a total of 2 cups) of grains and starchy vegetables per day. You can easily achieve this with gluten-free options like rice, quinoa, corn, amaranth, oats, buckwheat, potatoes, and sweet potatoes.

However, if you experience symptoms when you eat wheat, barley, and rye, it's wise to do a little further investigating before embarking on a completely gluten-free diet. At the very least, you should first rule out both celiac disease and wheat allergy by getting appropriate tests through your health-care provider. Then, it might be a good idea to explore a low-FODMAP diet before assuming that gluten is the issue.

Please note that some health-care practitioners use tests that measure the level of IgG antibodies in your blood to determine if you have an allergy. While it's common to do this, this is not a correct use of IgG testing. IgG will provide information on what sorts of protein fragments are in your blood, but they cannot diagnose a food allergy.

DEALING WITH IRRITABLE BOWEL SYNDROME: THE LOW-FODMAP DIET

Irritable bowel syndrome (IBS) is a cluster of symptoms affecting the large intestine. It can cause cramping, bloating, and diarrhea. IBS isn't life-threatening, but it can greatly impact quality of life. It's a frustrating problem, because no one knows what causes it and there are no tests to diagnosis it. It's relatively common, too, affecting as much as 15 percent of the population.

One theory is that people with IBS are sensitive to certain carbohydrates. Some of these carbohydrates are poorly digested and some are not digested at all. Others, like lactose in milk or the sugar fructose, are digested by some but not all people. Like the fermentable fiber that supports a healthy population of bacteria in the large intestine, these carbohydrates travel to the colon intact, where they are fermented by bacteria, resulting in gas production. They can also pull water into the lower intestines, creating an uncomfortable feeling of distension. Most people experience very little discomfort from this if they notice it at all. But people with IBS may be hypersensitive to the effects of water and gas in their lower intestines.

The carbohydrates responsible for this effect are collectively known as FODMAPs. Studies suggest that many people with IBS can benefit from reducing or eliminating certain FODMAPs in their diets, and a low-FODMAP diet has been created by researchers at Monash University in Australia.[10]

The low-FODMAP diet limits many foods that are common in vegan diets. This creates a challenge but not an insurmountable one. A quick search on the internet reveals that many vegans have successfully used this diet to reduce their symptoms of IBS.

The FODMAP Family of Foods

The term FODMAP is an acronym for **F**ermentable **O**ligosaccharides, **D**isaccharides, **M**onosaccharides, and **P**olyols. They include:

Galactans: These are oligosaccharides (short chains of sugars) that are abundant in beans. Humans lack the enzymes to break down these sugars, so no one can digest them. That's why beans can cause gas even in people who don't suffer from IBS as we talked about earlier.

Fructans: Another type of oligosaccharide, these are chains of the simple sugar fructose. Fructans are found in artichokes, garlic, onions, leeks, wheat, rye, and barley. Certain types of fructans called inulin and FOS are sometimes added to foods for their prebiotic effects.

Lactose: A disaccharide—two simple sugars linked together—found in milk and other dairy foods. Since vegan diets don't contain dairy foods, it's not an issue.

Fructose: A simple sugar (also called a monosaccharide) found in table sugar, high-fructose corn syrup, and fruits. The ratio of fructose to glucose (another monosaccharide) is more important than the total amount of fructose in the diet since this ratio affects absorption. As a result, some fruits that are high in fructose, like apples, pears, watermelon, and mango, can be worse for IBS symptoms than plain old table sugar, which is half fructose and half glucose. Agave nectar is also higher in fructose than table sugar.

Polyols: Also called sugar alcohols, these include sorbitol, xylitol, and mannitol. They're used in sugarless gums and candies. They also occur naturally in some fruits like apples, apricots, avocado, cherries, nectarines, pears, plums, and prunes.

Eating a Low-FODMAP Diet

These carbohydrates are not unhealthy, and in fact, they may have health benefits, especially in lowering risk for colon cancer. It wouldn't be possible to eliminate them completely (unless you ate an all-meat diet) but, if you suffer from IBS, a low-FODMAP diet can help you determine if you need to reduce some of these carbohydrates.

The FODMAP approach limits these fermentable carbs for several weeks to see if IBS symptoms improve. If you feel better after avoiding these foods, it's a good indication that you are sensitive to one or more of these carbohydrates. The next step is to gradually add foods back one at a time to see which carbohydrates are a problem for you.

The table on page 272 shows foods you can eat during the elimination phase of a FODMAP diet and the foods you should avoid. After six to eight weeks, if your symptoms have improved, you can start to add back high-FODMAP foods to determine which FODMAPs are the source of your discomfort. Make sure you start with small quantities. You may be able to tolerate ¼ cup of high-FODMAP beans but not ½ cup.

It's also important to test one type of fermentable carbohydrate at a time. This isn't always as straightforward as it might seem. For example, an apple provides two different types of FODMAPS: fructose and polyols (sugar alcohols). If you eat an apple and it causes intestinal discomfort, you won't know which of those FODMAPs is the problem. Instead, choose apricots to test your sensitivity to polyols and mangos to determine whether you are sensitive to fructose. We recommend working with a dietitian and keeping a food diary as you begin to add FODMAPs back to your diet.

FODMAP RESOURCES

You'll find a wealth of information on the FODMAP diet on the internet, including tips from vegans. Here are a few that we recommend:

- Monashfodmap.com which is the official FODMAP site
- *Monash Uni Low FODMAP Diet* phone app
- https://www.katescarlata.com/ A website by a registered dietitian that is devoted to digestive health. Includes resources for vegans.
- *The Low-FODMAP Diet Step by Step: A Personalized Plan to Relieve the Symptoms of IBS and Other Digestive Disorders* by Kate Scarlata and Dédé Wilson
- *Low FODMAP and Vegan: What to Eat When You Can't Eat Anything* by Jo Stepaniak

	Low FODMAP Foods (Eat these during the elimination phase)	High FODMAP Foods (Avoid these during the elimination phase)
Legumes	Tofu, tempeh, peanut butter, small amounts (¼ cup per meal) of canned butter beans, lima beans, chickpeas, lentils Pea and rice protein isolates	All except for small quantities of canned butter beans, lima beans, chickpeas, lentils (sprouted beans may be tolerated) Textured vegetable protein (TVP) Veggie meats made with soy protein
Nuts and seeds	Macadamias, peanuts, pecans, pine nuts, pumpkin seeds, sesame seeds, sunflower seeds, walnuts Limit almonds and hazelnuts to fewer than ten nuts per serving.	Cashews, pistachios
Vegetables	Bok choy, green beans, bell peppers, Brussels sprouts, carrot, chicory leaves, collards, cucumber, eggplant, endive, fennel bulb, fennel leaves, kale, lettuce, radicchio, okra, spring onion (green tops only), parsnip, potatoes, radish, spaghetti squash, baby spinach, Swiss chard, tomatoes, turnip, water chestnuts, zucchini	Artichokes, asparagus, beetroot, celery, garlic, leek bulb, onions (all), Savoy cabbage, sugar snap peas, sweet corn Pickled onions and beets may be tolerated
Fruit	Limit fruit to one serving per meal. Choose well-ripened fruit since it's lower in fructose. Banana, blueberries, cantaloupe, grapes, kiwi, lemon, mandarin oranges, honeydew melon, navel oranges, papaya, pineapple, raspberries, rhubarb, starfruit, strawberries	Apples, apricots, avocado, blackberries, boysenberry, cherries, currants, dates, figs, goji berries, grapefruit, lychee, mango, nectarines, peaches, pears, persimmon, plums, pomegranate, watermelon Canned and dried fruit
Grains	Quinoa, rice, rice noodles, oats, polenta, rice crackers, gluten-free bread (less than one slice per meal)	All wheat-containing products, almond meal, barley, rye
Milks and other beverages	Almond milk, soymilk made from soy protein (but not from whole soybeans) Black or green tea, coffee, weak herbal tea, ½ cup orange juice	Soymilk made from whole soybeans (this is true of most commercial soymilk), milks with added carrageenan Chamomile tea, fruit juices
Sweeteners	Stevia, brown sugar, raw sugar, white sugar, maple syrup, rice malt syrup, marmalade, sucralose	Agave, high-fructose corn syrup (HFCS), fructose, jam, anything sweetened with an ingredient ending in "ol" (like mannitol)
Snacks	Dark chocolate, corn chips, popcorn	
Condiments	Black and green olives, seaweed, coconut milk, miso, Marmite, nutritional yeast, "Vegg" egg yolk, EnerGEgg Replacer, agar-agar	Tahini, chutney, pickles, relish, salsa, commercial salad dressings, garlic or onion powder

continues

continued

Oils	Avocado, canola, coconut, olive, peanut, rice bran, sesame, sunflower, soy oils	
Alcohol	Beer, wine, gin, vodka, whiskey	Port and other fortified wines, brandy, champagne, rum

SAMPLE LOW-FODMAP MENU

Most people who are sensitive to some FODMAPs can still eat others. But even in the unlikely event that you can't tolerate any of these foods, you can still eat a vegan diet. Low-FODMAP foods include tofu, tempeh, peanut butter, many nuts and seeds, many fruits and vegetables, added fats, plenty of condiments, and gluten-free grains. You can also have small amounts of certain beans.

Here is one example of a low-FODMAP menu.

BREAKFAST

▸ Oatmeal with almond milk, blueberries, and chopped walnuts
▸ Coffee or tea
▸ Gluten-free toast with peanut butter

LUNCH

▸ Vegetable soup with potatoes, tomatoes, green beans, ¼ cup well-cooked lentils
▸ Salad with oil and vinegar dressing
▸ Banana

DINNER

▸ Tofu or tempeh sautéed with zucchini, bok choy, and spinach seasoned with ginger, miso, and sesame oil
▸ Quinoa or brown rice

SNACKS

▸ Rice cakes with sunflower seed butter
▸ Popcorn
▸ Gluten-free pretzels

CHAPTER 17

A Compassionate Approach to Weight and Dieting

A popular question is whether or not a vegan diet promotes weight loss. The research suggests that vegans often have lower BMIs and less body fat than meat-eaters and lacto-ovo vegetarians and that a vegan diet can be effective for weight loss.[1-3] That's encouraging news for anyone who wants to drop some weight, but we do need to be cautious in how we talk about this. It's not true that going vegan guarantees that you'll effortlessly shed pounds. Conflating veganism with a weight-loss diet may result in disappointment for new vegans who don't see their weight change, and it could be a reason why some people become disenchanted with veganism. A belief that "the right" vegan diet is a guarantee of a slender body can also create a toxic environment for vegans with larger bodies.

BODY SHAMING AND WEIGHT STIGMA

Weight stigma is a form of discrimination and stereotyping toward someone who has a larger body. It's frequently expressed through body shaming, which involves messages that are critical of the way certain bodies look. Weight stigma and body shaming contribute to a culture of shame about bodies that don't fit a certain standard. They are the result of simplistic and inaccurate beliefs about diet and obesity including the idea that you can determine a person's health status from their body size.

Weight stigma is born out of a culture that shares constant reminders about the obesity "crisis" or "epidemic," and that positions obesity as a burden on society and the economy. Both the dieting industry and public health efforts encouraging weight loss contribute to problems of weight stigma and body shaming, and the irony is that body shaming does not encourage weight loss. It is instead associated with a greater likelihood of weight gain.[4,5]

When people feel stigmatized and shamed about their weight, they are more likely to suffer from depression and anxiety and engage in disordered eating. They may be less likely to exercise. If they have been shamed about their weight by health-care providers, they may shy away from getting needed medical care including screenings for cancer and other chronic illnesses.[4,5]

On the surface, a promise of weight loss may seem like a useful way to draw more people to veganism. But suggesting that weight loss is "easy" provided you eat the "right" vegan diet creates a simplistic narrative that leads to blame and stigma. It suggests that we know the one and only way to produce weight loss—a belief that is naïve at best.

Increasingly, health professionals, social scientists, and the media are calling for a response to the implicit bigotry of body shaming and weight stigma. As advocates for a more just and compassionate world, we vegans have a clear place in these efforts.

Among vegans, body shaming has the tendency to alienate those whose bodies don't fit a particular ideal about what good vegan health looks like. This includes vegans with higher weights or with a disability as well as those whose bodies show natural signs of aging. How we talk about vegan diets as they relate to health and weight can go a long way toward alleviating this problem. Here are a few suggestions:

- Don't suggest that a vegan diet guarantees weight loss or is an easy way to lose weight.
- Be thoughtful about the pro-vegan media you share. Avoid those that show headless torsos of people with larger bodies, or that contrast lean vegans with meat-eaters. Note that these media, especially when aimed at shaming meat-eaters, sometimes masquerade as humor.
- Don't assume that everyone wants to lose weight.
- Don't make assumptions about someone's health or what they eat based on their weight.
- Avoid using phrases like "junk food vegan" and "cupcake vegan."
- Use neutral terms like "larger body" or "higher weight" rather than "overweight" or "obese."
- Praise other vegans for what they are doing to live a more compassionate life and/or promote vegan values rather than for how they look. Don't equate vegan diets with appearance or attractiveness.

WEIGHT LOSS AND HEALTH

Statistically, a high BMI is linked to greater risk for chronic diseases like heart disease, cancer, and type 2 diabetes. It's a little complicated, though. For one thing, where you carry fat on your body impacts risk. Visceral fat, the fat that surrounds your organs, is related to waist circumference and is more likely to raise risk for hypertension and diabetes than the fat that sits around hips and thighs.

Risk is also not quite so straightforward on an individual basis. While there are health risks attributed to body size at high or low ends of the BMI range it's not true that only people whose BMIs are within the "normal" range can be healthy. People with high body fat who engage in healthful behaviors can have optimal levels of blood cholesterol and blood pressure. One study of 43,000 subjects found that nearly a third of those whose BMIs fell in the obese range were healthy based on their fitness level, blood pressure, and cholesterol and triglyceride levels.[6]

Nor is it true that weight loss is the only way to improve health. In Chapter 15 we saw that people who followed the DASH diet could lower their blood pressure without losing weight. And even where weight loss is associated with improved health, it doesn't take much to have an effect. A small loss of 5 to 7 percent of weight—as little as ten pounds for someone who weighs two hundred pounds—can reduce risk of developing diabetes.[7]

Some researchers also argue that body size is less important than the stigma attached to it in determining health risks. Weight stigma can result in depression and anxiety, which are linked to greater inflammation in the body, raising risk for chronic disease. And although it's an area of debate, it's possible that weight cycling, or yo-yo dieting, which is sometimes a response to societal pressures to lose weight, promotes risk of hypertension and high LDL-cholesterol.[8]

ACHIEVING YOUR BEST WEIGHT

A multitude of factors affect weight; some are under your control and some aren't. Since we don't have a clear understanding of all these factors, it's no wonder that weight loss is often elusive.

Or more correctly, it is *permanent* weight loss that can be elusive. People are often good at shedding pounds but less successful in keeping the weight off. One reason is that many diets are short-term endeavors. People drop twenty pounds by changing their eating habits and then gradually morph back into old behaviors. But even a diligent dieter who is in it for the long term may find that weight eventually refuses to budge or it starts creeping back on. That's because smaller bodies burn fewer calories. Weight loss also promotes metabolic changes that are part of the body's defenses against starvation and that conserve calories, furthering hindering fat breakdown.[9] This means that as weight drops, so do your calorie needs. As a result, achieving an "ideal" weight—whether you're aiming for a particular BMI or a particular clothing size—often means a constant struggle with food and calories.

A more compassionate and realistic approach to weight management is to let go of the concept of "ideal" weight and instead embrace what the Canadian Obesity Network defines as "best weight."[10]

Your best weight is *whatever weight you achieve while living the healthiest lifestyle that you can truly enjoy.* You may be able to white knuckle it down to some deeply desired number on the scale through a starvation diet or by giving up every single food you love, but that's neither healthy nor enjoyable. And so that's not your best weight.

The concept of best weight embraces commitments to healthy behaviors, enjoyment around food choices, body positivity, and bodily autonomy. It's a focus that chooses to ignore external messages about what you should weigh and lets you make your own decision on what is the right weight for you. You are the only person who can determine what your best weight is. Given the health risks associated with weight stigma, learning to embrace this approach might have health benefits on its own.

The strategies and tips we provide in this chapter are meant to give you options for diet and lifestyle choices that can help you achieve or maintain your best weight. They will also enhance your health at any body size.

Before we look at those choices, though, we need to clear up some confusion about carbohydrates and fats and weight loss.

LOW-FAT OR LOW-CARB: DOES IT MATTER?

"Eat all you want and still lose weight!" You've probably seen plenty of those diets. As long as you avoid all high-fat foods, the pounds will simply melt away. Or just avoid carbs and watch the numbers on the scale plummet.

It's true that people have successfully lost weight on each of these approaches. Some studies have found that low-carb diets are associated with improved weight loss but others suggest that any difference between low-carbohydrate and low-fat diets disappears after a few months.[11-13] When researchers compared four popular diets—Atkins,

Ornish, Weight Watchers, and the Zone—they found that as long as people stuck to them, any of the diets produced weight loss. Subjects were least likely to adhere to Atkins (extremely low-carb) or Ornish (extremely low-fat).[14] In another large study, called DIETFITS, there was no difference in weight loss between people following a low-carbohydrate or a low-fat diet.[15]

Since fat has more than twice the calories as an equivalent amount of carbohydrate or protein, very low fat diets offer an effective way to reduce calorie intake. Diets that restrict whole categories of foods, like nuts, avocados, and oils, also make it harder to eat too many calories since people tend to eat less when their diet is less varied. But some higher-fat foods could actually help with weight control. Nuts are among the highest-fat plant foods but including a daily serving or two of these foods (preferably as whole nuts rather than nut butter) is linked to lower levels of body fat. Nuts have a strong satiety effect and their consumption may give a boost to the enhanced metabolism that normally occurs after a meal.[16,17] It also appears that not all of the calories in nuts are available to the body.[18]

Foods that are high in monounsaturated fats like olive and canola oils could be beneficial for reducing abdominal fat, possibly by increasing energy metabolism after a meal.[19] In a study at Brown University, women who added three tablespoons of olive oil to a reduced-calorie plant-based diet lost more weight than women eating a low-fat diet. All of the women in the study had a chance to try the olive oil diet and most preferred it, saying that they were less hungry and enjoyed their food more.[20]

This isn't to suggest a free-for-all with plant fats. Dousing your foods with oil or snacking on nuts all day can lead to excessive calorie intake. But there is no reason to think that you need to remove all high-fat foods and oils from your diet in order to lose weight. Given their health benefits, and the enjoyment that they can add to meals, including some of these foods in your menus can be a part of the strategy that lets you find your personal best weight, built on healthful and enjoyable foods.

Carbohydrates are good for you, too, when you get them mostly from beans, whole grains, vegetables, and fruits. Their high-fiber content can create a feeling of fullness. We saw in Chapter 16 that the effects of high-fiber diets on gut bacteria may promote weight loss.

When all is said and done, neither fat nor carbohydrates are off-limits for people who want to lose weight. Choosing healthful foods that you enjoy is more important than trying to minimize one of these nutrients.

FOOD CHOICES FOR ACHIEVING BEST WEIGHT

These are not rules about how you must eat to lose weight, but rather suggestions for making choices with a focus on health, satiety, and individual preferences. Whether your goal is to lose weight, prevent weight gain, or get healthier, these ideas can help.

Find the mix of carbohydrates and fats that works for you. Vegan diets can fit either a low-fat or low-carbohydrate approach, as well as a range of options in between. Low-carbohydrate vegan diets are built around nuts, seeds, vegetables, avocado, soyfoods, and added fats with moderate servings of beans and fruits, and limited grains. Low-fat vegan diets make generous use of grains, beans, fruits and vegetables while limiting nuts, seeds, soyfoods, avocado, and added fats. Either approach is healthy.

Eat plenty of protein. Ramping up protein intake can help protect bones and muscle during weight loss, especially if it's accompanied by exercise.[21] Protein is also more satiating than either carbohydrates or fats. Consuming it along with carbohydrates helps slow the release of glucose into the blood, providing a steadier source of energy. A high-protein meal can also increase the rate at which your body burns calories immediately afterward since it takes more work to digest and absorb protein than either carbohydrates or fats. Aim to include at least one serving of food from the legume group in the food guide in Chapter 10 in every meal and snack.

Choose foods with high satiety value. Protein and fiber are the dynamic duo for satiety and beans are among the few foods that are rich in both. Adding beans to your menus can promote modest weight loss even if you aren't focusing on calories.[22] Australian researchers asked subjects to make one simple change to their diet: eat four cans of chickpeas every week for twelve weeks. The subjects ended up replacing some of the grains in their diets with the chickpeas, and the result was a small weight loss.[23] And given the many health benefits of these foods, eating more beans is a good idea for everyone.[24]

Eat plenty of high-volume foods. Eating foods with a high water and fiber content helps create a feeling of fullness. The vegan foods with the highest bulk to calorie ratio are vegetables and fruits, followed by whole grains and beans. Make half your plate vegetables and fruits at every meal and include these foods in snacks, too. It's a good way to fill up on low-calorie foods, but don't try to fool your body with a diet of "rabbit food." You still need protein to create true satiety.

Satisfy your thirst with water. It's free and has no calories, so swapping out juices and sodas for water is an easy way to limit calorie intake. Most adults need about 4 to 6 cups of water per day, although that's a number that varies depending on climate and activity. Plain coffee, green and black tea, and herbal tea are also calorie-free beverages that can contribute to your fluid intake. There is some evidence that diet sodas confuse metabolic processes in a way that leads to weight gain, despite their lack of calories. The research is inconsistent, and these beverages are a better choice than sugary sodas, but until we have more information, we'd recommend limiting them to a serving or so a day if you consume them at all.

Be moderate with alcohol. This is always good advice under any circumstances. While moderate intake of one to two drinks per day doesn't appear to be a problem, excessive alcohol intake can contribute to weight gain.[25] And while we're on the topic of recreational substances, there is little evidence that cannabis ("the munchies" notwithstanding) is linked to weight gain except in low-weight individuals.[26] Possible explanations are that people choose calorie-free cannabis over calorie-laden alcohol. Or that medical marijuana users experience fewer aches and pains and are able to exercise more.[27] It's definitely an area where we need more research, which will most likely be forthcoming over the next decade.

Limit ultra-processed foods. While there is no established definition of "ultra-processed," these foods are usually identified as products that often have long lists of refined ingredients, are high in salt or sugar, and low in fiber. Sometimes they're manufactured to be "hyper-palatable," which encourages people to eat more of them. Examples are sodas, packaged cookies and pastries, some brands of chips, instant noodles, and some ready-to-eat meals. One group of researchers found that it's easy to consume more calories when you build meals around ultra-processed foods. The researchers offered the subjects three very large meals a day, allowing them to eat as much, or as little, as they wished. When the meals consisted almost entirely of ultra-processed foods, the subjects ate about five hundred calories more per day.[28]

The study showed what might happen when people eat these foods all day long, but it doesn't suggest that you need to eliminate these foods from your diet. And it doesn't mean that all processed foods are a problem. More gently processed foods like tofu, plant milks, canned and frozen beans and vegetables, prepared spaghetti sauce, and precooked grains can play important roles in vegan diets. Veggie meats can be valuable for boosting protein intake to protect muscles and bones during weight loss. And many ready-to-eat vegan products are actually packed with healthy ingredients. The best advice is to choose foods most often that are a good source of fiber and to limit commercial sweets and snacks.

FIND YOUR EATING STYLE: INTUITIVE OR PREEMPTIVE

Intuitive eating is a nondiet approach that teaches you to honor biological signals of hunger—and to eat in response to them. Instead of trying to control or ignore hunger the goal is to eat when you are hungry, without waiting until you are *too* hungry, which can result in reaching for the quickest-energy, high-calorie foods and then overeating. Intuitive eating aims to help you rebuild trust around your food choices, rather than making those choices according to external rules. It can be especially valuable for those who have dealt with eating disorders. For more on intuitive eating, we recommend this website from vegan dietitian Taylor Wolfram: http://www.wholegreenwellness.com/honor-bodys-hunger/.

A different approach uses preemptive eating to prevent hunger. This strategy involves eating a protein-rich meal or snack every several hours to preempt hunger, making it easier to manage dietary choices.

The two approaches share the goal of preventing the kind of hunger that can cause you to overeat. Eating mindfully is a good fit for either one. It's easy to eat more than you realize when you're glued to the TV or computer screen. Paying attention to the food you're eating allows you to tune in to appetite and satiety.

IT'S NOT JUST THE FOOD

Exercise, rest, and stress management are all crucial for good health and may help with weight loss or maintenance as well. Exercise makes cells more responsive to insulin, lowers blood pressure and cholesterol, and reduces inflammation. It improves sleep and can help with depression and anxiety. Aerobic activities like walking, running, dancing, biking, and cross-country skiing are good for cardiovascular health. Resistance training with free weights or machines strengthens muscles and helps protect bones. Both types of exercise are important for good health and resistance training is crucial if you are actively losing weight or if you are over the age of fifty.

Make sure you get adequate rest as well. Most adults need seven hours or more of sleep per night and getting enough can help prevent weight gain. If you find yourself hungrier on the day following a poor night's sleep, it isn't just your imagination. Lack of sleep can affect satiety hormones and drive up hunger.

Finally, depression and anxiety are linked to inflammation and weight gain. See page 252 for tips on lifestyle strategies to decrease depression.

WHEN YOU WANT TO GAIN WEIGHT

It may be a less common issue, but for some, getting enough calories to maintain their desired body weight is a challenge. Being underweight is associated with higher rates of mortality and it raises the risk for osteoporosis. In women, having too little body fat can make it difficult to conceive a baby. In older men and women, it is often associated with poor muscle strength, which can lead to frailty and disability.

Genetics influence body size and can be a factor for both lower and higher body weights. Smoking or drug use contribute to underweight and so does depression. Cancer treatment and long-term illnesses can cause weight loss, too.

If you have a low body weight because you find it difficult to eat enough calories, it's likely that you're at risk for nutrient deficiencies. Eating foods that are good sources of nutrients, including fortified foods, is valuable for ensuring adequate nutrition as you strive to gain weight, but it's fine to have some calorie-rich treats as well. Here are some tips for gaining weight:

- Eat more frequently. This is especially important if you find that you get full quickly. Eat five to six smaller meals during the day rather than two or three large meals.
- Try smoothies and shakes. Add protein powder and small amounts of nut butters to fruit smoothies to increase their calorie content.
- Snack on calorie-dense foods. If you're away from home during the day, carry snacks like nut butter with crackers, dried fruit,

energy bars, and mixed nuts. Granola with plant milk and fruit makes an energy-rich afternoon snack.

- Add extras. Stir cashew cream (soaked cashews blended with olive oil and lemon juice) or vegan sour cream into soups. Add nuts and avocado to salads.
- Sauté vegetables in small amounts of oil.
- Enjoy healthy treats. Top a bowl of fruit with a small scoop of vegan ice cream or stir granola and fruit into vegan yogurt. Or add chocolate-flavored plant milks to smoothies.
- Look for ways to choose higher-calorie foods. Cook oatmeal in full-fat soymilk since it's usually higher in calories than other plant milks. Choose extra-firm tofu, which is more calorie-dense than soft tofu.
- Include some refined grains in meals like white rice or white pasta to cut down on the satiating effects of fiber.
- If you're too busy to cook, stock the kitchen with convenience foods like precooked grains (frozen or in shelf-stable packages) and keep veggie meats on hand in the freezer.
- Try eating out of larger bowls to make your portions look smaller.
- Eat plenty of protein and carbohydrate since both are important for maintaining muscles.
- Engage in strength training to help you gain weight by building muscle. This might also improve your appetite.

EATING DISORDERS AND VEGAN DIETS

Eating disorders are serious and often fatal illnesses that are associated with severe disturbances in eating behaviors and the thoughts and emotions related to those behaviors.

The three common eating disorders are anorexia nervosa, bulimia nervosa, and binge-eating disorder. People with anorexia nervosa have an extreme fear of gaining weight and see themselves as overweight even if they are dangerously thin. They practice exceptionally restricted eating and often excessive exercise in a relentless pursuit of thinness. Bulimia nervosa involves frequent uncontrollable episodes of eating unusually large amounts of food followed by purging such as forced vomiting, laxatives, diuretics, or excessive exercise. The most common eating disorder, however, is binge-eating disorder in which people experience periods of overeating that is not followed by purging.

Eating disorders run in families and are linked to a complex interplay among genetic, biological, behavioral, psychological, and social factors. In most cases, eating disorders require a comprehensive intervention involving mental health counseling, medical monitoring, and nutrition counseling. Medications like antidepressants are sometimes useful, too.

Although eating disorders occur at any age and in both males and females, they are most common among teenage girls and young women. While some research suggests that eating disorders are more common among vegetarians and vegans, it appears that this is because teenage girls and young women sometimes adopt a vegetarian or vegan diet as a way to manage and disguise unhealthy food behavior.[29] That is, the eating disorder comes first and a vegan diet is merely one of many tools used to control calorie intake.[30] But healthy girls who become vegan or are raised in vegan households are no more likely than anyone else to develop an eating disorder. A vegan diet is not a sign of an eating disorder.

Research suggests that women who adopt vegetarian diets for ethical reasons are at lower risk for eating disorders than those who choose to limit animal foods for health, and especially for weight loss.[30-32] In fact, there is evidence that vegans are less likely to develop restricted eating behavior than those eating other plant-based diets like lacto-ovo vegetarians, semi-vegetarians, and flexitarians. This is most likely because health and dieting are more likely to be the motivations behind semi-vegetarian and flexitarian diets.[33,34] And it's interesting to learn that the incidence of disordered or restrictive eating seems to decline the longer a person follows a vegetarian diet.[34] That might suggest that those who follow it for the long term are less likely to be motivated by weight loss.

But even when ethics is the motivating factor, messages about vegan diets, weight loss, and healthy eating can sometimes morph into problematic attitudes toward food. Vegan diets that place extensive restrictions on food choices and suggest a need to make your diet as "clean" as possible may raise risk for unhealthy attitudes toward diet and food choices.

VEGAN DIETS AND RESTRICTIVE EATING

Limiting ultra-processed foods and concentrated sweets is a good idea for everyone. Beans, whole grains, fruits, vegetables, nuts, seeds and healthy fats are the foundation of a diet that maximizes the chance of attaining your best weight and good health. That doesn't mean you can never have a cupcake.

Labeling a food as forbidden or completely off-limits puts you just a step away from guilt and self-recrimination and can lead to anxiety and fear around food choices. If you slip up and eat that food, you've "fallen off the wagon." You might believe you've cheated or done something bad. It's a relationship with food that casts you as power-less in the face of temptation and assigns value to food as all-powerful. Giving yourself permission to eat those foods turns that dynamic on its head. While it may be beneficial to avoid foods that trigger over-eating in the short term, dietitians who specialize in eating disorders often recommend reintroducing these foods into your diet. The goal is to "normalize" all foods.

The concept of forbidden foods also spins a false narrative about diet and health. Your body is not so precarious or fragile that your health will fail if you don't eat only whole foods. Rigid ideas about which foods are allowed and which aren't can lead to binge eating and disordered eating.

A preoccupation with food that results in extreme attention to food choices and preparation and never-ending efforts at dietary improve-ment is part of a pattern that has been dubbed *orthorexia*.[35] It's true that veganism itself involves considerable attention to food choices and preparation. But there is a world of difference between eliminat-ing foods from your diet that cause harm to animals versus a belief that even small amounts of fats, sugar, and processed foods will damage your health.

An interest in the kind of healthy eating that we promote in this book is not orthorexia. But vegan messages suggesting that all added fats, food additives, nonorganic foods, processed foods, veggie meats and cheeses, or cooked foods are off-limits may invite unhealthy attitudes toward food. They can also invite criticisms of vegan diets. There are many instances where popular bloggers or fitness celebrities followed ultra-restrictive patterns, only to forsake their vegan diet when they started to feel unwell. Their followers and the media may believe that a vegan diet was at fault rather than a pattern of excessive dietary restriction.

Using care in how we talk about food can help minimize unhealthy practices and attitudes in relation to it. Describing certain foods as "toxic" can create anxiety around those foods, and labeling those who eat less healthy food as "junk food vegans" shames others based on their eating habits. Using terminology like "clean eating," can encourage an unhealthy relationship with food and promote fear of certain foods.

A better approach is to share helpful, evidence-based messages about a vegan diet as a healthy and responsible choice built on a foundation of whole plant foods while also including convenience products, treats, and favorite foods.

SETTING REALISTIC GOALS FOR HEALTHY LIVING

Whatever it means to you to live the most health-promoting lifestyle, chances are you can't do it every day. If you are overwhelmed by what you believe you need to do to enjoy good health, simply set a few priorities. Get a good night's sleep, go for a half-hour walk, and eat eight or more servings of fruits and vegetables plus a cup or two of beans every day. Build habits one at a time, keeping in mind that your goal is a healthy lifestyle that you enjoy.

AFTERWORD
Vegan for Life

Our aim in writing this book has been to give you the knowledge and tools that will make your vegan diet healthy, practical, and enjoyable. Choosing a diet that is packed with nutritious health-supporting foods, while also allowing your favorite foods and treats is empowering for anyone. We believe that it is even more so for vegans.

When it comes to diet, there are some things that are well within our control. For example, with the information in this book, you can feel certain about meeting nutrient needs on your vegan diet. And by eating a balanced vegan diet, avoiding tobacco, managing stress, exercising regularly, and getting appropriate medical screenings, you can be confident that you are doing your best to protect your health. But there is no diet in the world that can guarantee a slender body for everyone or that can promise complete protection from disease. Some things are in fact beyond our control.

But even if vegans get sick or the numbers on the scale don't budge, a vegan diet never stops being the best choice you could possibly make. It offers benefits that go far beyond health and personal well-being. Being vegan for life doesn't just impact your life, it impacts the lives of animals and the environment. It impacts the lives of future generations who will inhabit this planet.

To be vegan is to make choices every single day that are meaningful—to enact your values, inspire compassion, protect the earth, and respect your body. There is no other diet that can promise as much.

ACKNOWLEDGMENTS

From Jack and Ginny

Ten years ago, when we were working on the first edition of *Vegan for Life*, we had the good fortune to find our way to Renée Sedliar at Da Capo Press. We're grateful that she believed in our book from the start and that she gave us the opportunity to write this second edition. We couldn't ask for a more encouraging, enthusiastic, and skillful editor.

Thank you to our project manager, Cisca Schreefel, for piloting our book through production, and to Martha Whitt for her meticulous copy editing and enthusiasm for our manuscript. And to designers Terri Sirma and Trish Wilkinson for their talent and artistry.

Graphic designer and animal advocate Jenna White created the food guide for this book with the utmost patience, always willing to make "just one more change." Thank you to Dr. Reed Mangels, RD, for her generous help with our chapters on vegan diets in pregnancy and childhood.

As always, we are grateful to our agent Angela Miller for her ongoing support and for encouraging us to consider an update of this book.

From Jack

Thank you, Ginny, for your truly extraordinary commitment to making *Vegan for Life* the best it could be. Thank you, Alex, for your love and support and all you do to make this a better world for animals. Thank you to my family and friends for all your support and the sacrifices you've made to enable me to dedicate my life to animal advocacy. And thank you to all the staff, volunteers, and donors of Vegan Outreach for your dedication to moving the world beyond eating animals.

From Ginny

Thank you as always to my community of vegan health professionals who bring an ethic of compassion and a commitment to scientific integrity to this work that we do together. In addition to Jack, who continues to inspire me with his commitment to ethics and science, I'm grateful for the support and friendship of Reed Mangels, PhD, RD; Anya Todd, MS, RD; Taylor Wolfram, MS, RD; Matt Ruscigno, MPH, RD; David Weinman, MS, RD; and Ed Coffin, RD. I'm also indebted to my community of animal advocates in western Massachusetts, especially the members of Berkshire Voters for Animals.

I'm forever thankful to my parents, Willie Schrenk Kisch and Bill Kisch, who are temporarily gone from my sight but always in my heart. As always, I'm blessed to be married to Mark Messina, who still holds me accountable for every single thing I say about nutrition, still makes me laugh, and continues to be the best cat dad in the world.

REFERENCES

Introduction: Going Vegan for Life

1. Melina V, Craig W, Levin S. Position of the Academy of Nutrition and Dietetics: Vegetarian diets. *J Acad Nutr Diet.* 2016; 116:1970–1980.

Chapter 1. Why Vegan?

1. Compassion over Killing Investigations. http://cok.net/inv/.

2. Duncan I. Animal welfare issues in the poultry industry: Is there a lesson to be learned? *JAAWS.* 2001; 4:207–221.

3. United Egg Producers. Complete Guidelines for Cage and Cage-free Housing. https://uepcertified.com/wp-content/uploads/2015/08/UEP-Animal-Welfare -Guidelines-20141.pdf.

4. Webster AB. Welfare implications of avian osteoporosis. *Poult Sci.* 2004; 83:184–192.

5. Zuidhof MJ, Schneider BL, Carney VL, Korver DR, Robinson FE. Growth, efficiency, and yield of commercial broilers from 1957, 1978, and 2005. *Poult Sci.* 2014; 93:2970–2982.

6. Knowles TG, Kestin SC, Haslam SM, Brown SN, Green LE, Butterworth A, Pope SJ, Pfeiffer D, Nicol CJ. Leg disorders in broiler chickens: Prevalence, risk factors and prevention. *PLoS One.* 2008; 3:e1545.

7. Byrnes J. Raising pigs by the calendar at Maplewood Farm. *Hog Farm Management.* 1976; September:30–31.

8. Highlights of Swine 2006 Part III: Reference of Swine Health, Productivity, and General Management in the United States, 2006, Animal and Plant Health Inspection Service, USDA. March 2008. http://www.aphis.usda.gov/animal _health/nahms/swine/index.shtml.

9. Pork Checkoff. Online Farm Euthanasia of Swine: Recommendations for the Producer. https://www.aasv.org/aasv/documents/SwineEuthanasia.pdf.

10. Bekoff M. Killing "Happy" Pigs Is "Welfarish" and Isn't Just Fine. *Psychology Today,* May 7, 2015. https://www.psychologytoday.com/us/blog/animal-emotions /201505/killing-happy-pigs-is-welfarish-and-isnt-just-fine.

11. USDA Economic Research Service. The Changing Landscape of U.S. Milk Production. 2002. https://www.ers.usda.gov/webdocs/publications/47162/17864_sb978_1_.pdf?v=41056 (page 2).

12. USDA. Milk: Production Per Cow by Year. https://www.nass.usda.gov/Charts_and_Maps/Milk_Production_and_Milk_Cows/cowrates.php

13. Rogers D. Strange Noises Turn Out to Be Cows Missing Their Calves. Daily News. October 23, 2013. https://www.newburyportnews.com/news/local_news/strange-noises-turn-out-to-be-cows-missing-their-calves/article_d872e4da-b318-5e90-870e-51266f8eea7f.html.

14. Ask a Farmer: Use of Antibiotics in Cattle Feedlots. 2013. https://beefrunner.com/2013/11/18/ask-a-farmer-use-of-antibiotics-in-cattle-feedlots/.

15. Blackmore W. They Tested the Air Around Livestock Farms, and What It Contained Will Make You Gag. Take Part. 2015. http://www.takepart.com/article/2015/01/23/antibiotic-resistance-downwind-feedlots.

16. Edwards-Callaway LN, Walker J, Tucker CB. Culling decisions and dairy cattle welfare during transport to slaughter in the United States. *Front Vet Sci.* 2018; 5:343.

17. Humane Society of the United States. The Welfare of Animals in the Veal Industry. September 5, 2008. http://www.humanesociety.org/assets/pdfs/farm/hsus-the-welfare-of-animals-in-the-veal-industry.pdf.

18. Grandin T. Recommended Captive Bolt Stunning Techniques for Cattle. www.grandin.com/humane/cap.bolt.tips.html.

19. Vogel K, Grandin T. 2008 Restaurant Animal Welfare and Humane Slaughter Audits in Federally Inspected Beef and Pork Slaughter Plants in the U.S. and Canada. http://www.grandin.com/survey/2008.restaurant.audits.html; and Livestock Slaughter 2008 Summary, United States Department of Agriculture: Economics, Statistics, and Market Information System. http://usda.mannlib.cornell.edu/usda/nass/LiveSlauSu//2000s/2009/LiveSlauSu-03-06-2009.pdf.

20. USDA National Agricultural Statistics Service. Poultry Slaughter 2018. https://www.nass.usda.gov/Publications/Todays_Reports/reports/psla1018.pdf.

21. Jabr F. It's Official: Fish Feel Pain. January 8, 2018. https://www.smithsonianmag.com/science-nature/fish-feel-pain-180967764/.

22. Krantz R. "Wild-Caught," "Organic," "Grass-Fed": What Do All These Animal Welfare Labels Actually Mean? *Vox.* January 30, 2019. https://www.vox.com/future-perfect/2019/1/30/18197688/organic-cage-free-wild-caught-certified-humane.

23. Cornucopia Institute. Scrambled Eggs: Separating Factory Farm Production from Authentic Organic Production. https://www.cornucopia.org/scrambled-eggs-separating-factory-farm-egg-production-from-authentic-organic-agriculture/.

24. Farm Animal Sanctuary Directory. https://www.vegan.com/?s=sanc.

25. Singer P. *Animal Liberation: A New Ethic for Our Treatment of Animals.* Harper Collins; 1975.

26. Wuebbles DJ, Fahey DW, Hibbard KA, et al. Executive summary. In Wuebbles DJ, Fahey DW, Hibbard KA, Dokken DJ, Stewart BC, Maycock TK,

eds. *Climate Science Special Report: Fourth National Climate Assessment, Volume 1.* Washington, DC: US Global Change Research Program; 2017:12–34.

27. Lappé FM. *Diet for a Small Planet.* Ballantine Books, 1971.

28. Reijnders L, Soret S. Quantification of the environmental impact of different dietary protein choices. *Am J Clin Nutr.* 2003; 78:664S–668S.

29. Sabate J, Soret S. Sustainability of plant-based diets: back to the future. *Am J Clin Nutr.* 2014; 100 Suppl 1:476S–482S.

30. Scarborough P, Appleby PN, Mizdrak A, Briggs AD, Travis RC, Bradbury KE, Key TJ. Dietary greenhouse gas emissions of meat-eaters, fish-eaters, vegetarians and vegans in the UK. *Clim Change.* 2014; 125:179–192.

31. Environmental Protection Agency. Estimated Animal Agriculture Nitrogen and Phosphorus from Manure. https://www.epa.gov/nutrient-policy-data/estimated-animal-agriculture-nitrogen-and-phosphorus-manure.

32. Harwatt H, Sabaté J, Eshel G, Soret S, Ripple W. Substituting beans for beef as a contribution toward US climate change targets. *Clim Change.* 2017; 143:261.

33. Goldstein B, Moses R, Sammons N, Birkved M. Potential to curb the environmental burdens of American beef consumption using a novel plant-based beef substitute. *PLoS One.* 2017; 12:e0189029.

Chapter 3. Understanding Vegan Nutrition Needs

1. Mangels R, Messina V, Messina M. *The Dietitian's Guide to Vegetarian Diets.* 3rd ed. Sudbury, MA: Jones and Bartlett, 2011.

2. Davey GK, Spencer EA, Appleby PN, Allen NE, Knox KH, Key TJ. EPIC-Oxford: Lifestyle characteristics and nutrient intakes in a cohort of 33, 883 meat-eaters and 31, 546 non meat-eaters in the UK. *Public Health Nutr.* 2003; 6:259–269.

3. Rizzo NS, Jaceldo-Siegl K, Sabate J, Fraser GE. Nutrient profiles of vegetarian and nonvegetarian dietary patterns. *J Acad Nutr Diet.* 2013; 113:1610–1619.

4. Sobiecki JG, Appleby PN, Bradbury KE, Key TJ. High compliance with dietary recommendations in a cohort of meat eaters, fish eaters, vegetarians, and vegans: Results from the European Prospective Investigation into Cancer and Nutrition—Oxford study. *Nutr Res.* 2016; 36:464–477.

Chapter 4. Plant Protein

1. Young VR, Pellett PL. Plant proteins in relation to human protein and amino acid nutrition. *Am J Clin Nutr.* 1994; 59:1203S–1212S.

2. Lappé FM. *Diet for a Small Planet.* Ballantine Books, 1971.

3. Fuller MF, Reeds PJ. Nitrogen cycling in the gut. *Annu Rev Nutr.* 1998; 18:385–411.

4. WHO Technical Report Series 935: Protein and Amino Acid Requirements in Human Nutrition. https://www.who.int/nutrition/publications/nutrientrequirements/WHO_TRS_935/en/.

5. Elango R, Humayun MA, Ball RO, Pencharz PB. Evidence that protein requirements have been significantly underestimated. *Curr Opin Clin Nutr Metab Care.* 2010; 13:52–57.

6. Sarwar G. Digestibility of protein and bioavailability of amino acids in foods: Effects on protein quality assessment. *World Rev Nutr Diet.* 1987; 54:26–70.

7. Leidy HJ, Clifton PM, Astrup A, et al. The role of protein in weight loss and maintenance. *Am J Clin Nutr.* 2015; 101:1320S–1329S.

8. Buendia JR, Bradlee ML, Singer MR, Moore LL. Diets higher in protein predict lower high blood pressure risk in Framingham Offspring Study adults. *Am J Hypertens.* 2015; 28:372–379.

9. Rizzoli R, Biver E, Bonjour JP, Coxam V, et al. Benefits and safety of dietary protein for bone health: An expert consensus paper endorsed by the European Society for Clinical and Economical Aspects of Osteopororosis, Osteoarthritis, and Musculoskeletal Diseases and by the International Osteoporosis Foundation. *Osteoporos Int.* 2018; 29:1933–1948.

10. Martone AM, Marzetti E, Calvani R, et al. Exercise and protein intake: A synergistic approach against sarcopenia. *Biomed Res Int.* 2017; Article ID 2672435. https://www.hindawi.com/journals/bmri/2017/2672435/cta/.

11. Paddon-Jones D, Rasmussen BB. Dietary protein recommendations and the prevention of sarcopenia. *Curr Opin Clin Nutr Metab Care.* 2009; 12:86–90.

12. Bauer J, Biolo G, Cederholm T, et al. Evidence-based recommendations for optimal dietary protein intake in older people: A position paper from the PROT-AGE Study Group. *J Am Med Dir Assoc.* 2013; 14:542–559.

13. Richter CK, Skulas-Ray AC, Champagne CM, Kris-Etherton PM. Plant protein and animal proteins: Do they differentially affect cardiovascular disease risk? *Adv Nutr.* 2015; 6:712–728.

14. Richard DM, Dawes MA, Mathias CW, Acheson A, Hill-Kapturczak N, Dougherty DM. L-Tryptophan: Basic metabolic functions, behavioral research and therapeutic indications. *Int J Tryptophan Res.* 2009; 2:45–60.

Chapter 5. Eating for Healthy Bones: Calcium and Vitamin D

1. Eaton SB, Nelson DA. Calcium in evolutionary perspective. *Am J Clin Nutr.* 1991; 54:281S–287S.

2. Konner M, Eaton SB. Paleolithic nutrition: Twenty-five years later. *Nutr Clin Pract.* 2010; 25:594–602.

3. Mangels R, Messina V, Messina M. *The Dietitian's Guide to Vegetarian Diets.* 3rd ed. Sudbury, MA: Jones and Bartlett, 2011.

4. Sobiecki JG, Appleby PN, Bradbury KE, Key TJ. High compliance with dietary recommendations in a cohort of meat eaters, fish eaters, vegetarians, and vegans: Results from the European Prospective Investigation into Cancer and Nutrition—Oxford study. *Nutr Res.* 2016; 36:464–477.

5. Rizzo NS, Jaceldo-Siegl K, Sabate J, Fraser GE. Nutrient profiles of vegetarian and nonvegetarian dietary patterns. *J Acad Nutr Diet.* 2013; 113:1610–1619.

6. Feskanich D, Willett WC, Stampfer MJ, Colditz GA. Milk, dietary calcium, and bone fractures in women: A 12-year prospective study. *Am J Public Health.* 1997; 87:992–997.

7. Bischoff-Ferrari HA, Dawson-Hughes B, Baron JA, et al. Calcium intake and hip fracture risk in men and women: A meta-analysis of prospective cohort studies and randomized controlled trials. *Am J Clin Nutr.* 2007; 86:1780–1790.

8. Abelow BJ, Holford TR, Insogna KL. Cross-cultural association between dietary animal protein and hip fracture: A hypothesis. *Calcif Tissue Int.* 1992; 50:14–18.

9. Wetzsteon RJ, Hughes JM, Kaufman BC, et al. Ethnic differences in bone geometry and strength are apparent in childhood. *Bone.* 2009; 44:970–975.

10. Faulkner KG, Cummings SR, Black D, Palermo L, Gluer CC, Genant HK. Simple measurement of femoral geometry predicts hip fracture: The study of osteoporotic fractures. *J Bone Miner Res.* 1993; 8:1211–1217.

11. Lee DH, Jung KY, Hong AR, et al. Femoral geometry, bone mineral density, and the risk of hip fracture in premenopausal women: A case control study. *BMC Musculoskelet Disord.* 2016; 17:42.

12. Kwan MM, Tsang WW, Lin SI, Greenaway M, Close JC, Lord SR. Increased concern is protective for falls in Chinese older people: The chopstix fall risk study. *J Gerontol A Biol Sci Med Sci.* 2013; 68:946–953.

13. Russell-Aulet M, Wang J, Thornton JC, Colt EW, Pierson RN, Jr. Bone mineral density and mass in a cross-sectional study of white and Asian women. *J Bone Miner Res.* 1993; 8:575–582.

14. Bow CH, Cheung E, Cheung CL, et al. Ethnic difference of clinical vertebral fracture risk. *Osteoporos Int.* 2012; 23:879–885.

15. Cao JJ, Pasiakos SM, Margolis LM, et al. Calcium homeostasis and bone metabolic responses to high-protein diets during energy deficit in healthy young adults: A randomized controlled trial. *Am J Clin Nutr.* 2014; 99:400–407.

16. Cao JJ, Johnson LK, Hunt JR. A diet high in meat protein and potential renal acid load increases fractional calcium absorption and urinary calcium excretion without affecting markers of bone resorption or formation in postmenopausal women. *J Nutr.* 2011; 141:391–397.

17. Kerstetter JE, O'Brien KO, Insogna KL. Dietary protein affects intestinal calcium absorption. *Am J Clin Nutr.* 1998; 68:859–865.

18. Fenton TR, Lyon AW, Eliasziw M, Tough SC, Hanley DA. Meta-analysis of the effect of the acid-ash hypothesis of osteoporosis on calcium balance. *J Bone Miner Res.* 2009; 24:1835–1840.

19. Calvez J, Poupin N, Chesneau C, Lassale C, Tome D. Protein intake, calcium balance and health consequences. *Eur J Clin Nutr.* 2012; 66:281–295.

20. Beasley JM, LaCroix AZ, Larson JC, et al. Biomarker-calibrated protein intake and bone health in the Women's Health Initiative clinical trials and observational study. *Am J Clin Nutr.* 2014; 99:934–240.

21. Munger RG, Cerhan JR, Chiu BC. Prospective study of dietary protein intake and risk of hip fracture in postmenopausal women. *Am J Clin Nutr.* 1999; 69:147–152.

22. Pedone C, Napoli N, Pozzilli P, et al. Quality of diet and potential renal acid load as risk factors for reduced bone density in elderly women. *Bone.* 2010; 46:1063–1067.

23. Devine A, Dick IM, Islam AF, Dhaliwal SS, Prince RL. Protein consumption is an important predictor of lower limb bone mass in elderly women. *Am J Clin Nutr.* 2005; 81:1423–1428.

24. Schurch MA, Rizzoli R, Slosman D, Vadas L, Vergnaud P, Bonjour JP. Protein supplements increase serum insulin-like growth factor-I levels and attenuate proximal femur bone loss in patients with recent hip fracture: A randomized, double-blind, placebo-controlled trial. *Ann Intern Med.* 1998; 128:801–809.

25. Thorpe DL, Knutsen SF, Beeson WL, Rajaram S, Fraser GE. Effects of meat consumption and vegetarian diet on risk of wrist fracture over 25 years in a cohort of peri- and postmenopausal women. *Public Health Nutr.* 2008; 11:564–572.

26. Lousuebsakul-Matthews V, Thorpe DL, Knutsen R, Beeson WL, Fraser GE, Knutsen SF. Legumes and meat analogues consumption are associated with hip fracture risk independently of meat intake among Caucasian men and women: the Adventist Health Study-2. *Public Health Nutr* 2014; 17:2333–2343.

27. Thorpe MP, Evans EM. Dietary protein and bone health: Harmonizing conflicting theories. *Nutr Rev.* 2011; 69:215–230.

28. Ho-Pham LT, Nguyen ND, Nguyen TV. Effect of vegetarian diets on bone mineral density: A Bayesian meta-analysis. *Am J Clin Nutr.* 2009; 90: 943–950.

29. Appleby P, Roddam A, Allen N, Key T. Comparative fracture risk in vegetarians and nonvegetarians in EPIC-Oxford. *Eur J Clin Nutr.* 2007; 61:1400–1406.

30. Chiu JF, Lan SJ, Yang CY, et al. Long-term vegetarian diet and bone mineral density in postmenopausal Taiwanese women. *Calcif Tissue Int.* 1997; 60:245–249.

31. Weaver CM, Heaney RP, Connor L, Martin BR, Smith DL, Nielsen E. Bioavailability of calcium from tofu vs. milk in premenopausal women. *J Food Sci.* 2002; 68:3144–3147.

32. Weaver CM, Heaney RP, Nickel KP, Packard PI. Calcium bioavailability from high oxalate vegetables: Chinese vegetables, sweet potatoes and rhubarb. *J Food Sci.* 1997; 63:524–525.

33. Weaver CM, Plawecki KL. Dietary calcium: Adequacy of a vegetarian diet. *Am J Clin Nutr.* 1994; 59:1238S–1241S.

34. Weaver CM, Proulx WR, Heaney R. Choices for achieving adequate dietary calcium with a vegetarian diet. *Am J Clin Nutr.* 1999; 70:543S–548S.

35. Samelson EJ, Booth SL, Fox CS, et al. Calcium intake is not associated with increased coronary artery calcification: The Framingham Study. *Am J Clin Nutr.* 2012; 96:1274–1280.

36. Thacher TD, Clarke BL. Vitamin D insufficiency. *Mayo Clin Proc.* 2011; 86:50–60.

37. Holick MF, Binkley NC, Bischoff-Ferrari HA, et al. Evaluation, treatment, and prevention of vitamin D deficiency: An Endocrine Society clinical practice guideline. *J Clin Endocrinol Metab.* 2011; 96:1911–1930.

38. Armas LA, Hollis BW, Heaney RP. Vitamin D_2 is much less effective than vitamin D_3 in humans. *J Clin Endocrinol Metab.* 2004; 89:5387–5391.

39. Holick MF, Biancuzzo RM, Chen TC, et al. Vitamin D_2 is as effective as vitamin D_3 in maintaining circulating concentrations of 25-hydroxyvitamin D. *J Clin Endocrinol Metab.* 2008; 93:677–681.

40. Lehmann U, Hirche F, Stangl GI, Hinz K, Westphal S, Dierkes J. Bioavailability of vitamin D(2) and D(3) in healthy volunteers: A randomized placebo-controlled trial. *J Clin Endocrinol Metab.* 2013; 98:4339–4345.

41. Webb AR, Kline L, Holick MF. Influence of season and latitude on the cutaneous synthesis of vitamin D_3: Exposure to winter sunlight in Boston and Edmonton will not promote vitamin D_3 synthesis in human skin. *J Clin Endocrinol Metab.* 1988 Aug; 67(2):373–378.

42. Specker BL, Valanis B, Hertzberg V, Edwards N, Tsang RC. Sunshine exposure and serum 25-hydroxyvitamin D concentrations in exclusively breast-fed infants. *J Pediatr.* 1985; 107:372–376.

43. Clemens TL, Adams JS, Henderson SL, Holick MF. Increased skin pigment reduces the capacity of skin to synthesise vitamin D_3. *Lancet.* 1982; 1:74–76.

44. Holick MF, Matsuoka LY, Wortsman J. Age, vitamin D, and solar ultraviolet. *Lancet.* 1989;2:1104–1105.

45. Tucker KL, Hannan MT, Chen H, Cupples LA, Wilson PW, Kiel DP. Potassium, magnesium, and fruit and vegetable intakes are associated with greater bone mineral density in elderly men and women. *Am J Clin Nutr.* 1999; 69:727–736.

46. Ruiz-Ramos M, Vargas LA, Fortoul Van der Goes TI, Cervantes-Sandoval A, Mendoza-Nunez VM. Supplementation of ascorbic acid and alpha-tocopherol is useful to preventing bone loss linked to oxidative stress in elderly. *J Nutr Health Aging.* 2010; 14:467–472.

47. Feskanich D, Weber P, Willett WC, Rockett H, Booth SL, Colditz GA. Vitamin K intake and hip fractures in women: A prospective study. *Am J Clin Nutr.* 1999; 69:74–79.

48. Booth SL, Broe KE, Gagnon DR, et al. Vitamin K intake and bone mineral density in women and men. *Am J Clin Nutr.* 2003; 77:512–516.

Chapter 6. Vitamin B_{12}

1. van den Berg H, Dagnelie PC, van Staveren WA. Vitamin B_{12} and seaweed. *Lancet.* 1988; 1:242–243.

2. Carmel R, Karnaze DS, Weiner JM. Neurologic abnormalities in cobalamin deficiency are associated with higher cobalamin "analogue" values than are hematologic abnormalities. *J Lab Clin Med.* 1988; 111:57–62.

3. Merchant RE, Phillips TW, Udani J. Nutritional supplementation with *Chlorella pyrenoidosa* lowers serum methylmalonic acid in vegans and vegetarians with a suspected vitamin B(1)(2) deficiency. *J Med Food.* 2015; 18:1357–1362.

4. Mozafar A, Oertli JJ. Uptake of a microbially-produced vitamin (B_{12}) by soybean roots. *Plant Soil.* 1992; 139:23–30.

5. Bito T, Ohishi N, Hatanaka Y, et al. Production and characterization of cyanocobalamin-enriched lettuce (*Lactuca sativa* L.) grown using hydroponics. *J Agric Food Chem.* 2013; 61:3852–3858.

6. Van Dam F, Van Gool WA. Hyperhomocysteinemia and Alzheimer's disease: A systematic review. *Arch Gerontol Geriatr.* May–June 2009; 48(3):425–430. Epub 2008 May 13.

7. Walters MJ, Sterling J, Quinn C, et al. Associations of lifestyle and vascular risk factors with Alzheimer's brain biomarker changes during middle age: A 3-year longitudinal study in the broader New York City area. *BMJ Open.* Nov 25, 2018; 8(11):e023664.

8. Douaud G, Refsum H, de Jager CA, et al. Preventing Alzheimer's disease-related gray matter atrophy by B-vitamin treatment. *Proc Natl Acad Sci U S A.* June 4, 2013; 110(23):9523–9528. DOI: 10.1073/pnas.1301816110. Epub May 20, 2013.

9. Molloy AM, Kirke PN, Troendle JF, et al. Maternal vitamin B_{12} status and risk of neural tube defects in a population with high neural tube defect prevalence and no folic acid fortification. *Pediatrics.* March 2009; 123(3):917–923.

10. Krivosikova Z, Krajcovicova-Kudlackova M, Spustova V, et al. The association between high plasma homocysteine levels and lower bone mineral density in Slovak women: The impact of vegetarian diet. *Eur J Nutr.* 2010; 49(3):147–153.

11. Herrmann W, Obeid R, Schorr H, et al. Enhanced bone metabolism in vegetarians: The role of vitamin B_{12} deficiency. *Clin Chem Lab Med.* 2009; 47(11): 1381–1387.

12. Martí-Carvajal AJ, Solà I, Lathyris D, Dayer M. Homocysteine-lowering interventions for preventing cardiovascular events. *Cochrane Database Syst Rev.* Aug 17, 2017; 8:CD006612.

13. Norris J. Mild B_{12} deficiency-elevated homocysteine. www.veganhealth .org/b12/hcy.

14. Pawlak R, Parrott SJ, Raj S, Cullum-Dugan D, Lucus D. How prevalent is vitamin B(12) deficiency among vegetarians? *Nutr Rev.* Feb 2013; 71(2):110–117.

15. Pawlak R, Lester SE, Babatunde T. The prevalence of cobalamin deficiency among vegetarians assessed by serum vitamin B_{12}: A review of literature. *Eur J Clin Nutr.* 2016; 70:866.

16. Kwok T, Chook P, Qiao M, et al. Vitamin B-12 supplementation improves arterial function in vegetarians with subnormal vitamin B-12 status. *J Nutr Health Aging.* 2012; 16(6):569–573.

17. Allen LH. How common is vitamin B-12 deficiency? *Am J Clin Nutr.* 2009; 89:693S–696S.

18. Opinion of the Scientific Panel on Food Additives, Flavourings, Processing Aids and Materials in Contact with Food (AFC) on hydrocyanic acid in flavourings and other food ingredients with flavouring properties. *The EFSA Journal.* 2004:105.

19. Hokin BD, Butler T. Cyanocobalamin (vitamin B-12) status in Seventh-Day Adventist ministers in Australia. *Am J Clin Nutr.* 1999; 70:576S–578S.

20. Mason R. paleovegan.blogspot.com/2010/08Afarensis-may-have-used -stone-tool-so.html.

21. Billings T. http://www.beyondveg.com/billings-t/comp-anat/comp-anat-9e .shtml.

Chapter 7. Fats: Making the Best Choices

1. Mangels R, Messina V, Messina M. *The Dietitian's Guide to Vegetarian Diets.* 3rd ed. Sudbury, MA: Jones and Bartlett, 2011.

2. Keys A, Menotti A, Karvonen MJ, et al. The diet and 15-year death rate in the Seven Countries Study. *Am J Epidemiol.* 1986; 124:903–915.

3. Welch AA, Bingham SA, Khaw KT. Estimated conversion of alpha-linolenic acid to long chain n-3 polyunsaturated fatty acids is greater than expected in non fish-eating vegetarians and non fish-eating meat-eaters than in fish-eaters. *J Hum Nutr Diet.* 2008; 21:404.

4. Kornsteiner M, Singer I, Elmadfa I. Very low n-3 long-chain polyunsaturated fatty acid status in Austrian vegetarians and vegans. *Ann Nutr Metab.* 2008; 52:37–47.

5. Mann N, Pirotta Y, O'Connell S, Li D, Kelly F, Sinclair A. Fatty acid composition of habitual omnivore and vegetarian diets. *Lipids.* 2006; 41:637–646.

6. Mozaffarian D, Wu JH. Omega-3 fatty acids and cardiovascular disease: Effects on risk factors, molecular pathways, and clinical events. *J Am Coll Cardiol.* 2011; 58:2047–2067.

7. Mente A, de Koning L, Shannon HS, Anand SS. A systematic review of the evidence supporting a causal link between dietary factors and coronary heart disease. *Arch Intern Med.* 2009; 169:659–669.

8. Aung T, Halsey J, Kromhout D, et al. Associations of omega-3 fatty acid supplement use with cardiovascular disease risks: Meta-analysis of 10 trials involving 77,917 individuals. *JAMA Cardiol.* 2018; 3:225–234.

9. Abdelhamid AS, Brown TJ, Brainard JS, et al. Omega-3 fatty acids for the primary and secondary prevention of cardiovascular disease. *Cochrane Database Syst Rev.* 2018; 11:CD003177.

10. Kromhout D. Omega-3 fatty acids and coronary heart disease: The final verdict? *Curr Opin Lipidol.* 2012; 23:554–559.

11. Jung UJ, Torrejon C, Tighe AP, Deckelbaum RJ. n-3 Fatty acids and cardiovascular disease: Mechanisms underlying beneficial effects. *Am J Clin Nutr.* 2008; 87:2003S–2009S.

12. Rosell MS, Lloyd-Wright Z, Appleby PN, Sanders TA, Allen NE, Key TJ. Long-chain n-3 polyunsaturated fatty acids in plasma in British meat-eating, vegetarian, and vegan men. *Am J Clin Nutr.* 2005; 82:327–334.

13. Sanders TA, Roshanai F. Platelet phospholipid fatty acid composition and function in vegans compared with age- and sex-matched omnivore controls. *Eur J Clin Nutr.* 1992; 46:823–831.

14. Reddy S, Sanders TA, Obeid O. The influence of maternal vegetarian diet on essential fatty acid status of the newborn. *Eur J Clin Nutr.* 1994; 48:358–368.

15. Krajcovicova-Kudlackova M, Simoncic R, Bederova A, Klvanova J. Plasma fatty acid profile and alternative nutrition. *Ann Nutr Metab.* 1997; 41:365–370.

16. Agren JJ, Tormala ML, Nenonen MT, Hanninen OO. Fatty acid composition of erythrocyte, platelet, and serum lipids in strict vegans. *Lipids.* 1995; 30: 365–369.

17. Mezzano D, Munoz X, Martinez C, et al. Vegetarians and cardiovascular risk factors: Hemostasis, inflammatory markers and plasma homocysteine. *Thromb Haemost.* 1999; 81:913–917.

18. Mezzano D, Kosiel K, Martinez C, et al. Cardiovascular risk factors in vegetarians: Normalization of hyperhomocysteinemia with vitamin B(12) and reduction of platelet aggregation with n-3 fatty acids. *Thromb Res.* 2000; 100:153–160.

19. Key TJ, Fraser GE, Thorogood M, et al. Mortality in vegetarians and non-vegetarians: Detailed findings from a collaborative analysis of 5 prospective studies. *Am J Clin Nutr.* 1999; 70:516S–524S.

20. Crowe FL, Appleby PN, Travis RC, Key TJ. Risk of hospitalization or death from ischemic heart disease among British vegetarians and nonvegetarians: Results from the EPIC-Oxford cohort study. *Am J Clin Nutr.* 2013; 97:597–603.

21. Burdge GC, Calder PC. Conversion of alpha-linolenic acid to longer-chain polyunsaturated fatty acids in human adults. *Reprod Nutr Dev.* 2005; 45:581–597.

22. Burdge GC, Jones AE, Wootton SA. Eicosapentaenoic and docosapentaenoic acids are the principal products of alpha-linolenic acid metabolism in young men*. *Br J Nutr.* 2002; 88:355–363.

23. Emken EA, Adlof RO, Gulley RM. Dietary linoleic acid influences desaturation and acylation of deuterium-labeled linoleic and linolenic acids in young adult males. *Biochim Biophys Acta.* 1994; 1213:277–288.

24. Gerster H. Can adults adequately convert alpha-linolenic acid (18:3n-3) to eicosapentaenoic acid (20:5n-3) and docosahexaenoic acid (22:6n-3)? *Int J Vitam Nutr Res.* 1998; 68:159–173.

25. Liou YA, King DJ, Zibrik D, Innis SM. Decreasing linoleic acid with constant alpha-linolenic acid in dietary fats increases (n-3) eicosapentaenoic acid in plasma phospholipids in healthy men. *J Nutr.* 2007; 137:945–952.

26. Wien M, Rajaram S, Oda K, Sabate J. Decreasing the linoleic acid to alpha-linolenic acid diet ratio increases eicosapentaenoic acid in erythrocytes in adults. *Lipids.* 2010; 45:683–692.

27. Fokkema MR, Brouwer DA, Hasperhoven MB, Martini IA, Muskiet FA. Short-term supplementation of low-dose gamma-linolenic acid (GLA), alpha-linolenic acid (ALA), or GLA plus ALA does not augment LCP omega 3 status of Dutch vegans to an appreciable extent. *Prostaglandins Leukot Essent Fatty Acids* 2000; 63:287–292.

28. Wood KE, Mantzioris E, Gibson RA, Ramsden CE, Muhlhausler BS. The effect of modifying dietary LA and ALA intakes on omega-3 long chain polyunsaturated fatty acid (n-3 LCPUFA) status in human adults: A systematic review and commentary. *Prostaglandins Leukot Essent Fatty Acids.* 2015; 95:47–55.

29. Sanders TA, Younger KM. The effect of dietary supplements of omega 3 polyunsaturated fatty acids on the fatty acid composition of platelets and plasma choline phosphoglycerides. *Br J Nutr.* 1981; 45:613–616.

30. Ghafoorunissa IM. n-3 Fatty acids in Indian diets: Comparison of the effects of precursor (alpha-linolenic acid) vs. product (long chain n-3 polyunsaturated fatty acids). *Nutr Res.* 1992; 12:569–582.

31. FAO report 91 Fats and fatty acids in human nutrition: Report of an expert consultation. *Food and Nutrition Paper* 91. FAO of the UN, Rome 2010.

32. Pinto AM, Sanders TA, Kendall AC, et al. A comparison of heart rate variability, n-3 PUFA status and lipid mediator profile in age- and BMI-matched middle-aged vegans and omnivores. *Br J Nutr*. 2017; 117:669–685.

33. Allés B, Baudry J, Mejean C, et al. Comparison of sociodemographic and nutritional characteristics between self-reported vegetarians, vegans, and meat-eaters from the NutriNet-Sante Study. *Nutrients*. 2017; 9(9):1023. https://www.ncbi.nlm.nih.gov/pmc/articles/PMC5622783/.

34. Rizzo NS, Jaceldo-Siegl K, Sabate J, Fraser GE. Nutrient profiles of vegetarian and nonvegetarian dietary patterns. *J Acad Nutr Diet*. 2013; 113:1610–1619.

35. Lloyd-Wright Z, Preston R, Gray R, et al. Randomized placebo controlled trial of a daily intake of 200 mg docasahexanoic acid in vegans. Abstract in *Proc Nutr Soc*. 2003; 62:42a.

36. Conquer JA, Holub BJ. Supplementation with an algae source of docosahexaenoic acid increases (n-3) fatty acid status and alters selected risk factors for heart disease in vegetarian subjects. *J Nutr*. 1996; 126:3032–3039.

37. Lipoeto NI, Agus Z, Oenzil F, Wahlqvist M, Wattanapenpaiboon N. Dietary intake and the risk of coronary heart disease among the coconut-consuming Minangkabau in West Sumatra, Indonesia. *Asia Pac J Clin Nutr*. 2004; 13:377–384.

38. Khaw KT, Sharp SJ, Finikarides L, et al. Randomised trial of coconut oil, olive oil or butter on blood lipids and other cardiovascular risk factors in healthy men and women. *BMJ Open*. 2018; 8:e020167.

Chapter 8. Vitamins and Minerals: Maximizing Vegan Sources

1. Baker RD, Greer FR. Diagnosis and prevention of iron deficiency and iron-deficiency anemia in infants and young children (0–3 years of age). *Pediatrics*. 2010; 126:1040–1050.

2. Miller EM. Iron status and reproduction in US women: National Health and Nutrition Examination Survey, 1999–2006. *PLoS One*. 2014; 9:e112216.

3. Mei Z, Cogswell ME, Looker AC, et al. Assessment of iron status in US pregnant women from the National Health and Nutrition Examination Survey (NHANES), 1999–2006. *Am J Clin Nutr*. 2011; 93:1312–1320.

4. Mangels R, Messina V, Messina M. *The Dietitian's Guide to Vegetarian Diets*. 3rd ed. Sudbury, MA: Jones and Bartlett, 2011.

5. Haddad EH, Berk LS, Kettering JD, Hubbard RW, Peters WR. Dietary intake and biochemical, hematologic, and immune status of vegans compared with nonvegetarians. *Am J Clin Nutr*. 1999; 70:586S–593S.

6. Rizzo NS, Jaceldo-Siegl K, Sabate J, Fraser GE. Nutrient profiles of vegetarian and nonvegetarian dietary patterns. *J Acad Nutr Diet*. 2013; 113:1610–1619.

7. Davey GK, Spencer EA, Appleby PN, Allen NE, Knox KH, Key TJ. EPIC-Oxford: Lifestyle characteristics and nutrient intakes in a cohort of 33,883 meat-eaters and 31,546 non meat-eaters in the UK. *Public Health Nutr*. 2003; 6:259–269.

8. Monsen ER, Balintfy JL. Calculating dietary iron bioavailability: Refinement and computerization. *J Am Diet Assoc*. 1982; 80:307–311.

9. Seshadri S, Shah A, Bhade S. Haematologic response of anaemic preschool children to ascorbic acid supplementation. *Hum Nutr Appl Nutr*. 1985; 39:151–154.

10. Oliveira MA, Osorio MM. [Cow's milk consumption and iron deficiency anemia in children]. *J Pediatr (Rio J)*. 2005; 81:361–367.

11. Haider LM, Schwingshackl L, Hoffmann G, Ekmekcioglu C. The effect of vegetarian diets on iron status in adults: A systematic review and meta-analysis. *Crit Rev Food Sci Nutr*. 2018; 58:1359–1374.

12. Śliwińska A, Luty J, Aleksandrowicz-Wrona E, Malgorzewicz S. Iron status and dietary iron intake in vegetarians. *Adv Clin Exp Med*. 2018; 27:1383–1389.

13. Cook JD, Dassenko SA, Lynch SR. Assessment of the role of nonheme-iron availability in iron balance. *Am J Clin Nutr*. 1991; 54:717–722.

14. Lonnerdal B. Soybean ferritin: Implications for iron status of vegetarians. *Am J Clin Nutr*. 2009; 89:1680S–1685S.

15. Rushton DH. Nutritional factors and hair loss. *Clin Exp Dermatol*. 2002; 27:396–404.

16. Sobiecki JG, Appleby PN, Bradbury KE, Key TJ. High compliance with dietary recommendations in a cohort of meat eaters, fish eaters, vegetarians, and vegans: Results from the European Prospective Investigation into Cancer and Nutrition—Oxford study. *Nutr Res*. 2016; 36:464–477.

17. Bath SC, Hill S, Infante HG, Elghul S, Nezianya CJ, Rayman MP. Iodine concentration of milk-alternative drinks available in the UK in comparison with cows' milk. *Br J Nutr*. 2017; 118:525–532.

18. Ma W, He X, Braverman L. Iodine Content in milk alternatives. *Thyroid*. 2016; 26:1308–1310.

19. Vance K, Makhmudov A, Jones RL, Caldwell KL. Re: "Iodine Content in Milk Alternatives" by Ma et al. (*Thyroid* 2016; 26:1308–1310). *Thyroid*. 2017; 27:748–749.

20. Lighttowler HJ, Davis GJ. The effect of self-selected dietary supplements on micronutrient intakes in vegans. *Proc Nutr Soc*. 1998; 58:35A.

21. Key TJA, Thorogood M, Keenant J, Long A. Raised thyroid stimulating hormone associated with kelp intake in British vegan men. *J Human Nutr Diet*. 1992; 5:323–326.

22. Brantsaeter AL, Knutsen HK, Johansen NC, et al. Inadequate iodine intake in population groups defined by age, life stage and vegetarian dietary practice in a Norwegian convenience sample. *Nutrients*. 2018; 10.

23. Draper A, Lewis J, Malhotra N, Wheeler E. The energy and nutrient intakes of different types of vegetarian: A case for supplements? [published erratum appears in Br J Nutr 1993 Nov;70(3):812]. *Br J Nutr*. 1993; 69:3–19.

24. Krajcovicova-Kudlackova M, Buckova K, Klimes I, Sebokova E. Iodine deficiency in vegetarians and vegans. *Ann Nutr Metab*. 2003; 47:183–185.

25. Leung AM, Lamar A, He X, Braverman LE, Pearce EN. Iodine status and thyroid function of Boston-area vegetarians and vegans. *J Clin Endocrinol Metab*. 2011; 96:E1303–1307.

26. Teas J, Pino S, Critchley A, Braverman LE. Variability of iodine content in common commercially available edible seaweeds. *Thyroid*. 2004; 14:836–841.

27. Leung AM, Pearce EN, Braverman LE. Iodine content of prenatal multi-vitamins in the United States. *N Engl J Med*. 2009; 360:939–940.

28. Kopec RE, Cooperstone JL, Schweiggert RM, et al. Avocado consumption enhances human postprandial provitamin A absorption and conversion from a novel high-beta-carotene tomato sauce and from carrots. *J Nutr.* 2014; 144: 1158–1166.

29. Booth SL. Roles for vitamin K beyond coagulation. *Annu Rev Nutr.* 2009; 29:89–110.

30. Booth SL, Tucker KL, Chen H, et al. Dietary vitamin K intakes are associated with hip fracture but not with bone mineral density in elderly men and women. *Am J Clin Nutr.* 2000; 71:1201–1208.

31. Sanders TA, Roshanai F. Platelet phospholipid fatty acid composition and function in vegans compared with age- and sex-matched omnivore controls. *Eur J Clin Nutr.* 1992; 46:823–831.

32. Geleijnse JM, Vermeer C, Grobbee DE, et al. Dietary intake of menaquinone is associated with a reduced risk of coronary heart disease: The Rotterdam Study. *J Nutr.* 2004; 134:3100–3105.

33. Beulens JW, Bots ML, Atsma F, et al. High dietary menaquinone intake is associated with reduced coronary calcification. *Atherosclerosis.* 2009; 203:489–493.

34. Nimptsch K, Rohrmann S, Kaaks R, Linseisen J. Dietary vitamin K intake in relation to cancer incidence and mortality: Results from the Heidelberg cohort of the European Prospective Investigation into Cancer and Nutrition (EPIC-Heidelberg). *Am J Clin Nutr.* 2010; 91:1348–1358.

35. Conly JM, Stein K, Worobetz L, Rutledge-Harding S. The contribution of vitamin K_2 (menaquinones) produced by the intestinal microflora to human nutritional requirements for vitamin K. *Am J Gastroenterol.* 1994; 89:915–923.

36. Judd PA, Long A, Butcher M, Caygill CP, Diplock AT. Vegetarians and vegans may be most at risk from low selenium intakes. *BMJ.* 1997; 314:1834.

37. Larsson CL, Johansson GK. Dietary intake and nutritional status of young vegans and omnivores in Sweden. *Am J Clin Nutr.* 2002; 76:100–106.

Chapter 9. Soyfoods in Vegan Diets

1. Hughes GJ, Ryan DJ, Mukherjea R, et al. Protein digestibility-corrected amino acid scores (PDCAAS) for soy protein isolates and concentrate: Criteria for evaluation. *J Agric Food Chemistry.* 2011; 59(23):12707–12712.

2. Weaver CM, Heaney RP, Connor L, et al. Bioavailability of calcium from tofu vs. milk in premenopausal women. *J Food Sci.* 2002; 67:3144–3147.

3. Zhao Y, Martin BR, Weaver CM. Calcium bioavailability of calcium carbonate fortified soymilk is equivalent to cow's milk in young women. *J Nutr.* 2005; 135(10):2379–2382.

4. Lonnerdal B. Soybean ferritin: Implications for iron status of vegetarians. *Am J Clin Nutr.* 2009; 89(5):1680S–1685S.

5. Lonnerdal B, Bryant A, Liu X, et al. Iron absorption from soybean ferritin in nonanemic women. *Am J Clin Nutr.* 2006; 83(1):103–107.

6. Oseni T, Patel R, Pyle J, et al. Selective estrogen receptor modulators and phytoestrogens. *Planta Med.* 2008; 74(13):1656–1665.

7. Speirs V, Carder PJ, Lane S, et al. Oestrogen receptor beta: What it means for patients with breast cancer. *The Lancet Oncology.* 2004; 5(3):174–181.

8. Setchell KD, Brown NM, Lydeking-Olsen E. The clinical importance of the metabolite equol: A clue to the effectiveness of soy and its isoflavones. *J Nutr.* 2002; 132(12):3577–3584.

9. Sekikawa A, Ihara M, Lopez O, et al. Effect of S-equol and soy isoflavones on heart and brain. *Curr Cardiol Rev.* 2018; 15:114–135.

10. Wu GD, Compher C, Chen EZ, et al. Comparative metabolomics in vegans and omnivores reveal constraints on diet-dependent gut microbiota metabolite production. *Gut.* 2016; 65(1):63–72.

11. Setchell KD, Cole SJ. Method of defining equol-producer status and its frequency among vegetarians. *J Nutr.* 2006;136(8):2188–2193.

12. Hod R, Kouidhi W, Ali Mohd M, et al. Plasma isoflavones in Malaysian men according to vegetarianism and by age. *Asia Pac J Clin Nutr.* 2016; 25(1): 89–96.

13. Jenkins DJ, Mirrahimi A, Srichaikul K, et al. Soy protein reduces serum cholesterol by both intrinsic and food displacement mechanisms. *J Nutr.* 2010; 140(12):2302S–2311S.

14. Anderson JW, Bush HM. Soy protein effects on serum lipoproteins: A quality assessment and meta-analysis of randomized, controlled studies. *J Am Coll Nutr.* 2011; 30(2):79–91.

15. Zhan S, Ho SC. Meta-analysis of the effects of soy protein containing isoflavones on the lipid profile. *Am J Clin Nutr.* 2005; 81(2):397–408.

16. Jenkins DJ, Kendall CW, Faulkner D, et al. A dietary portfolio approach to cholesterol reduction: Combined effects of plant sterols, vegetable proteins, and viscous fibers in hypercholesterolemia. *Metabolism.* 2002; 51:1596–1604.

17. Desroches S, Mauger JF, Ausman LM, et al. Soy protein favorably affects LDL size independently of isoflavones in hypercholesterolemic men and women. *J Nutr.* 2004; 134(3):574–579.

18. Li SH, Liu XX, Bai YY, et al. Effect of oral isoflavone supplementation on vascular endothelial function in postmenopausal women: A meta-analysis of randomized placebo-controlled trials. *Am J Clin Nut.*2010; 91(2):480–486.

19. Lambert MNT, Hu LM, Jeppesen PB. A systematic review and meta-analysis of the effects of isoflavone formulations against estrogen-deficient bone resorption in peri- and postmenopausal women. *Am J Clin Nutr.* 2017; 106(3):801–811.

20. Wei P, Liu M, Chen Y, et al. Systematic review of soy isoflavone supplements on osteoporosis in women. *Asian Pac J Trop Med.* 2012; 5(3):243–248.

21. Zhang X, Shu XO, Li H, et al. Prospective cohort study of soy food consumption and risk of bone fracture among postmenopausal women. *Arch Intern Med.* 2005; 165(16):1890–1895.

22. Koh WP, Wu AH, Wang R, et al. Gender-specific associations between soy and risk of hip fracture in the Singapore Chinese Health Study. *Am J Epidemiol.* 2009; 170(7):901–909.

23. Taku K, Melby MK, Kronenberg F, et al. Extracted or synthesized soybean isoflavones reduce menopausal hot flash frequency and severity: Systematic review

and meta-analysis of randomized controlled trials. *Menopause.* 2012; 19(7): 776–790.

24. Bitto A, Arcoraci V, Alibrandi A, et al. Visfatin correlates with hot flashes in postmenopausal women with metabolic syndrome: Effects of genistein. *Endocrine.* 2017; 55(3):899–906.

25. Setchell KD, Brown NM, Zhao X, et al. Soy isoflavone phase II metabolism differs between rodents and humans: Implications for the effect on breast cancer risk. *Am J Clin Nutr.* 2011; 94(5):1284–1294.

26. EFSA. EFSA ANS Panel (EFSA Panel on Food Additives and Nutrient Sources Added to Food). 2015. Scientific opinion on the risk assessment for peri- and post-menopausal women taking food supplements containing isolated isoflavones. *EFSA J.* 2015; 13(10):4246 (342 pp).

27. Rock CL, Doyle C, Demark-Wahnefried W, et al. Nutrition and physical activity guidelines for cancer survivors. *CA Cancer J Clin.* 2012; 62(4):242–274.

28. American Institute for Cancer Research. Soy is safe for breast cancer survivors. http://www.aicr.org/cancer-research-update/november_21_2012/cru-soy-safehtml.

29. World Cancer Research Fund International. Continuous Update Project Report: Diet, Nutrition, Physical Activity, and Breast Cancer Survivors. 2014. www.wcrf.org/sites/default/files/Breast-Cancer-Survivors-2014-Report.pdf.

30. Messina M, Hilakivi-Clarke L. Early intake appears to be the key to the proposed protective effects of soy intake against breast cancer. *Nutr Cancer.* 2009; 61(6):792–798.

31. Baglia ML, Zheng W, Li H, et al. The association of soy food consumption with the risk of subtype of breast cancers defined by hormone receptor and HER2 status. *Int J Cancer.* 2016; 139(4):742–748.

32. Applegate CC, Rowles JL, Ranard KM, et al. Soy consumption and the risk of prostate cancer: An updated systematic review and meta-analysis. *Nutrients.* 2018; 10(1).

33. Grainger EM, Moran NE, Francis DM, et al. A novel tomato-soy juice induces a dose-response increase in urinary and plasma phytochemical biomarkers in men with prostate cancer. *J Nutr.* 2019; 149(1):26–35.

34. White LR, Petrovitch H, Ross GW, et al. Brain aging and midlife tofu consumption. *J Am Coll Nutr.* 2000; 19(2):242–255.

35. Soni M, Rahardjo TB, Soekardi R, et al. Phytoestrogens and cognitive function: A review. *Maturitas.* 2014; 77(3):209–220.

36. Chuang SY, Lo YL, Wu SY, et al. Dietary patterns and foods associated with cognitive function in Taiwanese older adults: The cross-sectional and longitudinal studies. *J Am Med Dir Assoc.* 2019.

37. Zajac IT, Herreen D, Bastiaans K, et al. The effect of whey and soy protein isolates on cognitive function in older Australians with low vitamin B_{12}: A randomised controlled crossover trial. *Nutrients.* 2018;11(1).

38. Huser S, Guth S, Joost HG, et al. Effects of isoflavones on breast tissue and the thyroid hormone system in humans: A comprehensive safety evaluation. *Arch Toxicol.* 2018; 92(9):2703–2748.

39. Messina M, Redmond G. Effects of soy protein and soybean isoflavones on thyroid function in healthy adults and hypothyroid patients: A review of the relevant literature. *Thyroid.* 2006; 16(3):249–258.

40. Alekel DL, Genschel U, Koehler KJ, et al. Soy Isoflavones for Reducing Bone Loss study: Effects of a 3-year trial on hormones, adverse events, and endometrial thickness in postmenopausal women. *Menopause.* 2015; 22(2):185–197.

41. Bitto A, Polito F, Atteritano M, et al. Genistein aglycone does not affect thyroid function: Results from a three-year, randomized, double-blind, placebo-controlled trial. *J Clin Endocrinol Metab.* 2010; 95(6):3067–3072.

42. Food Labeling: Health Claims; Soy Protein and Coronary Heart Disease. A Proposed Rule by the Food and Drug Administration on 10/31/2017. https://www.federalregister.gov/documents/2017/10/31/2017-23629/food-labeling-health-claims-soy-protein-and-coronary-heart-disease.

43. EFSA ANS Panel (EFSA Panel on Food Additives and Nutrient Sources Added to Food), 2015. Scientific opinion on the risk assessment for peri- and post-menopausal women taking food supplements containing isolated isoflavones. *EFSA J.* 13(10):4246 (342 pp).

44. Sathyapalan T, Manuchehri AM, Thatcher NJ, et al. The effect of soy phytoestrogen supplementation on thyroid status and cardiovascular risk markers in patients with subclinical hypothyroidism: A randomized, double-blind, crossover study. *J Clin Endocrinol Metab.* 2011; 96(5):1442–1449.

45. Sathyapalan T, Dawson AJ, Rigby AS, et al. The effect of phytoestrogen on thyroid in subclinical hypothyroidism: Randomized, double blind, crossover study. *Front Endocrinol (Lausanne).* 2018; 9:531.

46. Hamilton-Reeves JM, Vazquez G, Duval SJ, et al. Clinical studies show no effects of soy protein or isoflavones on reproductive hormones in men: Results of a meta-analysis. *Fertil Steril.* 2010; 94(3):997–1007.

47. Haun CT, Mobley CB, Vann CG, et al. Soy protein supplementation is not androgenic or estrogenic in college-aged men when combined with resistance exercise training. *Scientific Reports.* 8, Article number 11151 (2018). https://www.nature.com/articles/s41598-018-29591-4.

48. Sathyapalan T, Rigby AS, Bhasin S, et al. Effect of soy in men with type 2 diabetes mellitus and subclinical hypogonadism: A randomized controlled study. *J Clin Endocrinol Metab.* 2017; 102(2):425–433.

49. Messina M. Soybean isoflavone exposure does not have feminizing effects on men: A critical examination of the clinical evidence. *Fertil Steril.* 2010; 93(7):2095–2104.

50. Chavarro JE, Toth TL, Sadio SM, et al. Soy food and isoflavone intake in relation to semen quality parameters among men from an infertility clinic. *Hum Reprod.* 2008; 23(11):2584–2590.

51. Beaton LK, McVeigh BL, Dillingham BL, et al. Soy protein isolates of varying isoflavone content do not adversely affect semen quality in healthy young men. *Fertil Steril.* 2010; 94(5):1717–1722.

52. Mitchell JH, Cawood E, Kinniburgh D, et al. Effect of a phytoestrogen food supplement on reproductive health in normal males. *Clin Sci (Lond).* 2001; 100(6):613–618.

53. Messina M, Watanabe S, Setchell KD. Report on the 8th International Symposium on the Role of Soy in Health Promotion and Chronic Disease Prevention and Treatment. *J Nutr.* 2009; 139(4):796S–802S.

54. Nagino T, Kaga C, Kano M, et al. Effects of fermented soymilk with *Lactobacillus casei* Shirota on skin condition and the gut microbiota: A randomised clinical pilot trial. *Beneficial Microbes.* 2018; 9(2):209–218.

55. Jenkins G, Wainwright LJ, Holland R, et al. Wrinkle reduction in postmenopausal women consuming a novel oral supplement: A double-blind placebo-controlled randomized study. *Int J Cosmet Sci.* 2014; 36(1):22–31.

56. Messina M, Nagata C, Wu AH. Estimated Asian adult soy protein and isoflavone intakes. *Nutr Cancer.* 2006; 55(1):1–12.

Chapter 11. A Healthy Start:
Vegan Diets in Pregnancy and Breastfeeding

1. Carter JP, Furman T, Hutcheson HR. Preeclampsia and reproductive performance in a community of vegans. *South Med J.* 1987; 80:692–697.

2. Piccoli GB, Clari R, Vigotti FN, et al. Vegan-vegetarian diets in pregnancy: Danger or panacea? A systematic narrative review. *BJOG.* 2015; 122:623–633.

3. Melina V, Craig W, Levin S. Position of the Academy of Nutrition and Dietetics: Vegetarian diets. *J Acad Nutr Diet.* 2016; 116:1970–1980.

4. Chavarro JE, Rich-Edwards JW, Rosner BA, Willett WC. Diet and lifestyle in the prevention of ovulatory disorder infertility. *Obstet Gynecol.* 2007; 110: 1050–1058.

5. Anderson K, Nisenblat V, Norman R. Lifestyle factors in people seeking infertility treatment: A review. *Aust N Z J Obstet Gynaecol.* 2010; 50:8–20.

6. Parazzini F, Chiaffarino F, Surace M, et al. Selected food intake and risk of endometriosis. *Hum Reprod.* 2004; 19:1755–1759.

7. Visioli F, Hagen TM. Antioxidants to enhance fertility: Role of eNOS and potential benefits. *Pharmacol Res.* 2011; 64:431–437.

8. Rich-Edwards JW, Spiegelman D, Garland M, et al. Physical activity, body mass index, and ovulatory disorder infertility. *Epidemiology.* 2002; 13: 184–190.

9. Kiddy DS, Hamilton-Fairley D, Bush A, et al. Improvement in endocrine and ovarian function during dietary treatment of obese women with polycystic ovary syndrome. *Clin Endocrinol (Oxf).* 1992; 36:105–111.

10. Payne M, Stephens T, Lim K, Ball RO, Pencharz PB, Elango R. Lysine requirements of healthy pregnant women are higher during late stages of gestation compared to early gestation. *J Nutr.* 2018; 148:94–99.

11. CDC: https://www.cdc.gov/mmwr/preview/mmwrhtml/00019479.htm.

12. Institute of Medicine. Food and Nutrition Board. *Dietary Reference Intakes: Thiamin, Riboflavin, Niacin, Vitamin B$_6$, Folate, Vitamin B$_{12}$, Pantothenic Acid, Biotin, and Choline.* Washington, DC: National Academy Press; 1998.

13. CDC: https://www.cdc.gov/mmwr/preview/mmwrhtml/00051880.htm.

14. King JC. Determinants of maternal zinc status during pregnancy. *Am J Clin Nutr.* 2000; 71:1334S–1343S.

15. Nishiyama S, Mikeda T, Okada T, Nakamura K, Kotani T, Hishinuma A. Transient hypothyroidism or persistent hyperthyrotropinemia in neonates born to mothers with excessive iodine intake. *Thyroid.* 2004; 14:1077–1083.

16. Guan H, Li C, Li Y, et al. High iodine intake is a risk factor of post-partum thyroiditis: Result of a survey from Shenyang, China. *J Endocrinol Invest.* 2005; 28:876–881.

17. Lakin V, Haggarty P, Abramovich DR, et al. Dietary intake and tissue concentration of fatty acids in omnivore, vegetarian and diabetic pregnancy. *Prostaglandins Leukot Essent Fatty Acids.* 1998; 59:209–220.

18. Middleton P, Gomersall JC, Gould JF, Shepherd E, Olsen SF, Makrides M. Omega-3 fatty acid addition during pregnancy. *Cochrane Database Syst Rev.* 2018; 11:CD003402.

19. Carlson SE. Docosahexaenoic acid supplementation in pregnancy and lactation. *Am J Clin Nutr.* 2009; 89:678S–684S.

20. Koletzko B, Lien E, Agostoni C, et al. The roles of long-chain polyunsaturated fatty acids in pregnancy, lactation and infancy: Review of current knowledge and consensus recommendations. *J Perinat Med.* 2008; 36:5–14.

21. Simopoulos AP. Essential fatty acids in health and chronic disease. *Am J Clin Nutr.* 1999; 70:560S–569S.

22. Steele NM, French J, Gatherer-Boyles J, Newman S, Leclaire S. Effect of acupressure by Sea-Bands on nausea and vomiting of pregnancy. *J Obstet Gynecol Neonatal Nurs.* 2001; 30:61–70.

23. Matthews A, Dowswell T, Haas DM, Doyle M, O'Mathuna DP. Interventions for nausea and vomiting in early pregnancy. *Cochrane Database Syst Rev.* 2010:CD007575.

24. Somogyi A, Beck H. Nurturing and breast-feeding: Exposure to chemicals in breast milk. *Environ Health Perspect.* 1993; 101:S45–52.

25. Hergenrather J, Hlady G, Wallace B, Savage E. Pollutants in breast milk of vegetarians. *N Engl J Med.* 1981; 304:792.

26. Pawlak R, Vos P, Shahab-Ferdows S, Hampel D, Allen LH, Perrin MT. Vitamin B-12 content in breast milk of vegan, vegetarian, and nonvegetarian lactating women in the United States. *Am J Clin Nutr.* 2018; 108:525–531.

Chapter 12. Raising Vegan Children and Teens

1. AAP. Breastfeeding and the Use of Human Milk. https://pediatrics.aappublications.org/content/129/3/e827.full#content-block.

2. Mendez MA, Anthony MS, Arab L. Soy-based formulae and infant growth and development: A review. *J Nutr.* 2002; 132: 2127–2130.

3. Bhatia J, Greer F. Use of soy protein-based formulas in infant feeding. *Pediatrics.* 2008; 121:1062–1068.

4. Koplin JJ, Allen KJ. Optimal timing for solids introduction: Why are the guidelines always changing? *Clin Exp Allergy.* 2013; 43:826–834.

5. Huh SY, Rifas-Shiman SL, Taveras EM, Oken E, Gillman MW. Timing of solid food introduction and risk of obesity in preschool-aged children. *Pediatrics.* 2011; 127:e544–551.

6. Perez-Escamilla R, Segura-Perez S, Lott M, on behalf of the RWJF HER Expert Panel on Best Practices for Promoting Healthy Nutrition, Feeding Patterns, and Weight Status for Infants and Toddlers from Birth to 24 Months. Feeding Guidelines for Infants and Young Toddlers: A Responsive Parenting Approach. Durham, NC: Healthy Eating Research, 2017. http://healthyeating research.org.

7. Mennella JA, Reiter AR, Daniels LM. Vegetable and fruit acceptance during infancy: Impact of ontogeny, genetics, and early experiences. *Adv Nutr.* 2016; 7:211S–219S.

8. Gupta RS, Warren CM, Smith BM, et al. Prevalence and severity of food allergies among US adults. *JAMA Netw Open.* Published online January 4, 2019, 2(1):e185630.

9. Verrill L, Bruns R, Luccioli S. Prevalence of self-reported food allergy in U.S. adults: 2001, 2006, and 2010. *Allergy Asthma Proc.* 2015; 36(6):458–467.

10. Soller L, Ben-Shoshan M, Harrington DW, et al. Overall prevalence of self-reported food allergy in Canada. *J Allergy Clin Immunol.* 2012; 130(4): 986–988.

11. McGowan EC, Keet CA. Prevalence of self-reported food allergy in the National Health and Nutrition Examination Survey (NHANES) 2007–2010. *J Allergy Clin Immunol.* 2013; 132(5):1216–1219 e5.

12. Fleischer DM, Sicherer S, Greenhawt M, et al. Consensus communication on early peanut introduction and prevention of peanut allergy in high-risk infants. *Pediatr Dermatol.* 2016; 33:103–106.

13. AAP. American Academy of Pediatrics Recommends No Fruit Juice for Children Under 1 Year. https://www.aap.org/en-us/about-the-aap/aap-press -room/Pages/American-Academy-of-Pediatrics-Recommends-No-Fruit-Juice -For-Children-Under-1-Year.aspx.

14. Messina M, Hilakivi-Clarke L. Early intake appears to be the key to the proposed protective effects of soy intake against breast cancer. *Nutr Cancer.* 2009; 61:792–798.

Chapter 13. Vegan Diets for People over Fifty

1. Balan E, Decottignies A, Deldicque L. Physical activity and nutrition: Two promising strategies for telomere maintenance? *Nutrients.* 2018; 10:1942. DOI: 10.3390/nu10121942.

2. Martone AM, Marzetti E, Calvani R, et al. Exercise and protein intake: A synergistic approach against sarcopenia. *Biomed Res Int.* 2017; Article ID 2672435.

3. Paddon-Jones D, Rasmussen BB. Dietary protein recommendations and the prevention of sarcopenia. *Curr Opin Clin Nutr Metab Care.* 2009; 12:86–90.

4. Bauer J, Biolo G, Cederholm T, et al. Evidence-based recommendations for optimal dietary protein intake in older people: A position paper from the PROT-AGE Study Group. *J Am Med Dir Assoc.* 2013; 14:542–559.

5. Houston DK, Nicklas BJ, Ding J, et al. Dietary protein intake is associated with lean mass change in older, community-dwelling adults: The Health, Aging, and Body Composition (Health ABC) Study. *Am J Clin Nutr.* 2008; 87:150–155.

6. Munger RG, Cerhan JR, Chiu BC. Prospective study of dietary protein intake and risk of hip fracture in postmenopausal women. *Am J Clin Nutr.* 1999; 69:147–152.

7. Haub MD, Wells AM, Tarnopolsky MA, Campbell WW. Effect of protein source on resistive-training-induced changes in body composition and muscle size in older men. *Am J Clin Nutr.* 2002; 76:511–517.

8. Holick MF. Vitamin D: A d-lightful solution for health. *J Investig Med.* 2011; 59:872–880.

9. Allen LH. How common is vitamin B-12 deficiency? *Am J Clin Nutr.* 2009; 89:693S–696S.

10. IOM/FNB (Institute of Medicine/Food and Nutrition Board). Dietary Reference Intakes for Energy, Carbohydrate, Fiber, Fat, Protein and Amino Acids: A Report of the Panel on Micronutrients, Subcommittee on Upper Reference Levels of Nutrients and Interpretation and Uses of Dietary Reference Intakes and the Standing Committee on the Scientific Evaluation of Dietary Reference Intakes (Uncorrected Prepublication Version). Washington, DC: The National Academy Press, 2002.

11. Glem P, Beeson WL, Fraser GE. The incidence of dementia and intake of animal products: Preliminary findings from the Adventist Health Study. *Neuroepidemiology* 1993; 12:28–36.

12. Smith AD, Smith SM, de Jager CA, et al. Homocysteine-lowering by B vitamins slows the rate of accelerated brain atrophy in mild cognitive impairment: A randomized controlled trial. *PLoS One.* 2010; 5:e12244.

13. Selhub J, Bagley LC, Miller J, Rosenberg IH. B vitamins, homocysteine, and neurocognitive function in the elderly. *Am J Clin Nutr.* 2000; 71:614S–620S.

14. Van Dam F, Van Gool WA. Hyperhomocysteinemia and Alzheimer's disease: A systematic review. *Arch Gerontol Geriatr.* 2009; 48:425–430.

15. Walters MJ, Sterling J, Quinn C, et al. Associations of lifestyle and vascular risk factors with Alzheimer's brain biomarker changes during middle age: A 3-year longitudinal study in the broader New York City area. *BMJ Open.* 2018; 8:e023664.

16. Rizzo NS, Jaceldo-Siegl K, Sabate J, Fraser GE. Nutrient profiles of vegetarian and nonvegetarian dietary patterns. *J Acad Nutr Diet.* 2013; 113:1610–1619.

17. Mangels R, Messina V, Messina M. *The Dietitian's Guide to Vegetarian Diets.* 3rd ed. Sudbury, MA: Jones and Bartlett, 2011.

18. Robinson JG, Ijioma N, Harris W. Omega-3 fatty acids and cognitive function in women. *Womens Health (Lond).* 2010; 6:119–134.

19. Liguori I, Russo G, Aran L, et al. Sarcopenia: Assessment of disease burden and strategies to improve outcomes. *Clin Interv Aging.* 2018; 13:913–927.

20. Domazetovic V, Marcucci G, Iantomasi T, Brandi ML, Vincenzini MT. Oxidative stress in bone remodeling: Role of antioxidants. *Clin Cases Miner Bone Metab.* 2017; 14:209–216.

21. Rao LG, Mackinnon ES, Josse RG, Murray TM, Strauss A, Rao AV. Lycopene consumption decreases oxidative stress and bone resorption markers in postmenopausal women. *Osteoporos Int.* 2007; 18:109–115.

22. Carlsen MH, Halvorsen BL, Holte K, et al. The total antioxidant content of more than 3100 foods, beverages, spices, herbs and supplements used worldwide. *Nutr J.* 2010; 9:3.

23. Hostmark AT, Lystad E, Vellar OD, Hovi K, Berg JE. Reduced plasma fibrinogen, serum peroxides, lipids, and apolipoproteins after a 3-week vegetarian diet. *Plant Foods Hum Nutr.* 1993; 43:55–61.

24. Krajcovicova-Kudlackova M, Valachovicova M, Paukova V, Dusinska M. Effects of diet and age on oxidative damage products in healthy subjects. *Physiol Res.* 2008; 57:647–651.

25. Appleby PN, Allen NE, Key TJ. Diet, vegetarianism, and cataract risk. *Am J Clin. Nutr* 2011; 93:1128–1135.

26. Morris MC. Nutritional determinants of cognitive aging and dementia. *Proc Nutr Soc.* 2012; 71:1–13.

27. Morris MC, Tangney CC, Wang Y, Sacks FM, Bennett DA, Aggarwal NT. MIND diet associated with reduced incidence of Alzheimer's disease. *Alzheimers Dement.* 2015; 11:1007–1014.

28. Busti F, Campostrini N, Martinelli N, Girelli D. Iron deficiency in the elderly population, revisited in the hepcidin era. *Front Pharmacol.* 2014; 5:83.

Chapter 14. Sports Nutrition for Vegans

1. Thomas DT, Erdman KA, Burke LM. Position of the Academy of Nutrition and Dietetics, Dietitians of Canada, and the American College of Sports Medicine: Nutrition and athletic performance. *J Acad Nutr Diet.* 2016; 116:501–528.

2. Kerksick CM, Wilborn CD, Roberts MD, et al. ISSN exercise & sports nutrition review update: Research & recommendations. *J Int Soc Sports Nutr.* 2018; 15:38.

3. Morton RW, Murphy KT, McKellar SR, et al. A systematic review, meta-analysis and meta-regression of the effect of protein supplementation on resistance training-induced gains in muscle mass and strength in healthy adults. *Br J Sports Med.* 2018; 52:376–384.

4. Churchward-Venne TA, Burd NA, Mitchell CJ, et al. Supplementation of a suboptimal protein dose with leucine or essential amino acids: Effects on myofibrillar protein synthesis at rest and following resistance exercise in men. *J Physiol.* 2012; 590:2751–2765.

5. Tang JE, Moore DR, Kujbida GW, Tarnopolsky MA, Phillips SM. Ingestion of whey hydrolysate, casein, or soy protein isolate: Effects on mixed muscle protein synthesis at rest and following resistance exercise in young men. *J Appl Physiol.* 2009; 107(3):987–992.

6. Messina M, Lynch H, Dickinson JM, Reed KE. No difference between the effects of supplementing with soy protein versus animal protein on gains in muscle mass and strength in response to resistance exercise. *Int J Sport Nutr Exerc Metab.* 2018; 28:674–685.

7. DellaValle DM. Iron supplementation for female athletes: Effects on iron status and performance outcomes. *Curr Sports Med Rep.* 2013; 12:234–239.

8. Kreider RB. Effects of creatine supplementation on performance and training adaptations. *Mol Cell Biochem.* 2003; 244:89–94.

9. Nelson AG, Arnall DA, Kokkonen J, Day R, Evans J. Muscle glycogen supercompensation is enhanced by prior creatine supplementation. *Med Sci Sports Exerc.* 2001; 33:1096–1100.

10. Shomrat A, Weinstein Y, Katz A. Effect of creatine feeding on maximal exercise performance in vegetarians. *Eur J Appl Physiol.* 2000; 82:321–325.

11. Butts J, Jacobs B, Silvis M. Creatine use in sports. *Sports Health.* 2018; 10:31–34.

12. Casey A, Greenhaff PL. Does dietary creatine supplementation play a role in skeletal muscle metabolism and performance? *Am J Clin Nutr.* 2000; 72:607S–617S.

13. Peeling P, Binnie MJ, Goods PSR, Sim M, Burke LM. Evidence-based supplements for the enhancement of athletic performance. *Int J Sport Nutr Exerc Metab.* 2018; 28:178–187.

14. Maughan RJ, Burke LM, Dvorak J, et al. IOC consensus statement: Dietary supplements and the high-performance athlete. *Int J Sport Nutr Exerc Metab.* 2018; 28:104–125.

15. Rebouche CJ, Bosch EP, Chenard CA, Schabold KJ, Nelson SE. Utilization of dietary precursors for carnitine synthesis in human adults. *J Nutr.* 1989; 119: 1907–1913.

16. Harris RC, Jones G, Hill, CA, et al. "The carnosine content of V Lateralis in vegetarians and omnivores," abstract in *FASEB Journal.* 2007; 769:20.

17. Salles Painelli V, Nemezio KM, Jessica A, et al. HIIT Augments muscle carnosine in the absence of dietary beta-alanine intake. *Med Sci Sports Exerc.* 2018; Epub ahead of print.

18. Hill CA, Harris RC, Kim HJ, et al. Influence of beta-alanine supplementation on skeletal muscle carnosine concentrations and high intensity cycling capacity. *Amino Acids.* 2007; 32:225–233.

19. Kendrick IP, Harris RC, Kim HJ, et al. The effects of 10 weeks of resistance training combined with beta-alanine supplementation on whole body strength, force production, muscular endurance and body composition. *Amino Acids.* 2008; 34:547–554.

20. Brisola GMP, Zagatto AM. Ergogenic effects of beta-alanine supplementation on different sports modalities: Strong evidence or only incipient findings? *J Strength Cond Res.* 2019; 33:253–282.

21. Weiss Kelly AK, Hecht S. The female athlete triad. *Pediatrics.* 2016; 138.

Chapter 15. Plant Food Advantages:
Reducing Chronic Disease with a Vegan Diet

1. Orlich MJ, Singh PN, Sabate J, et al. Vegetarian dietary patterns and mortality in Adventist Health Study 2. *JAMA Intern Med.* 2013; 173:1230–1238.

2. Spencer EA, Appleby PN, Davey GK, Key TJ. Diet and body mass index in 38,000 EPIC-Oxford meat-eaters, fish-eaters, vegetarians and vegans. *Int J Obes Relat Metab Disord.* 2003; 27:728–734.

3. Donaldson AN. The relation of protein foods to hypertension. *Calif West Med.* 1926; 24:328–331.

4. Fraser GE. Vegetarian diets: What do we know of their effects on common chronic diseases? *Am J Clin Nutr.* 2009; 89:1607S–1612S.

5. Pettersen BJ, Anousheh R, Fan J, Jaceldo-Siegl K, Fraser GE. Vegetarian diets and blood pressure among white subjects: Results from the Adventist Health Study-2 (AHS-2). *Public Health Nutr.* 2012; 15:1909–1916.

6. Appleby PN, Davey GK, Key TJ. Hypertension and blood pressure among meat eaters, fish eaters, vegetarians and vegans in EPIC-Oxford. *Public Health Nutr.* 2002; 5:645–654.

7. Appel LJ, Moore TJ, Obarzanek E, et al. A clinical trial of the effects of dietary patterns on blood pressure. DASH Collaborative Research Group. *N Engl J Med.* 1997; 336:1117–1124.

8. Steinberg D, Bennett GG, Svetkey L. The DASH diet, 20 years later. *JAMA.* 2017; 317:1529–1530.

9. Juraschek SP, Miller ER, 3rd, Weaver CM, Appel LJ. Effects of sodium reduction and the DASH diet in relation to baseline blood pressure. *J Am Coll Cardiol.* 2017; 70:2841–2848.

10. Appel LJ, Sacks FM, Carey VJ, et al. Effects of protein, monounsaturated fat, and carbohydrate intake on blood pressure and serum lipids: Results of the OmniHeart randomized trial. *JAMA.* 2005; 294:2455–2464.

11. Mente A, de Koning L, Shannon HS, Anand SS. A systematic review of the evidence supporting a causal link between dietary factors and coronary heart disease. *Arch Intern Med.* 2009; 169:659–669.

12. Siri-Tarino PW, Sun Q, Hu FB, Krauss RM. Meta-analysis of prospective cohort studies evaluating the association of saturated fat with cardiovascular disease. *Am J Clin Nutr.* 2010; 91:535–546.

13. Li Y, Hruby A, Bernstein AM, et al. Saturated fats compared with unsaturated fats and sources of carbohydrates in relation to risk of coronary heart disease: A prospective cohort study. *J Am Coll Cardiol.* 2015; 66:1538–1548.

14. Nettleton JA, Brouwer IA, Geleijnse JM, et al. Saturated fat consumption and risk of coronary heart disease and ischemic stroke: A science update. *Ann Nutr Metab.* 2017; 70:26–33.

15. Mangels R, Messina V, Messina M. *The Dietitian's Guide to Vegetarian Diets.* 3rd ed. Sudbury, MA: Jones and Bartlett, 2011.

16. Bradbury KE, Crowe FL, Appleby PN, Schmidt JA, Travis RC, Key TJ. Serum concentrations of cholesterol, apolipoprotein A-I and apolipoprotein B in a total of 1,694 meat-eaters, fish-eaters, vegetarians and vegans. *Eur J Clin Nutr.* 2014; 68:178–183.

17. Shah B, Newman JD, Woolf K, et al. Anti-inflammatory effects of a vegan diet versus the American Heart Association–recommended diet in coronary artery disease trial. *J Am Heart Assoc.* 2018; 7:e011367.

18. Key TJ, Fraser GE, Thorogood M, et al. Mortality in vegetarians and non-vegetarians: Detailed findings from a collaborative analysis of 5 prospective studies. *Am J Clin Nutr.* 1999; 70:516S–524S.

19. Rizzo NS, Jaceldo-Siegl K, Sabate J, Fraser GE. Nutrient profiles of vegetarian and nonvegetarian dietary patterns. *J Acad Nutr Diet.* 2013; 113:1610–1619.

20. Crowe FL, Appleby PN, Travis RC, Key TJ. Risk of hospitalization or death from ischemic heart disease among British vegetarians and nonvegetarians: Results from the EPIC-Oxford cohort study. *Am J Clin Nutr.* 2013; 97:597–603.

21. Pawlak R. Is vitamin B$_{12}$ deficiency a risk factor for cardiovascular disease in vegetarians? *Am J Prev Med.* 2015;48:e11–26.

22. Marti-Carvajal AJ, Sola I, Lathyris D, Salanti G. Homocysteine lowering interventions for preventing cardiovascular events. *Cochrane Database Syst Rev.* 2009:CD006612.

23. Ornish D, Brown SE, Scherwitz LW, Billings JH, Armstrong WT, Ports TA, McLanahan SM, Kirkeeide RL, Brand RJ, Gould KL. Can lifestyle changes reverse coronary heart disease? The Lifestyle Heart Trial. *Lancet* 1990; 336: 129–133.

24. Esselstyn CB, Jr., Gendy G, Doyle J, Golubic M, Roizen MF. A way to reverse CAD? *J Fam Pract.* 2014; 63:356–364b.

25. Estruch R, Ros E, Salas-Salvado J, et al. Primary prevention of cardiovascular disease with a Mediterranean diet supplemented with extra-virgin olive oil or nuts. *N Engl J Med.* 2018. Epub ahead of print.

26. Feig JE, Feig JL, Dangas GD. The role of HDL in plaque stabilization and regression: Basic mechanisms and clinical implications. *Coron Artery Dis.* 2016; 27:592–603.

27. Berryman CE, Fleming JA, Kris-Etherton PM. Inclusion of almonds in a cholesterol-lowering diet improves plasma HDL subspecies and cholesterol efflux to serum in normal-weight individuals with elevated LDL cholesterol. *J Nutr.* 2017; 147(8):1517–1523.

28. Berryman CE, Grieger JA, West SG, et al. Acute consumption of walnuts and walnut components differentially affect postprandial lipemia, endothelial function, oxidative stress, and cholesterol efflux in humans with mild hypercholesterolemia. *J Nutr.* 2013; 143:788–794.

29. Berrougui H, Ikhlef S, Khalil A. Extra virgin olive oil polyphenols promote cholesterol efflux and improve HDL functionality. *Evid Based Complement Alternat Med.* 2015; 2015:208062.

30. Vogel RA, Corretti MC, Plotnick GD. Effect of a single high-fat meal on endothelial function in healthy subjects. *Am J Cardiol.* 1997; 79:350–354.

31. Marchesi S, Lupattelli G, Schillaci G, et al. Impaired flow-mediated vasoactivity during post-prandial phase in young healthy men. *Atherosclerosis.* 2000; 153:397–402.

32. Bae JH, Bassenge E, Kim KB, Kim YN, Kim KS, Lee HJ, Moon KC, Lee MS, Park KY, Schwemmer M. Postprandial hypertriglyceridemia impairs endothelial function by enhanced oxidant stress. *Atherosclerosis.* 2001; 155:517–523.

33. Karatzi K, Stamatelopoulos K, Lykka M, et al. Sesame oil consumption exerts a beneficial effect on endothelial function in hypertensive men. *Eur J Prev Cardiol.* 2013; 20:202–208.

34. Moreno-Luna R, Munoz-Hernandez R, Miranda ML, et al. Olive oil polyphenols decrease blood pressure and improve endothelial function in young women with mild hypertension. *Am J Hypertens.* 2012; 25:1299–1304.

35. Cortes B, Nunez I, Cofan M, et al. Acute effects of high-fat meals enriched with walnuts or olive oil on postprandial endothelial function. *J Am Coll Cardiol.* 2006; 48:1666–1671.

36. Fuentes F, Lopez-Miranda J, Sanchez E, et al. Mediterranean and low-fat diets improve endothelial function in hypercholesterolemic men. *Ann Intern Med.* 2001; 134:1115–1119.

37. Chistiakov DA, Revin VV, Söbenin IA, Orekhov AN, Bobryshev YV. Vascular endothelium: Functioning in norm, changes in atherosclerosis and current dietary approaches to improve endothelial function. *Mini Rev Med Chem.* 2015; 15:338–350.

38. Shai I, Spence JD, Schwarzfuchs D, et al. Dietary intervention to reverse carotid atherosclerosis. *Circulation* 2010; 121:1200–1208.

39. Mayhew AJ, de Souza RJ, Meyre D, Anand SS, Mente A. A systematic review and meta-analysis of nut consumption and incident risk of CVD and all-cause mortality. *Br J Nutr.* 2016; 115:212–225.

40. Widmer RJ, Freund MA, Flammer AJ, et al. Beneficial effects of polyphenol-rich olive oil in patients with early atherosclerosis. *Eur J Nutr.* 2013; 52:1223–1231.

41. Augustin LS, Kendall CW, Jenkins DJ, et al. Glycemic index, glycemic load and glycemic response: An International Scientific Consensus Summit from the International Carbohydrate Quality Consortium (ICQC). *Nutr Metab Cardiovasc Dis.* 2015; 25:795–815.

42. Abete I, Parra D, Martinez JA. Energy-restricted diets based on a distinct food selection affecting the glycemic index induce different weight loss and oxidative response. *Clin Nutr.* 2008; 27:545–551.

43. Tonstad S, Butler T, Yan R, Fraser GE. Type of vegetarian diet, body weight, and prevalence of type 2 diabetes. *Diabetes Care.* 2009; 32:791–796.

44. Tonstad S, Stewart K, Oda K, Batech M, Herring RP, Fraser GE. Vegetarian diets and incidence of diabetes in the Adventist Health Study-2. *Nutr Metab Cardiovasc Dis.* 2013; 23:292–299.

45. Kahleova H, Dort S, Holubkov R, Barnard ND. A plant-based high-carbohydrate, low-fat diet in overweight individuals in a 16-week randomized clinical trial: The role of carbohydrates. *Nutrients.* 2018; 10:1302.

46. Barnard ND, Cohen J, Jenkins DJ, et al. A low-fat vegan diet and a conventional diabetes diet in the treatment of type 2 diabetes: A randomized, controlled, 74-wk clinical trial. *Am J Clin Nutr.* 2009; 89:1588S–1596S.

47. Barnard ND, Cohen J, Jenkins DJ, et al. A low-fat vegan diet improves glycemic control and cardiovascular risk factors in a randomized clinical trial in individuals with type 2 diabetes. *Diabetes Care* 2006; 29:1777–1783.

48. Lee YM, Kim SA, Lee IK, et al. Effect of a brown rice based vegan diet and conventional diabetic diet on glycemic control of patients with type 2 diabetes: A 12-week randomized clinical trial. *PLoS One.* 2016; 11:e0155918.

49. Kahleova H, Matoulek M, Malinska H, et al. Vegetarian diet improves insulin resistance and oxidative stress markers more than conventional diet in subjects with type 2 diabetes. *Diabet Med.* 2011; 28:549–559.

50. Kiecolt-Glaser JK, Derry HM, Fagundes CP. Inflammation: Depression fans the flames and feasts on the heat. *Am J Psychiatry.* 2015; 172:1075–1091.

51. Rienks J, Dobson AJ, Mishra GD. Mediterranean dietary pattern and prevalence and incidence of depressive symptoms in mid-aged women: Results from a large community-based prospective study. *Eur J Clin Nutr.* 2013; 67:75–82.

52. Psaltopoulou T, Sergentanis TN, Panagiotakos DB, Sergentanis IN, Kosti R, Scarmeas N. Mediterranean diet, stroke, cognitive impairment, and depression: A meta-analysis. *Ann Neurol.* 2013; 74:580–591.

53. Sanchez-Villegas A, Martinez-Gonzalez MA, Estruch R, et al. Mediterranean dietary pattern and depression: The PREDIMED randomized trial. *BMC Med.* 2013; 11:208.

54. Beezhold B, Radnitz C, Rinne A, DiMatteo J. Vegans report less stress and anxiety than omnivores. *Nutr Neurosci.* 2015; 18:289–296.

55. Beezhold BL, Johnston CS. Restriction of meat, fish, and poultry in omnivores improves mood: A pilot randomized controlled trial. *Nutr J.* 2012; 11:9.

56. Beezhold BL, Johnston CS, Daigle DR. Vegetarian diets are associated with healthy mood states: A cross-sectional study in Seventh-Day Adventist adults. *Nutr J.* 2010; 9:26.

57. Hibbeln JR, Northstone K, Evans J, Golding J. Vegetarian diets and depressive symptoms among men. *J Affect Disord.* 2018; 225:13–17.

58. Sanchez-Villegas A, Verberne L, De Irala J, et al. Dietary fat intake and the risk of depression: The SUN Project. *PLoS One.* 2011; 6:e16268.

59. Kyrozis A, Psaltopoulou T, Stathopoulos P, Trichopoulos D, Vassilopoulos D, Trichopoulou A. Dietary lipids and geriatric depression scale score among elders: The EPIC-Greece cohort. *J Psychiatr Res.* 2009; 43:763–769.

60. Glick-Bauer M, Yeh MC. The health advantage of a vegan diet: Exploring the gut microbiota connection. *Nutrients.* 2014; 6:4822–4838.

61. Key TJ, Appleby PN, Crowe FL, Bradbury KE, Schmidt JA, Travis RC. Cancer in British vegetarians: Updated analyses of 4,998 incident cancers in a cohort of 32,491 meat eaters, 8,612 fish eaters, 18,298 vegetarians, and 2,246 vegans. *Am J Clin Nutr.* 2014;100 Suppl 1:378S–385S.

62. Tantamango-Bartley Y, Jaceldo-Siegl K, Fan J, Fraser G. Vegetarian diets and the incidence of cancer in a low-risk population. *Cancer Epidemiol Biomarkers Prev.* 2013; 22:286–294.

63. Tantamango-Bartley Y, Knutsen SF, Knutsen R, et al. Are strict vegetarians protected against prostate cancer? *Am J Clin Nutr.* 2016; 103:153–160.

64. Chauveau P, Koppe L, Combe C, Lasseur C, Trolonge S, Aparicio M. Vegetarian diets and chronic kidney disease. *Nephrol Dial Transplant.* 2019; 34:199–207.

65. Noori N, Sims JJ, Kopple JD, et al. Organic and inorganic dietary phosphorus and its management in chronic kidney disease. *Iran J Kidney Dis.* 2010; 4:89–100.

66. Revedin A, Aranguren B, Becattini R, et al. Thirty thousand-year-old evidence of plant food processing. *Proc Natl Acad Sci U S A.* 2010; 107:18815–18819.

67. Henry AG, Brooks AS, Piperno DR. Microfossils in calculus demonstrate consumption of plants and cooked foods in Neanderthal diets (Shanidar III, Iraq; Spy I and II, Belgium). *Proc Natl Acad Sci U S A.* 2011; 108:486–491.

68. Konner M, Eaton SB. Paleolithic nutrition: Twenty-five years later. *Nutr Clin Pract.* 2010; 25:594–602.

69. Frassetto LA, Schloetter M, Mietus-Synder M, Morris RC, Jr., Sebastian A. Metabolic and physiologic improvements from consuming a paleolithic, hunter-gatherer type diet. *Eur J Clin Nutr.* 2009; 63:947–955.

70. Scientific American, https://www.scientificamerican.com/article/food-for-thought/.

71. Paoli A. Ketogenic diet for obesity: Friend or foe? *Int J Environ Res Public Health.* 2014; 11:2092–2107.

72. Hallberg SJ, McKenzie AL, Williams PT, et al. Effectiveness and safety of a novel care model for the management of type 2 diabetes at 1 year: An open-label, non-randomized, controlled study. *Diabetes Ther.* 2018; 9:583–612.

Chapter 16. Plant Foods and Digestive Health

1. Wen L, Duffy A. Factors influencing the gut microbiota, inflammation, and type 2 diabetes. *J Nutr.* 2017; 147:1468S–1475S.

2. Zmora N, Suez J, Elinav E. You are what you eat: Diet, health and the gut microbiota. *Nat Rev Gastroenterol Hepatol.* 2019; 16:35–56.

3. Wu GD, Compher C, Chen EZ, et al. Comparative metabolomics in vegans and omnivores reveal constraints on diet-dependent gut microbiota metabolite production. *Gut.* 2016; 65:63–72.

4. Koeth RA, Wang Z, Levison BS, et al. Intestinal microbiota metabolism of L-carnitine, a nutrient in red meat, promotes atherosclerosis. *Nat Med.* 2013; 19:576–585.

5. Zimmer J, Lange B, Frick JS, et al. A vegan or vegetarian diet substantially alters the human colonic faecal microbiota. *Eur J Clin Nutr.* 2012; 66:53–60.

6. Winham DM, Hutchins AM. Perceptions of flatulence from bean consumption among adults in 3 feeding studies. *Nutr J.* 2011; 10:128.

7. Biesiekierski JR, Peters SL, Newnham ED, Rosella O, Muir JG, Gibson PR. No effects of gluten in patients with self-reported non-celiac gluten sensitivity after dietary reduction of fermentable, poorly absorbed, short-chain carbohydrates. *Gastroenterology.* 2013; 145:320–8 e1–3.

8. Skodje GI, Sarna VK, Minelle IH, et al. Fructan, rather than gluten, induces symptoms in patients with self-reported non-celiac gluten sensitivity. *Gastroenterology.* 2018; 154:529–539 e2.

9. Schuppan D, Zevallos V. Wheat amylase trypsin inhibitors as nutritional activators of innate immunity. *Dig Dis.* 2015; 33:260–263.

10. Altobelli E, Del Negro V, Angeletti PM, Latella G. Low-FODMAP diet improves irritable bowel syndrome symptoms: A meta-analysis. *Nutrients.* 2017; 9:940.

Chapter 17. A Compassionate Approach to Weight and Dieting

1. Orlich MJ, Singh PN, Sabate J, et al. Vegetarian dietary patterns and mortality in Adventist Health Study 2. *JAMA Intern Med.* 2013; 173:1230–1238.

2. Spencer EA, Appleby PN, Davey GK, Key TJ. Diet and body mass index in 38,000 EPIC-Oxford meat-eaters, fish-eaters, vegetarians and vegans. *Int J Obes Relat Metab Disord.* 2003; 27:728–734.

3. Huang RY, Huang CC, Hu FB, Chavarro JE. Vegetarian diets and weight reduction: A meta-analysis of randomized controlled trials. *J Gen Intern Med.* 2016; 31:109–116.

4. Puhl R, Suh Y. Health consequences of weight stigma: Implications for obesity prevention and treatment. *Curr Obes Rep.* 2015; 4:182–190.

5. Tomiyama AJ, Carr D, Granberg EM, et al. How and why weight stigma drives the obesity "epidemic" and harms health. *BMC Med.* 2018; 16:123.

6. Ortega FB, Lee DC, Katzmarzyk PT, et al. The intriguing metabolically healthy but obese phenotype: Cardiovascular prognosis and role of fitness. *Eur Heart J.* 2013; 34:389–397.

7. Long-term effects of lifestyle intervention or metformin on diabetes development and microvascular complications over 15-year follow-up: The Diabetes Prevention Program Outcomes Study. *Lancet Diabetes Endocrinol.* 2015; 3:866–875.

8. Brown RE, Kuk JL. Consequences of obesity and weight loss: A devil's advocate position. *Obes Rev.* 2015; 16:77–87.

9. Hall KD, Kahan S. Maintenance of lost weight and long-term management of obesity. *Med Clin North Am.* 2018; 102:183–197.

10. http://www.drsharma.ca/obesity-best-weight.

11. Tobias DK, Chen M, Manson JE, Ludwig DS, Willett W, Hu FB. Effect of low-fat diet interventions versus other diet interventions on long-term weight change in adults: A systematic review and meta-analysis. *Lancet Diabetes Endocrinol.* 2015; 3:968–979.

12. Hession M, Rolland C, Kulkarni U, Wise A, Broom J. Systematic review of randomized controlled trials of low-carbohydrate vs. low-fat/low-calorie diets in the management of obesity and its comorbidities. *Obes Rev.* 2009; 10:36–50.

13. Nordmann AJ, Nordmann A, Briel M, et al. Effects of low-carbohydrate vs low-fat diets on weight loss and cardiovascular risk factors: A meta-analysis of randomized controlled trials. *Arch Intern Med.* 2006; 166:285–293.

14. Dansinger ML, Gleason JA, Griffith JL, Selker HP, Schaefer EJ. Comparison of the Atkins, Ornish, Weight Watchers, and Zone diets for weight loss and heart disease risk reduction: A randomized trial. *JAMA.* 2005; 293:43–53.

15. Gardner CD, Trepanowski JF, Del Gobbo LC, et al. Effect of low-fat vs low-carbohydrate diet on 12-month weight loss in overweight adults and the association with genotype pattern or insulin secretion: The DIETFITS randomized clinical trial. *JAMA.* 2018; 319:667–679.

16. Mattes RD, Dreher ML. Nuts and healthy body weight maintenance mechanisms. *Asia Pac J Clin Nutr.* 2010; 19:137–141.

17. Jackson CL, Hu FB. Long-term associations of nut consumption with body weight and obesity. *Am J Clin Nutr.* 2014;100 Suppl 1:408S–411S.

18. Baer DJ, Gebauer SK, Novotny JA. Walnuts consumed by healthy adults provide less available energy than predicted by the Atwater Factors. *J Nutr.* 2016; 146:9–13.

19. Liu X, Kris-Etherton PM, West SG, et al. Effects of canola and high-oleic-acid canola oils on abdominal fat mass in individuals with central obesity. *Obesity (Silver Spring)* 2016; 24:2261–2268.

20. Flynn MM, Reinert SE. Comparing an olive oil–enriched diet to a standard lower-fat diet for weight loss in breast cancer survivors: A pilot study. *J Womens Health (Larchmt).* 2010; 19:1155–1161.

21. Longland TM, Oikawa SY, Mitchell CJ, Devries MC, Phillips SM. Higher compared with lower dietary protein during an energy deficit combined with intense exercise promotes greater lean mass gain and fat mass loss: A randomized trial. *Am J Clin Nutr.* 2016; 103:738–746.

22. Kim SJ, de Souza RJ, Choo VL, Ha V, et al. Effects of dietary pulse consumption on body weight: A systematic review and meta-analysis of randomized controlled trials. *Am J Clin Nutr.* 2016; 103:1213–1223.

23. Pittaway JK, Robertson IK, Ball MJ. Chickpeas may influence fatty acid and fiber intake in an ad libitum diet, leading to small improvements in serum lipid profile and glycemic control. *J Am Diet Assoc.* 2008; 108:1009–1013.

24. Messina V. Nutritional and health benefits of dried beans. *Am J Clin Nutr.* 2014; 100 Suppl 1:437S–442S.

25. Traversy G, Chaput JP. Alcohol consumption and obesity: An update. *Curr Obes Rep.* 2015; 4:122–130.

26. Sansone RA, Sansone LA. Marijuana and body weight. *Innov Clin Neurosci.* 2014; 11:50–54.

27. Beulaygue IC, French MT. Got Munchies? Estimating the relationship between marijuana use and body mass index. *J Ment Health Policy Econ.* 2016; 19:123–140.

28. Hall KD. Ultra-processed diets cause excess calorie intake and weight gain: A one-month inpatient randomized controlled trial of ad libitum food intake. NutriXiv. Feb 11, 2019. doi.org/10.31232/osf.io/w3zh2.

29. Janelle KC, Barr SI. Nutrient intakes and eating behavior scores of vegetarian and nonvegetarian women. *J Am Diet Assoc.* 1995; 95:180–186, 189, quiz 187–188.

30. Bardone-Cone AM, Fitzsimmons-Craft EE, Harney MB, et al. The interrelationships between vegetarianism and eating disorders among females. *J Acad Nutr Diet.* 2012; 112:1247–1252.

31. Barthels F, Meyer F, Pietrowsky R. Orthorexic and restrained eating behaviour in vegans, vegetarians, and individuals on a diet. *Eat Weight Disord.* 2018; 23:159–166.

32. Timko CA, Hormes JM, Chubski J. Will the real vegetarian please stand up? An investigation of dietary restraint and eating disorder symptoms in vegetarians versus non-vegetarians. *Appetite.* 2012; 58:982–990.

33. Forestell CA. Flexitarian diet and weight control: Healthy or risky eating behavior? *Front Nutr.* 2018; 5:59.

34. Dittfeld A, Gwizdek K, Jagielski P, Brzek J, Ziora K. A Study on the relationship between orthorexia and vegetarianism using the BOT (Bratman Test for Orthorexia). *Psychiatr Pol.* 2017; 51:1133–1144.

35. Dunn TM, Bratman S. On orthorexia nervosa: A review of the literature and proposed diagnostic criteria. *Eat Behav.* 2016; 21:11.

INDEX